British Cardiology in the 20th Century

Springer
London
Berlin
Heidelberg
New York
Barcelona
Hong Kong
Milan
Paris
Singapore
Tokyo

Edited by
Mark E Silverman, Peter R Fleming, Arthur Hollman,
Desmond G Julian and Dennis M Krikler

British Cardiology in the 20th Century

With a Foreword by Walter Somerville

Springer

British Library Cataloguing in Publication Data
British cardiology in the 20th century
1. Cardiology – Great Britain – History – 20th century
I. Silverman, Mark E.
616.1'2'00941'0904

ISBN-13: 978-1-4471-1199-3

Library of Congress Cataloging-in-Publication Data
British cardiology in the 20th century/Mark E. Silverman . . . [*et al.*] (eds); with a foreword by Walter Somerville.
p. ; cm.
Includes bibliographical references and index.

ISBN-13: 978-1-4471-1199-3 e-ISBN-13: 978-1-4471-0773-6
DOI: 10.1007/978-1-4471-0773-6

1. Cardiology—Great Britain—History—20th century. I. Title:
British cardiology in the twentieth century. II. Silverman, Mark E.
[DNLM: 1. Cardiology—history—Great Britain. 2. History of Medicine,
20th Cent.—Great Britain. WG 11 FA1 B862 2000]
RC666.5.B75 2000 00–036574

Softcover reprint of the hardcover 1st edition 2000

Typeset by Florence Production Ltd, Stoodleigh, Devon

28/3830–543210 Printed on acid-free paper SPIN 10765440

Foreword

I have been accorded the honour of writing a foreword, meaning words said before something more significant that follows. I shall take the prerogative, at my mature age, to look backwards first. As I reflect upon the last century, I realise that our knowledge of cardiology, obscure in 1900, has been like a distant mountain whose magnificent features became more sharply outlined and appreciated as we have travelled through the century. In 1900, the origin of ischaemic chest pain, for example, was a total blur and we did not even know how to diagnose coronary thrombosis. I take great pleasure that certain major disorders which affected so many, so cruelly in the past have been tamed, and in some cases almost eradicated. Among other benefits this century has seen are the dramatic fall in incidence of rheumatic fever; the precise control of coagulation of blood; the discovery of effective treatments for hypertension, syphilis, and endocarditis, and the remarkable developments in safe surgery for acquired and congenital heart disease.

British cardiology can be justly proud of its many contributions to the clinical understanding and the science of cardiology in the 20th century. The teachings of Mackenzie, Lewis, Parkinson, Wood, Pickering, and many respectfully remembered others from this country spring immediately to my mind. British cardiology has been a discipline that is recognised as one of our strong scientific exports. That this progress has occurred here despite the prolonged havoc and disruption of two world wars is all the more noteworthy.

As I look forward, however, I wonder if our wisdom will increase as much as our knowledge has in the past. Coronary disease, thought to be uncommon in the early years of this century, has become an increasing menace to our lives despite many advances in diagnosis and treatment. Can molecular biology be a stepping stone to its solution? Will the determination of the genetic code help us to eradicate congenital heart disease and cardiomyopathy as we have successfully overcome other problems? What will we do about the care of our ageing and expanding population, tobacco related disease, and the pervasive toxins that threaten our environment and our health? Finally, I wonder whether the stethoscope, the precious tool of the cardiologist, will be replaced by the computer as the symbol of the doctor in the eyes of the patient.

This book was not, of course, designed to answer these questions. But it does provide a fine perspective from which to view British contributions to cardiology and to tell us how far we have come in our 20th century journey to learn about the mountain . . . which no longer seems so distant or so mysterious. The editors and authors are to be congratulated and thanked for this important historical document.

Walter Somerville

Honorary Physician
Middlesex Hospital, London
President British Cardiac
Society, 1976–81

October 1999

Preface

British Cardiology in the 20th Century came about through a happy combination of circumstances. In May 1998, I came to London from Atlanta, Georgia as a visiting academic at the Wellcome Institute for the History of Medicine to undertake research on Paul Wood. After a lengthy search of archival resources, it became apparent that, with a few notable exceptions, relatively little had been written about British cardiology in this century. Considering the historical importance of British cardiology, beginning with William Harvey and extending through James Mackenzie and Thomas Lewis into modern times, this void was rather surprising. The concept of coediting a multiauthored book devoted to 20th century cardiology was discussed with Peter Fleming, Arthur Hollman, Desmond Julian, and Dennis Krikler - all like minded cardiologist-historians - at an initial meeting at the British Cardiac Society on 21 October 1998.

After due consideration of the many obstacles such a book would encounter, the group agreed that the idea was worthy. The purposes of the book were defined, chapter subjects developed, and potential authors selected. Potential publishers were contacted and financial support was obtained. The authors responded with enthusiasm and scholarship and within a year a vivid history of British cardiology in the 20th century has emerged.

I am grateful to the Burroughs Wellcome Fund in Durham, North Carolina and to the Academic Unit and library staff at the Wellcome Institute for the History of Medicine who made it possible for me to participate in this fulfilling project.

Mark E Silverman

Preface

Contents

Chapter 1
British Cardiology 1900–50
Peter Fleming 1

Heart failure 1
Cardiac arrhythmias 7
Conduction defects 8
Electrocardiography 9
Ischaemic heart disease 10
Angina 10
Myocardial infarction 12
Chronic rheumatic heart disease 15
Infections of the heart 18
Hypertensive heart disease 18
Pulmonary heart disease 19
Congenital heart disease 20
Da Costa's syndrome and related conditions 20

The Development of the Speciality

Chapter 2
The Second World War and the NHS – the Framework for the Development of Cardiology
Geoffrey Rivett 27

Hospitals and specialists before the war 27
Planning for district hospitals 28
Speciality development 29
Development of cardiology and cardiac surgery 30
NHS organisation and specialist services 32
London issues 33
Equity, cost, and quality 34

Chapter 3
The Training, Number, and Distribution of Cardiologists
Douglas Chamberlain **38**
Training within the NHS 38
Introduction of formal training 42
Regulating numbers 45
Growth and geographical distribution 49

The Organisations Involved in the Growth of Cardiology

Chapter 4
Societies, Journals, and Books
Arthur Hollman **52**
The Cardiac Club 52
The British Cardiac Society 54
Other British cardiology organisations 62
Journals and books 63

Chapter 5
The British Heart Foundation
Desmond G Julian and Brian Pentecost **74**
Founding committee 74
Statement of purpose 75
Fundraising 75
Governance 77
The medical department 77
Research 77
Professorial chairs 78
Education 78
Cardiac care 80

Chapter 6
Part I. The National Heart Hospital: The First of its Kind
Mark E Silverman **83**
London hospitals prior to special hospitals 83
The rise of special hospitals 84
Special hospitals gain recognition 84
The origins of the National Heart Hospital 85
The Dr Eldridge Spratt melodrama 85
The hospital gains sound footing and respect 87
The Second World War period 88
The National Heart Hospital and Institute of Cardiology 89
Cardiac catheterization and cardiovascular surgery 89
Closure and rebirth of the Heart Hospital 90
Acknowledgements 90

Part II. The Institute of Cardiology and the National Heart and Lung Institute
Mark E Silverman and Aubrey Leatham **92**
Formation of special institutes for postgraduate education 92
National Heart Hospital 93
Institute of Cardiology 94
Formation of the National Heart and Lung Institute 98

Chapter 7
The Hammersmith Hospital and the Royal Postgraduate Medical School
Mark E Silverman, Arthur Hollman and Dennis M Krikler **103**
Foundation 103
Voluntary hospitals and research 104
The Hammersmith model 105
Cardiac catheterisation 105
The Second World War 106
Cardiac surgery 107
Further research 108

Diagnosis and Treatment in Cardiology

Chapter 8
Bedside Diagnosis
Aubrey Leatham **111**
Principles of examination 111
Development of the phonocardiogram 112
Studies on identifying components of the second heart sound 115
Studies on components and intensity of the first heart sound 118
Studies on early systolic sounds 120

Chapter 9
The Chest X Ray in Cardiac Diagnosis, 1930–60
Derek Gibson **123**
Early use of the chest *x* ray 123
Improvement in radiological methods 124
First techniques 125
Cardiac enlargement and the pulmonary blood vessels 127
Heart failure 128
Cardiac catheterisation helps interpretation 128
Investigating pulmonary blood flow and oedema 129
Pulmonary hypertension 130

Chapter 10
Electrocardiography, Electrophysiology, and Arrhythmias
Dennis M Krikler **133**
Electrocardiography 133
Intracardiac electrocardiography 138
Developments in surface electrocardiography 138
Antiarrhythmic therapy 139

Chapter 11
Cardiac Catheterisation
Malcolm Towers and Simon Davies **143**
Early work 143
The Paul Wood era 144
Work in the 1960s and 1970s 146
Angioplasty 150

Chapter 12
Nuclear Medicine and Cardiology
Peter J Ell **155**
The MRC medical cyclotron unit 156
Cardiac imaging 156
New tracers 158
Emission tomography 159
British Nuclear Cardiology Society 159
Cost-benefit analysis of scintigraphy 159

Chapter 13
Cardiovascular Magnetic Resonance
Donald B Longmore and S Richard Underwood **163**
Early days of imaging 163
CORDA 164
Brompton Magnetic Resonance Unit 164
Magnetic resonance spectroscopy 166
Coronary and myocardial perfusion imaging 166
Specialist societies 167

Chapter 14
The Development of Cardiac Ultrasound
Stewart Hunter **170**
Beginnings 170
Developments in the 1970s and 1980s 172
Importance in paediatric cardiology 173
Transoesophageal echo 173
Ultrasound's role in cardiology 174
The next millennium 174

Chapter 15

Prevention of Heart Disease

Ross Lorimer **176**

Rheumatic heart disease 176
Coronary heart disease 177
Epidemiological studies 179
Prevention 184
Decreasing mortality from coronary heart disease 186
Hypertension 187

Chapter 16

Cardiac Surgery

Tom Treasure **192**

Back to the beginning 193
Closing in on the heart 197
Specialisation develops 197
Next wave of valvular surgery 199
Disseminating information 201
Impact of hypothermia and stopping the circulation 202
Further developments in valve surgery 205
Transplantation 207
Coronary artery surgery 208
Issues of conflict and quality 209

Chapter 17

Cardiac Pacing

Aubrey Leatham and Ronald Gold **214**

Early Days of Pacing at St George's Hospital 214
From St George's to the National Heart Hospital 219
Recollections of Pacing from a Regional Centre 225

Chapter 18

Cardiac Rehabilitation

Helen Stokes **232**

Moving on from bed rest 232
Cardiac rehabilitation as a developing speciality 233
Cardiology and rehabilitation 234
Psychosocial factors in cardiac rehabilitation 235
Safety and effectiveness of rehabilitation services 235
Expansion of services 236
Reviewing service provision 238
Consumer involvement 239
Where are we now? 239

Chapter 19
Clinical Trials
Desmond G Julian and Stuart Pocock **242**
Prevention and treatment of thrombosis 242
β adrenergic blocking drugs, calcium antagonists, nitrates, and magnesium in and after myocardial infarction 245
Hypertension 246
Heart failure 247
The coronary care unit 248
Coronary artery bypass surgery and angioplasty 248
Lifestyle, diet, and lipid modifying drugs 249
Methodology of randomised clinical trials 250

Selected Cardiac Disorders

Chapter 20
Cardiovascular Pathology
Michael J Davies **255**
Morphology 255
Academic pathology 256
Atherosclerosis research 256
Cardiomyopathy and myocarditis 264
Reginald Hudson 264
Cardiovascular pathology in the 1990s 266

Chapter 21
Paediatric Cardiology
Gerald Graham and James Taylor **269**
Pioneers and pioneering procedures 269
Establishing paediatric cardiac units 272
Establishment of consultant posts 274
Professional associations 274
Development of a paediatric cardiac service 275
Academic units 279
Conclusions and prospects 279

Chapter 22
Grown Up Congenital Heart (GUCH) Services for Adolescents and Adults
Jane Somerville **281**
Development of paediatric cardiology and cardiac surgery 282
Establishing a service 282
Other aspects of GUCH 286
GUCH information and services across the world 288

Chapter 23
Rheumatic Fever
Edwin Besterman **290**
History 290
Murmurs 291
Cardiac dilatation 291
Chorea 292
Aetiology 292
Changing prevalence 292
Canadian Red Cross Memorial Hospital, Taplow 294
Treating rheumatic fever 297
Remaining problems 297

Chapter 24
Valvular Disease, Endocarditis, and Cardiomyopathy
Celia M Oakley **300**
Valvular heart disease in Britain 300
Infective endocarditis 303
Cardiomyopathy 304

Chapter 25
Hypertension
William A Littler **310**
Work of Pickering 310
Battle of the knights 312
Epidemiological studies 314
Benign and malignant hypertension 315
Early drug treatments 316
Trial ethics 317
Research at the Hammersmith in the 1950s and 1960s 318
β blockers 319
MRC trial of drug treatment in mild hypertension 320
Role of meta-analysis 321

Chapter 26
Atherosclerosis Research after the Second World War
Michael F Oliver **323**
Early post war history 323
Increasing incidence of coronary heart disease 324
Risk factors 325
The arterial wall 328
Thrombosis research 329
Lipid and lipoprotein research 331
Organisational developments 332
Cardiovascular survey methods 333

Major research developments after 1970 333
Clinical trials on the reduction or prevention of atheromatous coronary heart disease 336

Chapter 27
Clinical Coronary Heart Disease
Desmond G Julian **343**

Myocardial infarction – 1945–60 343
Myocardial infarction – 1960 onward 345
Unstable angina 349
Variant angina 351
Stable angina 351

Chapter 28
Leaders of British Cardiology
Arthur Hollman, Gaston E Bauer and Mark E Silverman **357**

Russell Claude Brock, Lord Brock of Wimbledon 357
Sir Thomas Lewis 360
Sir James Mackenzie 363
Sir John McMichael 367
Sir John Parkinson 370
Paul Hamilton Wood 374

Index 379

Contributors

Gaston E Bauer
Consultant Cardiologist, Royal North Shore Hospital, Sydney, Australia

Edwin Besterman
Consultant Cardiologist, University Hospital, University of West Indies, Jamaica; Honorary Consultant Cardiologist, St Mary's Hospital, London; Honorary Consultant Cardiologist, Royal Postgraduate Medical School, Hammersmith Hospital, London

Douglas Chamberlain
Honorary Consultant Cardiologist, Brighton Health Care NHS Trust, Sussex, England; Honorary Professor of Resuscitation Medicine, University of Wales College of Medicine, Cardiff

Michael J Davies
British Heart Foundation - Professor of Cardiovascular Pathology, St George's Hospital, London

Simon Davies
Consultant Cardiologist, Royal Brompton and Harefield NHS Trust, London

Peter J Ell
Professor of Nuclear Medicine, University of London; Director, Institute of Nuclear Medicine, University College London

Peter Fleming
Formerly Senior Lecturer in Medicine, Charing Cross and Westminster Medical School, London

Derek Gibson
Consultant Cardiologist, Royal Brompton and Harefield NHS Trust, London

Ronald Gold
Formerly Consultant Cardiologist, Freeman Hospital, Newcastle upon Tyne and Clinical Lecturer in Cardiology, University of Newcastle upon Tyne

Gerald Graham
Emeritus Consultant Clinical Physiologist, Great Ormond Street Hospital for Children NHS Trust

Arthur Hollman
Formerly Consultant Cardiologist, University College Hospital, London; Archivist, The British Cardiac Society

Stewart Hunter
Consultant in Paediatric Cardiology, Freeman Hospital, Newcastle upon Tyne and Honorary Senior Lecturer in Paediatrics, University of Newcastle upon Tyne

Desmond G Julian
Emeritus Professor of Cardiology, University of Newcastle upon Tyne and Former Medical Director, British Heart Foundation

Dennis M Krikler
Consultant Cardiologist; former Senior Lecturer in Cardiology, Royal Postgraduate Medical School, Hammersmith Hospital, London

Aubrey Leatham
Formerly Consultant Physician, St George's and National Heart Hospitals; formerly Dean of the Institute of Cardiology

William A Littler
Professor of Cardiovascular Medicine, University of Birmingham; Consultant Cardiologist, Queen Elizabeth Hospital, Birmingham

Donald B Longmore
Professor of Cardiovascular Magnetic Resonance, Brompton MR Enterprises, Royal Brompton Hospital, London

Ross Lorimer
Honorary Professor in Medicine and Medical Cardiology, University of Glasgow; Consultant Physician and Cardiologist, Royal Infirmary, Glasgow

Celia M Oakley
Consultant Cardiologist and Emeritus Professor of Clinical Cardiology, Imperial College School of Medicine, Hammersmith Hospital

Michael F Oliver
Professor Emeritus of Cardiology, University of Edinburgh; President, British Cardiac Society 1980–84

Brian Pentecost
Emeritus Professor of Cardiology, University of Birmingham and Former Medical Director, British Heart Foundation

Stuart Pocock
Professor of Medical Statistics, London School of Hygiene and Tropical Medicine, London

Anthony Rickards
Consultant Cardiologist, Royal Brompton Hospital; Vice Dean of the Institute of Cardiology

Geoffrey Rivett
Medical historian; formerly Senior Principal Medical Officer, Department of Heath, England

Mark E Silverman
Professor of Cardiology, Emory University and Chief of Cardiology, the Fuqua Heart Center, Piedmont Hospital, Atlanta, Georgia, USA

Jane Somerville
Emeritus Consultant Cardiologist, Royal Brompton Hospital, London; Consultant Cardiologist, Grown Up Congenital Heart (GUCH) Unit, Middlesex Hospital, London; Professor of Cardiology, Imperial College London School of Medicine

Helen Stokes
Project Officer, Education and Training for Cardiac Rehabilitation, Department of Health Studies University of York; Past President, British Association for Cardiac Rehabilitation

James Taylor
Consultant Paediatric Cardiologist, Great Ormond Street Hospital for Children NHS Trust

Malcolm Towers
Formerly Consultant Cardiologist, Harefield Hospital, Middlesex

S Richard Underwood
Professor of Cardiac Imaging, Imperial College School of Medicine, London

Introduction

> I have tried to tell you something of the men who built the barn and gathered the first ears of the amazing harvest that their successors reap in the vast field of cardiology. They were not saints, but simple, kindly men with a great sense of duty . . . they cared for suffering hearts and by their labours won the affection and gratitude of many.
>
> Robert Marshall. Early days in Westmoreland Street (The National Heart Hospital). *Br Heart J* 1964:26:140.

British Cardiology in the 20th Century is a compilation of essays written with the following goals in mind:

- To highlight British contributions to cardiology in the 20th century;
- To provide a history of some of the figures, institutions, and organisations which played an important part in British cardiology;
- To describe British practice and treatment for heart disease during the 20th century;
- To explain how the specialty evolved in Britain – including the effects of the National Health Service, the second world war, and changing ideas about professional development and training;
- To stimulate interest in and awareness of British cardiology in an international audience;
- To provide a reliable historical resource for current and future writers.

British Cardiology in the 20th Century is not intended to be a comprehensive, chronological story of the entire field of British cardiology. The format of the book was dictated by the mid-century acceleration in cardiology and its subsequent division into many subspecialty interests. Therefore, the first chapter covers 1900 to 1950, during which period cardiology, although undergoing great changes, was mostly unified. The next two chapters are devoted to the emergence of cardiology as a specialty, the organising influences of the second world war and the NHS, and the development of manpower planning and the training pathway for aspiring cardiologists. From then on, contributing authors have been asked to write a narration of their special interest. Thus, each chapter and its accompanying references and notes can be used as a separate resource. The editors considered that some overlap between chapters was desirable to widen the historical perspective.

It is recognised that these chapters are personal and selective. The editors wish to point out that in some chapters particular statements are made that they would not endorse. Inevitably, a number of institutions and individuals who have made valuable contributions to British cardiology do not receive appropriate recognition. For these omissions, we apologise. We have, however, tried to cover the subject as broadly as possible and are proud to publish this first tribute to British cardiology in the past century.

The editors express their gratitude to the authors who have undertaken such a formidable task; to our publisher, Springer-Verlag, for their commitment; and to Norma Pearce, our indispensable technical editor. Their splendid work and dedication in bringing this book to completion at the end of the 20th century is greatly appreciated. We are grateful to the British Heart Foundation, the British Cardiac Society, and the Fuqua Heart Center of Piedmont Hospital, Atlanta, Georgia for their generous financial support without which this book would not have been possible.

British Cardiology in the 20th Century is dedicated to "the men who built the barn . . . and the amazing harvest that their successors reap in the vast field of cardiology."

Mark E Silverman
Peter R Fleming
Arthur Hollman
Desmond G Julian
Dennis M Krikler

Chapter 1

British Cardiology 1900–50

Peter Fleming

During the first half of the period covered in this chapter – the "Mackenzie – Lewis era," in McMichael's words[1] – the correlation of clinical features with pathological changes found at post-mortem examination, which had been so fruitful for so long, came to be overshadowed by attempts to see clinical symptoms and signs in terms of disordered physiology. By the second decade of the century, this perception of heart disease was so different from what had gone before that clinicians talked of the "new cardiology."[2] From this predominance of function over structure in the minds of clinicians, the pendulum swung back somewhat in the second half of the period, although never so far as to displace pathophysiology as the basic science of cardiology.

Heart failure

Work of Mackenzie

One of the first physicians to advocate the study of cardiac function was James Mackenzie. Mackenzie was a general practitioner in Burnley, Lancashire for most of the first decade of the century; he had read deeply in physiology and had been influenced particularly by the work of Walter Gaskell,[3] whose studies in animals he tried to reproduce in humans. Mackenzie had been conducting research into heart disease since 1880 – at first by careful history and examination and then with graphic records of the venous and other pulses. He made many valuable observations, particularly on disorders of the cardiac rhythm, which are discussed below. However, Mackenzie regarded this research as subsidiary to his main purpose. This was the study of prognosis and, in particular, answering the questions, "What is heart failure and what are the symptoms by which it can be recognised?"

By the end of the 19th century, the concept of cardiac dilatation as a disease sui generis had been replaced by the idea that "compensation" for a valve lesion by cardiac hypertrophy might be lost and that "decompensation" might become manifest by symptoms such as dyspnoea and oedema due to back pressure in chambers proximal to the valve lesion. This emphasis on valve lesions as important precursors of heart failure was anathema to Mackenzie and his followers, for whom it was the state of the myocardium that mattered. The functions of the heart muscle could be defined in the physiological terms used by Gaskell – namely stimulus production, excitability, conductivity, contractility, and tonicity.[4] Exhaustion of the "reserve" of a function led to clinical manifestations, and exhaustion of contractility manifested itself as angina, palpitation, and (most characteristically) pulsus alternans. The features of exhaustion of tonicity (the function which keeps the heart in a state of slight contraction during diastole) were cardiac enlargement, dropsy, and enlargement of the liver. These features were not to be explained by back pressure but by "failure of the circulation in remote organs and tissues."[5] This uncompromising statement of the concept of "forward failure" became the standard teaching of the exponents of the new cardiology. Mackenzie also disagreed with many of his predecessors in his rejection of the concept of separate right and left heart failure.

During his years in Burnley, especially after 1902 when his first book, *The study of the pulse*, was published,[6] Mackenzie became acquainted (in person or by correspondence) with many admirers of his work. Thus, he began corresponding with Carel Wenckebach in 1902, and in 1904 arranged for Wenckebach's book on cardiac arrhythmias to be translated and published in Britain. His association with Arthur Keith of the London Hospital began in 1903,[7] and William Osler visited the "Galilee of Burnley" in 1905,[8] less than six months after taking up his appointment as regius professor at Oxford. Other visitors included Arthur Cushny, pharmacologist at University College, London,[9] Graham Steell of Manchester,[10] and John Hay of Liverpool.[11] Mackenzie collaborated with several of these, and many began to use his methods, notably the famous clinical polygraph, to study their patients with heart disease.

Those who came to know Mackenzie while he was still in Burnley were a rather select group. When he moved to London in 1907, Mackenzie was not at all well known to the physicians of the metropolis, even though he had already published over 50 papers (19 of them in the *British Medical Journal*) as well as a book. Thus, Sir Arthur Hurst, writing in 1949, said that Mackenzie "remained almost completely unknown in England until he moved to London in 1907,"[12] and the 25 year old John Parkinson heard about him for the first time when he was visiting Germany in 1910. The consequence of this delayed recognition was that Mackenzie's approach to heart disease, and the doctrines of the new cardiology in general, became known in London with little prior warning. The views of Mackenzie and his followers did not go unchallenged, and the sometimes acrimonious debate between the old and the new occupied much of the second decade of the century.

Nature of heart failure

One of the more contentious issues was the nature of heart failure. The standard description of backward failure adhered to by most 19th century physicians has been outlined above. However, there were complicating factors. For example, the words "heart failure" were not widely used until well into the 20th century, and even then they sometimes implied a condition resembling the modern cardiogenic shock. Thus, Osler in 1892 wrote of heart failure only in connection with the circulatory collapse of diphtheria or typhoid.[13] In addition, some thought that the oedema of heart failure was related as much to increased capillary permeability as to high venous pressure. This "tissue factor" was referred to by Graham Steell, a "new" cardiologist, who, despite saying how much he appreciated Mackenzie's work, wrote in the same textbook of "the systemic venous stasis in which all varieties of cardiac failure sooner or later express themselves."[14]

Although he made his own view quite clear, Mackenzie did not say much to oppose the backward failure theory in the first edition of his textbook in 1908.[4] However, that opinion persisted. In 1908, for example, Lauder Brunton published a series of lectures on the therapeutics of the circulation, in which he attributed all the clinical manifestations of heart failure to backward pressure.[15] Mackenzie used his Oliver-Sharpey Lectures in 1911 to attack this view,[16] and continued this assault in all subsequent editions of his textbook and in other writings. The term backward pressure was probably being used in two different senses. Mackenzie seems to have equated this concept with regurgitation through the mitral and tricuspid valves – that is, direct transmission of the ventricular pressure backwards. He said that this could not be occurring because the murmurs of valvular regurgitation were not present. However, others may have interpreted it as simply meaning a rise in pressure in the corresponding atrium and veins without necessarily any regurgitation of blood.

Controversy heats up

The controversies about the old and the new cardiology in general and the mechanisms of heart failure in particular really broke out after George Sutherland's Lumleian Lectures in 1917.[17] Sutherland was an enthusiastic convert to the views of Mackenzie and Thomas Lewis, and his lectures were a comprehensive review of all the new ideas in cardiology. He did not like the terms "right sided" and "left sided" failure, and he outdid Mackenzie in his condemnation of the back pressure theory. Perhaps more important historically than the lectures was the subsequent correspondence. Fred Smith of Northampton fired the first shot. He roundly condemned Sutherland and Mackenzie for failing to respect the views of their distinguished predecessors, and he stated categorically that "Failure of the heart causes venous congestion."[18] Mackenzie was never one to turn the other cheek, and a few weeks later denounced Smith as a reactionary. Seventeen other letters followed . . . and the argument raged to and fro. Sutherland never joined in the debate (he is said to have had "a strong element of Scottish reserve"[19]), but the correspondence ended with Mackenzie claiming that no current textbook, except presumably his own, gave an intelligent definition of heart failure.[20] Clifford Allbutt's rejoinder was that, of course, there could be no definition of "so loose and colloquial a phrase" as heart failure.[21] On the whole, Mackenzie and his friends seem to have won the argument in the short term, and in Mackenzie's obituary in 1925, it was stated that "His views on heart failure are now generally accepted.[22]

Fatigue and failure

In his wide-ranging lectures Sutherland had referred to dilatation of the heart, opposing the old view that it was due to a primary weakness of the myocardium. In that connection, he referred to the experiments of Ernest Starling and his colleagues.[23] They had used an isolated dog heart-lung preparation and had published their conclusions in two papers in 1914.[24][25] They had shown that when the inflow into the right atrium, and consequently the arterial output, was increased, there was a progressive rise in venous pressure. At a critical point in the curve describing the relationship between venous pressure and cardiac output, a further rise in venous pressure was associated with a fall in output. When this occurred, the heart was said to have become fatigued. In neither of their original papers was it suggested that the findings in the isolated heart-lung preparation could be applied to the intact human heart. However, in his later Linacre Lecture on the "Law of the heart," Starling ill-advisedly implied a similar relationship in man without the caveats that have subsequently been found necessary to prevent the simplistic equation of "fatigue" in the dog's heart with "failure" in man.[26] This unwise extrapolation beyond the scope of the data led to criticism from physicians and physiologists, some of whom said that the "law of the heart" applied only to the isolated heart and was simply a biological curiosity; others accused Starling of plagiarising Otto Frank's work of 1898. The whole subject of Starling's work and its application in clinical medicine is discussed in detail by George Pickering[27] and Carleton Chapman.[28]

Mackenzie's vigorous advocacy of the forward failure theory never varied and influenced thinking in this country until his death. However, the term "congestive heart failure," with its implication of backward failure, continued to be used in the Unites States. Also, Lewis, who never did any experimental work on heart failure, modified his general acceptance of Mackenzie's ideas by adding that backward failure did occur late in the course of the illness. He was certainly insistent that the measurement of venous pressure was an important observation and even made a film to demonstrate this. However, according to Pickering, who was working with Lewis in the 1930s, he does not seem to have applied Starling's ideas clinically. During that decade, further work in the United States delivered a powerful blow to the forward failure theory,[29] and it seems that the theory was thoroughly discredited by the late 1940s. In 1950, Paul Wood was able to write "By far the most important sign of right ventricular failure is a rise in systemic venous pressure."[30] Yet, at this very time, still further work overseas set the pendulum swinging once again.[31]

Remedies – bed rest, digitalis, and diuretics

In the early years of the century, the two most important remedies for heart failure were rest and digitalis. Absolute rest was prescribed in the most severe cases. Lewis described a bedstead consisting of three sections hinged together so that the patient's position, with trunk upright and legs dependent, could be adjusted for maximum comfort.[32]

The popularity of digitalis has fluctuated more than that of almost any other drug. For much of the 19th century, the dramatic effect of digitalis as a diuretic in heart failure led some physicians to use it cautiously, because they feared its toxicity, and others to prescribe it widely and over optimistically for conditions such as consumption, measles, and goitre. Fear of toxicity and disappointment at its failure to act as a panacea combined with a "general nihilistic view of therapeutics" reduced the use of digitalis.[33] By the beginning of the 20th century, the indications for digitalis were confined to heart failure, but the debate about its mode of action continued.

In 1904, while still in the United States, Cushny had shown in animals that digitalis acted directly in increasing the force of ventricular contraction. He had become convinced that the beneficial action of digitalis in heart failure was not directly attributable to slowing of the heart. In 1905, Cushny returned to Britain, to the chair of pharmacology at University College, and played an important part in the characterisation of atrial fibrillation (see pages 7–8).

Mackenzie soon showed that digitalis had its most dramatic effect when heart failure was complicated by this arrhythmia. He also became convinced, despite his close association with Cushny, that the sole mechanism of the improvement was the reduction in heart rate. Mackenzie thought that digitalis might also produce some improvement in heart failure with normal rhythm. He believed that in this case there might be no effect on the heart rate and the improvement might result from a direct diuretic effect on the kidneys. Lewis was even more convinced that digitalis had no effect on the force of ventricular contraction. In 1919, he wrote, "those who regard digitalis as a cardiac stimulant mistake its character. To the heart foxglove is not tonic but powerfully hypnotic. It extends the diastoles of the heart; it extends the period of sleep."[34]

Cushny continued to work on the actions of digitalis. He showed that any slowing of the heart rate in normal rhythm was vagal in origin, while in patients with atrial fibrillation it resulted from impaired atrioventricular conduction. In both cases, it increased the force of ventricular contraction. Cushny published an authoritative monograph on digitalis in 1925.[35]

The consequence of the vigorously expressed views of Mackenzie and Lewis was that digitalis was largely confined in Britain to treating heart failure in patients with atrial fibrillation. In continental Europe and

America, its use when the heart was in normal rhythm was commoner. Practice here did not change until 1939, when Clarence Gavey and John Parkinson published a paper in the first issue of the *British Heart Journal* showing that digitalis was beneficial in heart failure with normal rhythm, but its effect in atrial fibrillation was greater.[36] For the rest of the first half of the century, the standard teaching in Britain was that digitalis was indicated in almost all cases of heart failure and should generally be continued indefinitely.

Until the 1920s, when organic mercurial compounds such as mersalyl became available, purine derivatives such as theophylline and inorganic mercury salts such as calomel (mercurous chloride) were the most commonly used diuretics in heart failure. These were sometimes supplemented with physical drainage of oedema fluid via Southey's tubes or short skin incisions. These manoeuvres, together with venesection for acute pulmonary oedema, continued in use well into the 1950s.

Postural changes in output

Around the middle of the century, John McMichael and his colleagues showed how Starling's concepts applied in heart failure in man and elucidated many of the details of the mode of action of digitalis glycosides. McMichael's first publication in this field came from Edinburgh in 1938.[37] He used the acetylene method to study changes in cardiac output in response to changes in posture. McMichael found that cardiac output rose when normal subjects went from the standing to the lying position (that is, when the effective ventricular filling pressure rose), and that this response was virtually absent in patients in heart failure. McMichael moved to Hammersmith in 1939, and after a few years he resumed his studies using cardiac catheterisation and the Fick principle to measure cardiac output. Many of his subsequent papers were on the effects of digoxin on the behaviour of the failing heart. He found that these effects – a fall in venous pressure and a rise in cardiac output – were nearly identical to those of mechanical lowering of the right atrial pressure by venous-occluding cuffs on the thighs, suggesting that digoxin might act primarily on the veins.[38] This idea seemed to be confirmed by the fact that the changes in cardiac output were not constant whereas the fall in venous pressure was invariable. In 1947, and particularly in his Strickland Goodall Lecture to the Society of Apothecaries in 1948,[39] McMichael summarised his views by saying that the rise in venous pressure was compensating for deteriorating ventricular function early in failure, but later "seems to carry the heart over the top of the Starling curve."[40]

Other important ideas emerged from the work at Hammersmith, in particular the concept of low output and high output failure. Furthermore, as techniques improved and it became possible to study left ventricular function by catheterising the pulmonary artery, it became apparent that the idea that digoxin had a primary venodilator effect was wrong.[41] Relating right ventricular filling pressure to left ventricular output was clearly unhelpful. In addition, the view that either ventricle could fail independently of the other, which Mackenzie had opposed, was certainly correct. In 1952, in his Oliver-Sharpey Lectures,[42] McMichael discussed how different causes of heart disease resulted in different types of heart failure. That same year, in a contribution to Erik Warburg's festschrift, he said "In the very near future we shall possibly abandon the vague term 'cardiac failure' and analyse all our cardiacs in terms of their altered dynamics."[43]

Cardiac arrhythmias

Unlike the controversy over heart failure, which was not to be resolved for many years, the study of the arrhythmias produced a general consensus. During the first decade of the century, most of the common disorders of cardiac rhythm were described in terms that have largely stood the test of time. So quickly was the new teaching on arrhythmias accepted that this, together with disorders of conduction, became the commonest cardiological topic in the examination papers for membership of the Royal College of Physicians of London between 1910 and 1920 ... for the first, and only, time.

Towards the end of Mackenzie's time in general practice, a group was gathering in London with the members of which he was to become well acquainted. This group could have been found any day in 1907, around lunchtime, in an ABC Cafe in Tottenham Court Road. It included three men from the department of physiology at University College – Ernest Starling, William Bayliss, and their much younger colleague, Thomas Lewis; Arthur Cushny would probably have been there as well. Of these men, only Bayliss, although very distinguished in other fields, played no part in this history.

Thomas Lewis had qualified in 1905, and within two years had obtained two hospital appointments, written his first paper on the pulse, and had begun working in Starling's laboratory. That was in 1907, the year in which Mackenzie moved to London; they met the following year, with momentous consequences. Although paroxysmal tachycardia had been described as a clinical observation several times in the 19th century, the only form of cardiac arrhythmia clearly recognised by the turn of the century was the extrasystole. Several authors, including Mackenzie, had described this in the 1890s. Total irregularity of the heart, Hering's pulsus irregularis perpetuus, was also well known in 1900, but its precise nature was unclear. Mackenzie's first attempt to explain its mechanism as "auricular paralysis" followed his encounter with a patient with mitral stenosis whose pulse suddenly became fast and irregular and in whom all the evidence of atrial activity disappeared. Mackenzie changed his mind a little later when he discovered at post-mortem examination in a similar case that the atria were not atrophic but hypertrophied, suggesting increased activity in life. He then labelled the arrhythmia "nodal rhythm."

Meanwhile, Cushny and Edmunds had produced fibrillation of the atria in dogs and had noted a fast irregular pulse very similar to that in human cases of atrial fibrillation.[44] Cushny had tried without success to convince Mackenzie that the two conditions were identical. In 1909, Lewis, who had that year obtained his first electrocardiograph, published a paper entitled "Auricular fibrillation: a common clinical condition."[45] Only after this paper was published did he see the paper by Rothberger and Winterberg from Vienna which had predated his own by five months.

"Speed limit" of the heart

Other arrhythmias were characterised during these early years of the century. William Ritchie of Edinburgh described atrial flutter. He had recorded a polygraphic tracing in an unusual case of heart block in 1905. In 1910, he re-investigated this patient with his new electrocardiograph, and with William Jolly (later professor of physiology at Cape Town), wrote a paper in which they named the arrhythmia "auricular flutter."[46] Arthur Hertz (later, by deed poll, Sir Arthur Hurst) and Gordon Goodhart of Guy's Hospital described recordings of the venous pulse and the electrocardiogram in a similar case. Realising that the bundle of His could not conduct all the impulses at very fast atrial rates, they entitled their paper "The speed limit of the human heart."[47]

Lewis became the world authority on cardiac arrhythmias. He recorded a case of nodal tachycardia in 1909, although at first he did not recognise it.[48] In so doing, he incidentally disproved further Mackenzie's second theory of the mechanism of atrial fibrillation, and during the next three years firmly laid the foundations of the study of cardiac rhythm with the electrocardiograph. Lewis summarised his work in his three most influential books, *The mechanism of the heart beat* in 1911,[49] *Clinical disorders of the heart beat* in 1912,[50] and *Clinical electrocardiography* in 1913.[51] In his Oliver–Sharpey Lectures in 1921, Lewis proposed his theory that atrial flutter and fibrillation were due to a "circus movement" in which an impulse travelled in a circle around the orifices of the venae cavae.[52] This was challenged but the demonstration of the Wolff–Parkinson–White syndrome led indirectly to the reincarnation of the circus movement as "re-entry."[53]

Until the second decade of the century there was no effective treatment for the arrhythmias, apart from the incomparable effect of digitalis in controlling the ventricular rate in atrial fibrillation. During those years quinine and, later, quinidine were introduced; the latter was quite widely used to restore or maintain sinus rhythm until it was superseded by better drugs.

Conduction defects

The idea that the heart beat is due to an impulse spreading from a site in the region of the primitive sinus venosus through the atria to the ventricles derived from the work of Gaskell towards the end of the 19th century. Gaskell had been stimulated by George Romanes' work. Romanes had studied the waves of contraction passing along strips of the swimming bell of the medusa (a jellyfish), and described the inability of these impulses to pass an artificially narrowed section as "block."[54] As a result of Gaskell's work, the concepts of "pacemaker" and "block of conduction" entered cardiac physiology. Mackenzie and his followers could readily diagnose heart block from polygraphic tracings, and began to propose that this condition might be due to lesions of the bundle of His, first described in 1893. Arthur Keith, responding to Mackenzie's suggestions, eventually succeeded in finding the bundle in hearts which the latter had sent to him ... but only after many failures. In fact, at one time in 1906, he doubted its very existence.[55] In that year, John Hay and Stuart Moore also found the bundle, partly obliterated, in a case of heart block.[56] They made the important point that the marked variation in the severity of the conduction defect in their graphic records implied that some additional factor, perhaps vagal activity, might be playing a part in addition to the organic lesion. In 1907, Keith followed up his work on the bundle by a successful search, with Martin Flack, for the sinoatrial node; this proved similar in structure to the atrioventricular node which had been described some time before.[57]

Electrocardiography

The polygraph and the electrocardiograph produce records of mechanical movement – of a pen or a beam of light (at first) and a stylus (later) respectively. However, they are fundamentally different in the way in which the records are produced. The polygraph produces a mechanical record of mechanical events, acting essentially as an amplifier, while an electrocardiograph produces a mechanical record of electrical events and functions as a transducer.

Joel Howell has argued that Lewis, having "graduated" to the electrocardiograph from the polygraph, tended to regard the former as a sophisticated version of the latter and had not considered the possibility that it could provide information about the state of the myocardium.[58] This assertion is not strictly true as he had included a short discussion on the electrocardiographic features of right and left ventricular hypertrophy in his *Clinical electrocardiography* in 1913. In the same book, Lewis mentioned the "aberrant contractions" produced when one or other branch of the bundle of His failed to conduct an impulse, and referred to the similarity of the QRS complex in that case to that of a ventricular extrasystole. He began his detailed study of the excitation process in the dog's heart in 1914, using multiple electrodes on the outside and inside of the heart. In 1915, Lewis began his research on bundle branch block, also on dogs. Lewis' choice of the dog as his experimental animal was unfortunate, as its electrocardiographic pattern is very different from that in the human. Consequently, he mixed up right and left bundle branch block and chose to ignore conflicting anatomical and clinical evidence in man when it was presented to him. This mistake was not finally corrected until 1932, when Frank Wilson at Ann Arbor produced conclusive proof. Lewis was not easily convinced of his error and continued to express doubts for another 10 years. A detailed account of the history of bundle branch block has been given by Hollman.[59]

Chest leads

After Lewis had completed his work, the main thrust of research on the electrocardiogram shifted to America – in particular, to Wilson and his colleagues who "did for the analysis of the ventricular complex of the electrocardiogram what Lewis had done for the arrhythmias."[60] The main practical outcome of Wilson's work was the introduction of the chest leads. A joint committee of the newly founded Cardiac Society (not the British Cardiac Society until 1946) and the American Heart Association met in 1937 to discuss this development and to produce recommendations. The two national groups differed only in that the Americans favoured multiple chest leads and the British preferred a single lead at that time.

Ischaemic heart disease

At the beginning of the 20th century, two main issues concerning what is known today as ischaemic heart disease awaited resolution. The first was the nature and significance of angina and the second elucidation of the nature of the various myocardial lesions now recognised as manifestations of ischaemia. The problems were virtually the same as those Peter Latham had summarised over 50 years before. In 1845, he wrote, "angina pectoris has existed indeed where there has been ossification or obstruction of the coronary arteries, where there has been dilatation of the aorta, where there has been valvular unsoundness, or hypertrophy or atrophy, or softening or conversion of the heart's muscular substance into fat . . . And it has existed where no form of disease or disorganisation whatever has been found in the heart or in the blood vessels nearest to it."[61]

Angina

At the end of the 18th century, angina had been attributed to disease of the coronary arteries. This theory had never been wholly abandoned, but throughout the 19th century other possible causes had been suggested – as many as 80 according to one French author.[62] In 1897, William Osler gave and published seven lectures on this subject at Johns Hopkins Hospital.[63] Osler described two varieties of angina – true angina and false or pseudo-angina. He had seen 40 cases of the former and 20 of the latter, which was a heterogeneous collection of chest pains, mostly of psychological origin. Osler emphasised the rarity of true angina in hospital practice and the consequent paucity of morbid anatomical material. However, he had seen "anaemic infarcts" and "fibroid myocarditis" with the formation of aneurysm of the heart and was convinced that "in the vast majority of cases angina was associated with disease of the coronary arteries and of the myocardium." There were also, he said, other aetiological factors, none of which he felt he could exclude. For example, gout might play an important part, diabetes and syphilis were well recognised associations, angina might be a sequel of influenza and, of the recognised types of heart disease, aortic but not mitral valve disease, aortic aneurysm, and adherent pericardium were all associated with angina. Finally, "By far the most common heart disease with which angina is associated is chronic myocarditis." As for the precise mechanism of the pain, he was impressed with suggestions that it was analogous to intermittent claudication, but he also felt obliged to mention "cramp" of the heart muscle and distension and stretching of the heart walls as possible factors. Another possibility Osler considered was that the pain arose from the arteries themselves, likening angina to migraine.

Angina was also the subject of Osler's Lumleian Lectures to the Royal College of Physicians in 1910.[64] In these lectures he reiterated much that he had said 13 years before, once again emphasising the rarity of angina with the statement, astonishing today, that "I had reached the Fellowship before I saw a case in hospital or private practice." Osler had given up using the term pseudo-angina by then and discussed in more detail the myocardial lesions described below.

Uncertainty over its nature

Osler's publications have been considered at some length to indicate the uncertainty in the mind of one of the leaders of the profession in the early years of the century. The view that angina was not only associated with but was mainly a result of coronary artery disease gradually gained ground. However, others, no less distinguished, did not agree. Mackenzie emphasised that all the conditions related to angina, of which coronary artery disease was only one, operated by impairing the contractility of the heart. For him, angina was "evidence of the exhaustion of the function of contractility." Clifford Allbutt, regius professor at Cambridge, also held very different views. In a series of papers from 1894 onwards, culminating in his very influential book of 1915, *Diseases of arteries including angina pectoris*,[65] Allbutt proposed that angina was caused by "an atheromatous process of a severe kind, penetrating more deeply than usual, in the suprasigmoid section of the aorta." He realised that his was a minority view, referring to the majority as "orthodox coronarians," but he held to it firmly until the end of his long life in 1925. Allbutt also maintained that angina and myocardial infarction were quite different conditions. He believed that inflammation and distension of the pericardium over the infarct caused the pain of myocardial infarction.

Angina and intermittent claudication

Lewis and his colleagues finally disposed of myocardial spasm and the other current hypotheses of the mechanism of angina in the early 1930s. Having seen several patients with intermittent claudication, Lewis began investigating this condition with George Pickering. They soon proved conclusively that the mechanism of the pain was ischaemia that produced a chemical substance which they labelled "factor P." The next logical step was the investigation of angina; this Lewis delegated to Edward Wayne. The methods used to study intermittent claudication (which involved temporary arrest of the circulation in healthy limbs) could not be applied, but indirect methods were used to show that angina was so closely analogous to intermittent claudication as to justify the conclusion that the mechanisms were identical.

Wayne's wish to record the electrocardiogram during an episode of pain was not supported by Lewis.[66] In fact, Guy Bousfield had first used electrocardiography to investigate angina much earlier – in 1918.[67] A patient with aortic valve disease had an attack of angina while an electrocardiogram was being recorded. During the attack the electrocardiogram showed bundle branch block (thought to be right – but actually left); afterwards conduction was normal but the T wave in lead II became inverted.

Treatment

Throughout the first half of the century, the only effective treatment for angina was sublingual glyceryl trinitrate or, occasionally, inhaled amyl nitrite. With these drugs, patients were able to treat their attacks promptly or even use the agents prophylactically when about to exert themselves to an extent likely, from past experience, to cause pain. Longer acting nitrates such as sodium nitrite or pentaerythritol tetranitrate were available, but these were not very effective in preventing attacks. For this reason, attempts were made to reduce the oxygen requirements of the heart by total thyroidectomy. This practice was never popular as it merely replaced one set of intolerable symptoms with another.

Myocardial infarction

The rarity of angina in clinical practice has already been referred to. The situation with regard to myocardial infarction (to use the modern term) was similar. To most British physicians in the early 1920s, a diagnosis of coronary thrombosis, as the condition came to be called at first, was not so much rare as non-existent. Evan Bedford, who qualified in 1921, had never heard of it as a student.[68] Coronary thrombosis was equally unknown to Cookson in Birmingham in 1923, but he had seen one case of "status anginosus."[69] The rapid transition from this state of affairs to the situation in 1929 when Terence East and Curtis Bain could write that coronary thrombosis "has become easy to recognise at the bedside" has puzzled historians.[70] Parkinson and Bedford provided a probable solution in 1928: "Until recent years . . . (coronary thrombosis) was regarded as a terminal complication of angina pectoris, an event of pathological interest in relation to sudden death." Consequently, an unknown American physician could say that the attempt to make a clinical diagnosis of coronary thrombosis "was ridiculous because it was impossible."[71] This dogmatic statement stemmed from the idea that experimental ligation of a major coronary artery in animals was invariably fatal. This was not actually the case, but the 19th century concept that the heart could not survive such a severe insult died hard.

Diagnostic difficulties

The process whereby the views of clinicians were changed began in the 19th century, and by its end the pathology of myocardial infarction caused by coronary thrombosis was well understood. For reasons outlined above, this was of little interest to clinicians; the new cardiologists were further influenced by Mackenzie's view that morbid anatomy provided no useful information about the living heart in this context. Yet, a few physicians took a different view, believing that death was not inevitable after coronary thrombosis. For example, in 1910 Osler said "blocking of a branch (of a coronary artery) with fresh thrombus is very common in cases of sudden death in angina. . . . In patients who live some time the infarct may soften and pericarditis may be excited."[64] Osler regarded a pericardial rub in a patient with angina as good evidence that infarction had occurred, but even he seems not to have considered the possibility that a patient might make a full recovery after a coronary thrombosis. Certainly, most physicians regarded coronary thrombosis and myocardial infarction as post mortem findings in patients who had died from angina. Mackenzie was one of these and described such changes in several cases in *Angina pectoris*, published in 1923. But, as Samuel Levine said in 1929, "it is apparent that he (Mackenzie) had not made clinical diagnoses of coronary thrombosis in his practice."[72]

In Britain, the situation began to change in the 1920s. One of the first to diagnose coronary thrombosis was Evan Bedford, then a medical registrar at the Middlesex Hospital, who made the diagnosis in 1924 in a patient admitted with a diagnosis of "acute abdomen."[68] On 25 May 1925, the Cardiac Club, having paid tribute to the memory of Mackenzie (who had died four months previously) listened to two papers on clinical aspects of anaemic necrosis of the heart that would certainly have puzzled Sir James.[73][74] In the same year, John McNee of Glasgow published an important paper on coronary thrombosis, based largely on his experience in the United States where the condition was already well recognised.[75] Physicians would have read McNee's paper in the *Quarterly Journal of Medicine*. They would also probably have heard from the members of the Cardiac Club, meeting the day before the Association of Physicians, about this "very remarkable clinical syndrome" as McNee had called it. As a result of this wider dissemination of knowledge the censors of the Royal College of Physicians required candidates sitting the membership examination in 1927 to "Describe the clinical features of coronary thrombosis and discuss its prognosis." Yet, in 1928, when Ian Hill as a house physician in Edinburgh saw his first case of coronary thrombosis diagnosed by the young clinical tutor, Rae Gilchrist, his chief (unnamed) had never heard of the condition.[76]

Dawning of recognition

In his Harveian Oration of 1968, Bedford said "working at the London Hospital with Parkinson in 1926, I watched the epidemic spreading around the neighbourhood as local practitioners began to recognise coronary thrombosis."[68] In 1928, these two physicians published two papers that became very influential in Britain. In the first, they described the clinical features in 100 cases of coronary thrombosis; all varieties of presentation including crescendo angina culminating in infarction were detailed.[77] They tabulated the differential diagnosis from angina, including pyrexia and leucocytosis suggesting tissue necrosis. With regard to treatment Bedford and Parkinson insisted that absolute rest in bed for not less than a month was "imperative," and thought that return to ordinary life should be postponed for as long as possible.

The second paper by Parkinson and Bedford dealt with the electrocardiographic features of the condition.[78] Harold Pardee's description of the changes in the RS-T and T wave had been published in 1920, but few would have disagreed with McNee's statement in 1925 that "there is no special electrocardiogram characteristic of coronary thrombosis."[75] Parkinson and Bedford clarified the situation, describing the serial changes in the electrocardiogram during the stages of necrosis and healing.

Prevalence

By the 1930s, the increase in numbers of cases of coronary thrombosis was becoming obvious and physicians began to speculate whether this was a true rise or merely a reflection of better diagnostic skills. This debate has continued, with opinions ranging from a suggestion that coronary thrombosis is virtually a new disease (having been very rare indeed before the 20th century) to a belief that the incidence has changed little for several centuries relative to the population at risk. The latter idea was partly supported by Maurice Campbell. He quoted a rise in the crude death rate per million living from 27 in 1921 to 467 in 1940, and performed some ingenious but unconventional calculations to show that this rise could be largely explained by the marked change in age structure of the population.[79][80] On the other hand, Morris's study of post mortem records at the London Hospital showed an approximately sevenfold increase in the numbers of cases of coronary heart disease between 1907–14 and 1944–9 but a substantial decrease in the prevalence of coronary atheroma over the same period.[81] Further analysis of these somewhat puzzling figures is beyond the scope of this chapter.

Chronic rheumatic heart disease

For the first 40 years of the 20th century, valvular disease (which must have been mostly rheumatic) was the most common cause of death from heart disease. This preponderance, although genuine, must have resulted partly from the fact that for many doctors all that was required for this diagnosis was the finding of a murmur. The writers of textbooks on this condition – the most influential of which was Carey Coombs's *Rheumatic heart disease* of 1924[82] – tried to encourage a more discriminating attitude by lengthy discussions on the significance of various murmurs, particularly the frequently heard systolic murmurs. A history of rheumatic fever was an important point in favour of an organic cause for a murmur, but the converse argument, that a murmur suggested a rheumatic aetiology, was discouraged. Even Mackenzie spent some time on the analysis of murmurs in his textbook, but, typically, was more interested in fibrosis of the papillary muscles as evidence of myocardial damage than in the size and shape of the mitral orifice.

Mitral stenosis

Another physician had been more impressed with the narrowing of the mitral valve orifice. In 1902, Lauder Brunton described how he had opened stenotic mitral valves post mortem, and wondered about the feasibility of this procedure in live patients.[83] This challenge was not accepted until 1923, when Cutler and Levine reported the first operation for mitral stenosis. The reaction of British physicians to this development was not encouraging. Mackenzie thought it "a foolish thing to try to do,"[1] Carey Coombs believed that the operation could "never become a general method of treatment,"[84] and the younger physicians were more interested in therapeutic developments such as mercurial diuretics and quinidine.[85]. Henry Souttar of the London Hospital did not agree with them. He performed the first British operation for mitral stenosis in 1925, saying that "the problem is to a large extent mechanical."[86] The early operations were not, in fact, successful. After Cutler and Beck reported the unacceptably poor results in most of the 10 reported cases, no further operations on the mitral valve were performed for nearly 20 years. Lewis thought in 1944 that such surgery would "continue to fail."[87] How quickly this judgment was shown to be incorrect is described in chapter 16.

Infections of the heart

Infective endocarditis

Two important discoveries about infective endocarditis were made around the turn of the 19th century and are illustrated by comparing two papers by William Osler. In his Goulstonian Lectures of 1885, he discussed the microbial theory of the aetiology of the disease.[88] Osler did not find the evidence for this absolutely convincing because the imperfect microbiological techniques of the day gave inconclusive results; he thought, however, that the theory was "very attractive." Furthermore, the duration of the disease in his cases, although variable, was never very long. It was "scarcely two days" in the most severe, and two or three months in a very few cases. By 1909, Osler had become convinced that infection was the cause of the disease and identified the subacute variety which lasted between four and 13 months (in his cases).[89]

The infective aetiology had been established by such new techniques as blood culture. The main exponent of this in Britain was Thomas Horder, who described the technique in precise detail in 1905.[90] Horder subsequently became a leading authority on infective endocarditis. He gave a good account of the clinical features in 1908,[91] opened a discussion on infective endocarditis at the first general meeting of the Cardiac Club in 1922, and chose endocarditis as the subject of his Lumleian Lectures in 1926.[92] Horder led in trying to treat infective endocarditis with vaccines and specific antistreptococcal serum, but these, together with other remedies in the pre-antibiotic era, had no effect. The exception was the discovery that infection could be eradicated surgically. In December 1939, Oswald Tubbs ligated an infected ductus arteriosus and cured the infection.[93]

During and after the first world war the prevalence of infective endocarditis seemed to increase. Although this may have been partly because of a concomitant increase in rheumatic fever, endocarditis was quite common at this time in previously normal hearts. The Medical Research Council commissioned a report on the condition from Thomas Cotton, which he based on his investigations at Colchester and then University College Hospital.[94] He was the first to describe clubbing of the fingers in this condition.[95]. Cotton was Lewis' chief assistant at Colchester, having worked with him previously in 1913. After the war, Cotton returned to University College Hospital, and it may have been his influence that directed Lewis's attention to the subject of infective endocarditis – particularly as it affected bicuspid aortic valves. In 1923, Lewis and Grant published a paper in which they referred to the presumed bacteraemia that had led to the valvular infection,[96] and, in 1935, Okell and Elliott published an important paper on this subject.[97] These workers emphasised the frequency of bacteraemia after dental extractions, an observation that became important when antibiotic prophylaxis became available.

Although the antibiotic treatment of infective endocarditis began with the clinical trials of the 1940s, it is largely outside the period of this chapter. It was well reviewed by Ian Gray in 1987.[98]

Syphilitic heart disease

The advances in microbiology, which were crucial for the understanding of the aetiology and pathology of infective endocarditis, were equally important in the case of syphilis. This had been known for centuries as an important cause of aortic aneurysm, and aortic regurgitation was also frequently thought to be syphilitic in origin. With no means of confirming the clinical diagnosis, other forms of heart disease (notably myocardial fibrosis) were also easily attributed to syphilis.

The organism causing syphilis was identified in the first decade of the 20th century, and a reliable diagnostic test – the Wassermann reaction – was introduced. Syphilis was found to be a cause of heart disease in 15% of patients, and in some studies it was considered a cause of aortic regurgitation in as many as 75%. In the 1920s, the introduction of organic arsenicals together with improved public health measures reduced the incidence of the early stages of syphilis. However, because of the relatively long period before the cardiovascular lesions became manifest, these cases remained common for several years. Thus, Carey Coombs, in his Lumleian Lectures in 1930, reported that 5% of over 2000 cases of heart disease seen between 1918 and 1929 and 30% of his 130 cases of aortic regurgitation were definitely due to syphilis.[99] Campbell and Shackle reported similar findings in 1932.[100] Thereafter, the prevalence of cardiovascular syphilis began to decline, but even in the 1950s, syphilis was thought to be the commonest cause of isolated aortic regurgitation.

In his lectures, Coombs outlined his policy on treating cardiovascular syphilis – regular iodide and mercury with courses of organic arsenic "about twice in the year." In a thorough follow up of 1000 men with heart disease, Ronald Grant described how he had treated 175 men with syphilitic heart disease in an early form of controlled trial.[101] He followed these cases for 10 years or until death, giving one of three treatments:

- all three standard drugs;
- iodide alone;
- no specific treatment.

The latter two groups fared nearly equally well but markedly less well than the first group.

Diphtheritic myocarditis

Before the 20th century the diagnosis of diphtheria depended solely on clinical findings and many mild cases must have been confused with other varieties of sore throat. Identification of the causative organism at the end of the 19th century was quickly followed by the introduction of antitoxin. Thereafter myocarditis was recognised as a dangerous complication of diphtheria, with a death rate of around 10%. One of the earliest publications on the subject was by Hume and Clegg. They used the polygraph to investigate disorders of rhythm in cases of diphtheria.[102] Hume became something of an authority on the subject and introduced a discussion on the heart in diphtheria at the Cardiac Club in 1932.

Diphtheria continued to be a serious problem in the 1930s and 1940s, and large series of cases of myocarditis were published by Leete[103] and Neubauer.[104] Harold Cookson described how he had investigated 83 cases of diphtheria in a large outbreak in Dorset in 1943, and found that 63 of these had abnormal electrocardiograms.[69] After the second world war, active immunisation against diphtheria became almost universal in the United Kingdom and the incidence of the disease fell from over 55 000 cases per annum before the war to 51 in 1956. Diphtheritic myocarditis almost ceased to exist in this country.

Hypertensive heart disease

Throughout the 20th century it has been possible to measure the blood pressure in man with a fair degree of accuracy. Scipione Riva-Rocci invented his sphygmomanometer in 1896, and by 1901 instruments of this type were appearing in the Allen and Hanbury's catalogue. For the next 15 years or so, numerous physicians and instrument makers tried to improve on his design and British scientists played their part in this endeavour.[105] Among these, to mention a few, were Leonard Hill, Martin Flack, Charles Martin (whose instrument was the type favoured by Mackenzie), and George Oliver, who introduced auscultation of the Korotkov sounds to blood pressure measurement in Britain.[106] Physicians varied in the details of their technique of sphygmomanometry, and it was not until 1939 that the Cardiac Society and the American Heart Association produced a joint statement in an effort to standardise blood pressure measurement; even in this they were forced to agree to differ on the method of measuring the diastolic pressure.

At first there was some reluctance to include sphygmomanometry in the routine examination of a patient. Graham Steell made no mention of it in his textbook on heart disease in 1906,[14] and Mackenzie did not possess an instrument of his own until 1905.[107] Even in 1908, Mackenzie believed that "the trained finger is as yet the best guide we have in judging the pressure within an artery."[108] Physicians were uncertain about the importance of a raised blood pressure; cerebral haemorrhage and left ventricular failure were late and far from inevitable complications of hyperpiesia and many patients had no symptoms and led active lives. "Hyperpiesia" was the term coined by the classicist Clifford Allbutt in preference to the hybrid "hypertension," although, not for the first time, usage has triumphed over scholarship. Allbutt's main contribution to the subject was his definitive account of raised blood pressure in the absence of proteinuria, the condition known today as essential hypertension.[65]

Poor therapeutic outlook

Another reason for the lack of enthusiasm for measuring blood pressure was the complete inability of physicians to lower the pressure, even if it had been desirable, as some doubted. Suggestions for treatment were many, ranging from atropine and bromides through liver extract to extract of water melon seeds and yohimbine. All were useless, but sodium and potassium thiocyanate were in vogue in the 1940s and seemed to have some effect – this was, of course, before the days of clinical trials. The failure of medical treatment led to attempts at surgical relief. The outcomes of nephrectomy for unilateral renal disease and extensive sympathectomy were occasionally successful but rarely permanently so.

The bleak therapeutic outlook became bleaker in the 1930s, when the serious prognosis in some cases of hypertension became clearer – particularly in 1939, after Keith and colleagues at the Mayo Clinic described hypertensive retinopathy. It is worth pointing out in this account of British practice that the Mayo Clinic workers had, to some extent, been preceded by two British ophthalmologists, Marcus Gunn in 1896 and Foster Moore in 1916.[109] Therapeutics did not catch up with diagnosis and prognosis until the middle of the century when the modern era of effective treatment of hypertension began. The British contribution to this is described in chapter 25.

Pulmonary heart disease

Chronic bronchitis and emphysema have been known for many years as a common disease affecting middle aged and elderly people, especially men. Only comparatively recently was the heart failure that must have complicated many cases identified as a specific entity in mortality figures. Thus, Harold Cookson, a house physician in Birmingham in 1923, never made the diagnosis,[69] and John Parkinson and Clifford Hoyle were able to gather only 13 cases for their study of the heart in emphysema.[110] Similarly, Thomas Lewis had little to say about pulmonary heart disease in the third edition of his textbook on heart disease,[87] but McMichael, around the same time, had enough cases to show that the cardiac output in this condition was significantly higher than in the heart failure resulting from most other types of heart disease (see page 6).

It became clear in the 1950s that the prevalence of pulmonary heart disease varied in different parts of the country, and physicians working in industrial areas began to point out to their colleagues in areas with less air pollution that the condition was far from rare. Thus, Fulton reported in 1953 that heart failure in chronic pulmonary disease in Manchester was an important cause of morbidity and mortality in middle aged men.[111] The following year, Flint from Sheffield published a very thorough review of 300 cases of congestive heart failure seen in 1952–3.[112] He found that pulmonary heart disease was the most common cause overall (76 cases), and much the most common cause (64 out of 159 cases) in men. Flint had been working in Charles (later Sir Charles) Stuart-Harris's department, and a detailed account of chronic bronchitis, emphysema, and cor pulmonale was published from that department in 1957.[113]

Congenital heart disease

At the beginning of the 20th century, the study of congenital heart disease was largely confined to the pathological anatomy of the various lesions and attempts at the analysis of the processes which had brought them about. An important British contribution to this was made by Arthur Keith who left the London Hospital in 1908 to become curator of the museum of the Royal College of Surgeons. He published a series of papers culminating in his Hunterian Lectures of 1909.[114] He showed that in the early development of the mammalian heart, there was an extra chamber, the bulbus cordis, between the primitive ventricle and the truncus arteriosus. This normally became part of the right ventricle and, as Keith said "A large number of the very commonest malformations of the human heart are due to an arrest of the process which ends in the incorporation of the bulbus cordis in the right ventricle." Keith's work later became the basis of Russell Brock's study of the surgical anatomy of pulmonary stenosis.[115]

At the beginning of the century, and for several years later, clinicians found little to interest them in these pathological and embryological studies. Only once did congenital heart disease feature on the programme of the Cardiac Club. This was on 7 May 1934, when Wardrop Griffith showed several anatomical specimens[116] and Parkinson and Bedford mentioned atrial septal defect in a paper entitled "Diseases of the pulmonary artery." Clinical interest revived somewhat after the publication of Maude Abbott's *Atlas of congenital heart disease* in 1936.[117] This was swiftly followed by *Congenital heart disease*, written by James Brown of Grimsby.[118] [119] This was a very influential account of the clinical aspects of the various congenital lesions, with detailed correlation with the pathological features. In the second edition of his book, in 1950 (by which time the subject was expanding quickly) Brown decided to confine his account to those aspects with which he was familiar. The quality of this edition was such that it received an extremely laudatory review from Paul Wood, a prime mover in the advance of knowledge of congenital heart disease and never one to bestow praise on the undeserving. Brown's book was naturally superseded within a decade by publications based on modern methods of investigation and surgery, but it is a work of vast erudition and still worth reading . . . and not only by historians.

Da Costa's syndrome and related conditions

The constellation of symptoms and signs considered here was first described as a recognisable entity by Jacob Da Costa in 1871. His description was based on his experience in the American Civil War, and although the condition is common among civilians, it has always received more attention in wartime. Interest revived in August 1914 when many soldiers who had been in the retreat from Mons were invalided home with complaints of chest pain, breathlessness, palpitation, exhaustion, and giddiness. By 1915, Mackenzie had written a paper on "The recruit's heart" and suggested the establishment of a special hospital for the growing problem.[120] This idea was implemented the same year at Mount Vernon Hospital in Hampstead, where all soldiers with presumed heart disease were admitted. The differential diagnosis then was simple – it was VDH (valvular disease of the heart) if a murmur had been heard and DAH (disordered action of the heart) if there were no murmur. Lewis later stigmatised this classification as "preposterous."[34]

Soldier's heart

The hospital was directed by Allbutt, Osler, and Mackenzie, but the guiding spirit was Lewis, who was appointed to the permanent scientific staff of the Medical Research Committee in 1916.[121] Intensive study of DAH – by now being called "soldiers' heart" or "irritable heart" – led to various theories of its aetiology, such as infections or hyperthyroidism. Lewis thought the most likely explanation was that the condition was a sequel of some form of infection. He was the main author of an anonymous report to the Medical Research Committee in 1917 in which that view was put forward.[122] The report also suggested avoiding the use of any diagnostic term implying affection of the heart. The symptoms were regarded as "exaggerated manifestations of healthy responses to exercise" and the diagnostic term "effort syndrome" was proposed. The most effective treatment was found to be a combination of graded exercise and what today would be called psychotherapy. Also in 1917, the 250 beds at Hampstead were found to be insufficient and the unit moved to a 700 bed hospital at Colchester. In 1918, Lewis summarised the work of the unit in *The soldiers' heart and the effort syndrome*.[123]

The work at Hampstead and Colchester was also noteworthy as an early example of Anglo-American collaboration. Among several American medical officers who worked there with Lewis were Samuel Levine and Frank Wilson. These leaders-to-be of American cardiology, together with Paul White who worked with Lewis before the war, have recorded their happy recollections of this experience which was the beginning of several lifelong friendships.

Not so much a cardiac disorder . . .

After the war the difficult question of pensions was tackled by the appointment of a group of physicians as consultants to advise on the assessment of cases. Despite the insistence of Lewis and others that the effort syndrome was not a disease of the heart and that the word "heart" should not be used in any diagnostic terms, all the consultants were specialists in heart disease. Had the illogicality of this been recognised, the history of British cardiology might perhaps have taken a different course.[124] The absence of heart disease was confirmed by Ronald Grant in 1936 by a follow up study.[125] He reviewed 665 cases diagnosed as effort syndrome in 1916–18. Few patients were symptom-free but the death rate was low; there was little evidence of heart disease but a surprising number had developed pulmonary tuberculosis, which might seem to have been belated support for the infection theory.

. . . as a psychiatric one

In the second world war fewer cases of effort syndrome were diagnosed, although patients with the characteristic symptoms were probably still being seen and given different diagnostic labels. The fall in incidence was largely due to Paul Wood's Goulstonian Lectures of 1941,[126] which showed that effort syndrome was a misnomer. He analysed the symptoms and signs in 200 cases, and showed that the one feature they all had in common was an excessive reaction to emotion, especially fear – in the first place fear of danger and then fear of heart disease because of the symptoms themselves. Wood declared emphatically that the condition was a psychiatric disorder and advocated the use of the non-committal term "Da Costa's syndrome" as more appropriate. Good reviews of the history of this subject have been published by Joel Howell and by Oglesby Paul.[127] [128]

X disease

Mackenzie described X disease in his textbook on heart disease, and it was diagnosed by him almost as often as angina in the second decade of the century. It is, of course, not to be confused with syndrome X. Patients with X disease were often spare and thin, with what they called a "feeble circulation." They felt cold and ill after a cold bath and often had gastric or bowel complaints. Some were "sane and intelligent," others "peevish and irritable." Examination might reveal cold hands and feet, a slow pulse with marked sinus arrhythmia, and sometimes a remarkably low respiratory rate. There was often excessive "splashing" on examination of the abdomen and prominent hepatojugular reflux.

Mackenzie added a footnote to his description as follows: "I employ the term X disease for the reason that I do not know the nature of this complaint. Many physicians call members of this class "neurasthenia" and are content to leave the matter there . . . This is simply to give a complaint a name."[129] X disease appeared very commonly in Mackenzie's case notes of 1908–15,[130] but had disappeared almost completely from his records by 1918.

In conclusion

Readers are invited to draw their own conclusions from this sample of early 20th century British cardiology. They are also reminded that "the past is another country; they do things differently there."

Notes and references

1. McMichael J. *A transition in cardiology: the Mackenzie Lewis era. The Harveian oration of 1975.* London: Royal College of Physicians, 1976.
2. Lawrence C. Moderns and ancients: the "new cardiology" in Britain 1880–1930. In: Bynum WF, Lawrence C, Nutton V, eds. *The emergence of modern cardiology.* London: Wellcome Institute for the History of Medicine, 1985. (Med Hist, suppl 5).
3. Walter Holbrook Gaskell (1847–1914) worked with Carl Ludwig in Leipzig on the vasomotor activity of the autonomic nervous system. He continued this work on his return to Cambridge in 1875. There, in Michael Foster's department, he began his work on conduction of the cardiac impulse from sinus venosus to ventricle with delay at the sinoatrial and atrioventricular junctions. He also demonstrated that the initiation and propagation of the muscular contraction was an intrinsic property of the muscle cells and needed no nervous impulse to stimulate it.
4. Mackenzie J. *Diseases of the heart.* London: Froude, 1908:7.
5. Mackenzie J. *Disease of the heart.* London: Froude, 1908:197.
6. Mackenzie J. *The study of the pulse.* Edinburgh: Pentland, 1902.
7. Sir Arthur Keith (1866–1955) worked on the anatomy of anthropoid apes in Thailand, where he was medical officer of a gold mine. On returning to Britain, he was appointed demonstrator and, later, lecturer in anatomy at the London Hospital. He became a great friend of Mackenzie at whose suggestion he verified Tawara's work on the conducting system of the heart, and, with Martin Flack, discovered the sinoatrial node. In 1909, he left the London to become curator of the Hunterian Museum of the Royal College of Surgeons. His work in embryology led to his discovery that many congenital malformations of the right ventricular outflow tract were due to failure of absorption of the bulbus cordis. In 1913, he was elected a fellow of the Royal Society and was knighted in 1921. After retirement he became master of the Buckston Browne Research Farm at Downe in Kent and lived at Down House, Charles Darwin's home for 40 years.
8. The quotation "from the Galilee of Burnley in Lancashire comes a new teacher." From an anonymous review of Mackenzie's *Study of the pulse* in the *BMJ* 1902;2:250. This was almost certainly by Allbutt.
9. Arthur Robertson Cushny (1866–1926) a graduate of Aberdeen, had been professor of pharmacology at Ann Arbor, Michigan before returning to Britain in 1905 to the chair of pharmacology at University College, London. He did experimental work on the production of atrial fibrillation in dogs and convinced Mackenzie of the identity of this with the human arrhythmia. He became an authority on digitalis and published a monograph on this in 1925 (reference[35]).
10. Graham Steell (1851–1942) graduated at Edinburgh but spent most of his professional life at Manchester where he was assistant physician and, later, physician at the Royal Infirmary from 1883 until his retirement in 1911. He became the leading cardiologist in the north of England and is best remembered for his description of a pulmonary diastolic murmur in pulmonary hypertension due to mitral stenosis (Steell G. The murmur of high pressure in the pulmonary artery. *Med Chron Manchester* 1888–9;9:182–8).
11. John Hay (1873–1959) was an influential figure in the medical life of Liverpool for about half a century. He became a disciple of Mackenzie and frequently visited him. In 1907, he was appointed assistant physician to the Royal Infirmary and, in 1924, became professor of medicine at Liverpool University. He was a founder member of the Cardiac Club and gave the St Cyres lecture at the National Heart Hospital in 1933; his subject was "Certain aspects of coronary thrombosis."
12. Hurst A. *A twentieth century physician.* London: Arnold, 1949.
13. Osler W. *The principles and practice of medicine.* New York: Appleton, 1892.
14. Steell G. *Textbook on diseases of the heart.* Manchester: At the University Press, 1906:11.
15. Brunton L. *Therapeutics of the circulation.* London: Murray, 1908.
16. Mackenzie J. Heart failure. *BMJ* 1911;1:793–7, 858–63.
17. Sutherland GA. Modern aspects of the circulation. Lancet 1917;i:401–6, 437–42, 477–82.
18. Smith FJ. Letter. *Lancet* 1917;i:555.

19. Brown GH. *Lives of the fellows of the Royal College of Physicians of London 1826–1925*. London: Royal College of Physicians, 1955:454–5.
20. Mackenzie J. Letter. *Lancet* 1917;ii:255–7.
21. Allbutt TC. Letter. *Lancet* 1917;ii:405–6.
22. Anonymous. Sir James Mackenzie: obituary. *BMJ* 1925;1:242–4.
23. Ernest Henry Starling (1866–1927) qualified from Guy's in 1888, and within a year turned to physiology as a full time study. Dissatisfied with the facilities at Guy's, he began to visit University College and began his collaboration with William Bayliss, working on the microcirculation. In 1899, Starling succeeded Schafer in the chair of physiology, and later began his famous work on the factors determining the cardiac output. After a highly productive but turbulent career, he died while on a cruise to the West Indies.
24. Patterson SW, Starling EH. On the mechanical factors which determine the output of the ventricles. *J Physiol* 1914;48:357–79.
25. Patterson SW, Piper H, Starling EH. The regulation of the heart beat. *J Physiol* 1914;48:465–513.
26. Starling EH. *The Linacre Lecture on the law of the heart*. London: Longmans, 1918.
27. Pickering G. Starling and the concept of heart failure. *Circulation* 1960;21:323–31.
28. Chapman CB. Impact of the Starling concepts on clinical cardiology. *JAMA* 1963;183:352–7.
29. Harrison TR. *Failure of the circulation*. 2nd ed. London: Baillière, 1939.
30. Wood P. *Diseases of the heart and circulation*. London: Eyre and Spottiswoode, 1950:154–92.
31. The work of Jan Brod of Prague on renal blood flow in the early 1950s, for example, suggested that a modification of the forward failure theory might be correct.
32. Lewis T. A bedstead for use in treating cardiac patients suffering from congestive heart failure. *BMJ* 1928;2:997–9.
33. Holmstedt B, Liljestrand G. *Readings in pharmacology*. Oxford: Pergamon Press, 1963:57.
34. Lewis T. On cardinal principles in cardiological practice. *BMJ* 1919;2:621–5.
35. Cushny AR. *The actions and uses in medicine of digitalis and its allies*. London: Longmans, 1925.
36. Gavey CJ, Parkinson J. Digitalis in heart failure with normal rhythm. *Br Heart J* 1939;1:27–44.
37. McMichael J. The output of the heart in congestive failure. *Q J Med* 1938;7:331–53.
38. McMichael J, Sharpey-Schafer EP. The action of intravenous digoxin in man. *Q J Med* 1944;13:123–35.
39. McMichael J. Pharmacology of the failing human heart. *BMJ* 1948;2:927–33.
40. McMichael J. Circulatory failure studied by means of venous catheterization. *Adv Intern Med* 1947;2:64–101.
41. Bayliss RIS, Etheridge MJ, Hyman AL, Kelly HG, McMichael J, Reid EAS. The effect of digoxin on the right ventricular pressure in hypertensive and ischaemic heart failure. *Br Heart J* 1950;12:317–26.
42. McMichael J. Dynamics of heart failure. *BMJ* 1952;2:525–9, 578–82.
43. McMichael J. Some problems of heart failure. *Acta Med Scand* 1952; 142 (suppl 206):701–10.
44. Cushny AR, Edmunds CW. Paroxysmal irregularity of the heart and auricular fibrillation. *Am J Med Sci* 1907;133:66–77.
45. Lewis T. Auricular fibrillation: a common clinical condition. *BMJ* 1909;2:1528.
46. Jolly WA, Ritchie WT. Auricular flutter and fibrillation. *Heart* 1910;2:177–221.
47. Hertz AF, Goodhart GW. The speed limit of the human heart. *Q J Med* 1908; 2:213–8.
48. Hollman A. Thomas Lewis – the early years. *Br Heart J* 1981;46:233–44.
49. Lewis T. *The mechanism of the heart beat*. London: Shaw and Sons, 1911.
50. Lewis T. *Clinical disorders of the heart beat*. London: Shaw and Sons, 1912.
51. Lewis T. *Clinical electrocardiography*. London: Shaw and Sons, 1913.
52. Lewis T. The nature of flutter and fibrillation of the auricle. *Lancet* 1921;i:785–8, 845–8.
53. Wolff L, Parkinson J, White PD. Bundle-branch block with short P-R interval in healthy young people prone to paroxysmal tachycardia. *Am Heart J* 1930;5:685–704.
54. French RD. Darwin and the physiologists or the Medusa and modern cardiology. *J Hist Biol* 1970;3:253–74.
55. There is a full account of Keith's difficulties in his, at first unsuccessful, search for the bundle and the role that Mackenzie played in this. In: Mair A. *Sir James Mackenzie, MD 1853–1925. General practitioner*. Edinburgh: Churchill Livingstone, 1973:212–6.
56. Hay J, Moore SA. Stokes-Adams disease and cardiac arrhythmia. *Lancet* 1906;ii:1271–6.
57. Keith A, Flack M. The form and nature of the muscular connections between the primary divisions of the vertebrate heart. *J Anat Physiol* 1907;41:172–89.
58. Howell JD. Early perceptions of the electrocardiogram: from arrhythmia to infarction. *Bull Hist Med* 1984;58:83–98.
59. Hollman A. The history of bundle-branch block. In: Bynum WF, Lawrence C, Nutton V, eds. *The emergence of modern cardiology*. London: Wellcome Institute for the History of Medicine, 1985:82–102. (Med Hist, suppl no 5).

60. Hill I. Frank Wilson: obituary. *Br Heart J* 1953;15:259–60.
61. Latham PM. *Lectures on subjects connected with clinical medicine: comprising diseases of the heart.* Vol 2. London: Longmans, 1845:361–2.
62. Huchard H. *Traité clinique des maladies du coeur et de l'aorte.* 3rd ed. Paris: Duin, 1899.
63. Osler W. *Lectures on angina pectoris and allied states.* New York: Appleton, 1897.
64. Osler W. The Lumleian Lectures on angina pectoris. *Lancet* 1910;i:697–702, 839–44, 973–7.
65. Allbutt TC. *Diseases of the arteries including angina pectoris.* 2 vols. London: Macmillan, 1915.
66. Hollman A. *Sir Thomas Lewis: pioneer cardiologist and clinical scientist.* London: Springer, 1997:161.
67. Bousfield G. Angina pectoris: changes in the electrocardiogram during a paroxysm. *Lancet* 1918;ii:457–8.
68. Bedford DE. Harvey's third circulation: de circulo sanguinis in corde. *BMJ* 1968;2:273–7.
69. Cookson H. Thirty years of cardiology. *BMJ* 1957;1:659–62.
70. East CFT, Bain CWC. *Recent advances in cardiology.* London: Churchill, 1929:4.
71. Herrick JB. An intimate account of my early experience with coronary thrombosis. *Am Heart J* 1944;27:1–18.
72. Levine SA. *Coronary thrombosis: its various clinical features.* London: Baillière, 1929:3.
73. Gibson AG. The clinical aspects of ischaemic necrosis of the heart muscle. *Lancet* 1925;ii:1270–5.
74. Coombs CF, Hadfield G. Ischaemic necrosis of the cardiac wall. *Lancet* 1926;i:14–15.
75. McNee J. The clinical syndrome of thrombosis of the coronary arteries. *Q J Med* 1925;19:44–52.
76. Hill I. The wind of change in cardiology. *Practitioner* 1968;201:44–55.
77. Parkinson J, Bedford DE. Cardiac infarction and coronary thrombosis. *Lancet* 1928;i:4–11.
78. Parkinson J, Bedford DE. Successive changes in the electrocardiogram after cardiac infarction (coronary thrombosis). *Heart* 1928;14:195–239.
79. Campbell M. Death rate from diseases of the heart: 1876 to 1959. *BMJ* 1963;2:528–35.
80. Campbell M. The main cause of increased death rate from diseases of the heart: 1920 to 1959. *BMJ* 1963: 2:712–17
81. Morris JN. Recent history of coronary disease. *Lancet* 1951;i:1–7, 69–73.
82. Coombs CF. *Rheumatic heart disease.* Bristol: Wright, 1924.
83. Brunton L. Preliminary note on the possibility of treating mitral stenosis by surgical methods. *Lancet* 1902;i:352. Although cautious, the reaction to this paper in a leading article and correspondence was surprisingly encouraging.
84. Coombs CF. *Rheumatic heart disease.* Bristol: Wright, 1924:330.
85. Campbell M. The early operations for mitral stenosis. *Br Heart J* 1965;28:670–3.
86. Souttar HS. The surgical treatment of mitral stenosis. *BMJ* 1925;2:603–6.
87. Lewis T. *Diseases of the Heart.* 3rd ed. London: Macmillan, 1944:148.
88. Osler W. The Gulstonian lectures on malignant endocarditis. *BMJ* 1885;1:467–70, 522–6, 577–9.
89. Osler W. Chronic infectious endocarditis. *Q J Med* 1909;2:219–30.
90. Horder TJ. Observations upon the importance of blood-culture, with an account of the technique recommended. *Practitioner* 1905;75:611–22.
91. Horder TJ. Infective endocarditis. *Q J Med* 1909;2:289–324.
92. Horder TJ. Endocarditis. *Lancet* 1926;i:695–700, 745–50, 850–5.
93. Keele KD, Tubbs OS. Combined ligation of ductus arteriosus and sulphapyridine therapy in a case of influenzal endocarditis. *St Bartholomew's Hospital J* 1940;1:175–7.
94. Cotton TF. Observations on subacute infective endocarditis. *BMJ* 1920;2:851–4.
95. Cotton TF. Clubbed fingers as a sign of subacute infective endocarditis. *Heart* 1922;9:347–64.
96. Lewis T, Grant RT. Observations relating to subacute infective endocarditis. *Heart* 1923; 10:21–97.
97. Okell CC, Elliott SD. Bacteraemia and oral sepsis. *Lancet* 1935;ii:869–72.
98. Gray IR. Infective endocarditis 1937–1987. *Br Heart J* 1987;58:211–13.
99. Coombs CF. Syphilis of the heart and great vessels. *Lancet* 1930;ii:227–31, 281–6, 333–9.
100. Campbell M, Shackle JW. A note on aortic valvular disease with reference to aetiology and prognosis. *BMJ* 1932;1:328–30.
101. Grant RT. After histories for ten years of a 1000 men suffering from heart disease. *Heart* 1933;16:275–483.
102. Hume WE, Clegg SJ. A clinical and pathological study of the heart in diphtheria. *Q J Med* 1914;8:1–18. This paper was unusual in having no references, demonstrating the paucity of experience of the condition at this time.
103. Leete HM. The heart in diphtheria. *Lancet* 1938;i:136–9.
104. Neubauer C. Diphtheritic heart disorders in children. *BMJ* 1942;2:91–4.
105. Naqvi NH, Blaufox MD. *Blood pressure measurement.* London: Parthenon, 1998.
106. George Oliver (1841–1915) had been a student of William Sharpey at University College and, in 1904, founded the Oliver-Sharpey lectures at the Royal College of Physicians of London in his memory.
107. Mackenzie J. *Diseases of the heart.* 3rd ed. London: Froude, 1914.

108. Mackenzie J. *Diseases of the heart.* London: Froude, 1908:89.
109. Dollery C. Hypertension. *Br Heart J* 1987;58:179–84.
110. Parkinson J, Hoyle C. The heart in emphysema. *Q J Med* 1937;30:59–86.
111. Fulton RM. The heart in chronic pulmonary disease. *Q J Med* 1953;22:43–58.
112. Flint FJ. Cor pulmonale. Incidence and aetiology in an industrial city. *Lancet* 1954;ii:51–8.
113. Stuart-Harris CH, Hanley T. *Chronic bronchitis, emphysema and cor pulmonale.* Bristol: Wright, 1957.
114. Keith A. Malformations of the heart. *Lancet* 1909;ii:359–63, 433–5.
115. Brock R. *The anatomy of congenital pulmonary stenosis.* London: Cassell, 1957.
116. Campbell M. The British Cardiac Society and the Cardiac Club: 1922–1961. *Br Heart J* 1962;24:673–95.
117. Abbott ME. *Atlas of congenital cardiac disease.* New York: American Heart Association, 1936.
118. James William Brown (1897–1958) began his medical career, like Mackenzie, as a general practitioner. He became interested in school clinics for children with rheumatic and other forms of heart disease. His comprehensive records and mastery of the literature made him uniquely equipped to publish what was far and away the best clinical account of congenital heart disease of the pre-surgical era.
119. Brown JW. *Congenital heart disease.* London: John Bale, 1939.
120. Mackenzie J. The recruit's heart. *BMJ* 1915;2:807–8.
121. Not the Medical Research *Council* until 1920.
122. Medical Research Committee. Report upon soldiers returned as cases of "disordered action of the heart" (DAH) or "valvular disease of the heart" (VDH). London: Medical Research Committee, 1917. (MRC Special Report Series, no 8.).
123. Lewis T. *The soldier's heart and the effort syndrome.* London: Shaw and Sons, 1918.
124. See chapter 4 for the story of how the Cardiac Club and, later, the British Cardiac Society, grew out of the meetings of these specialists.
125. Grant RT. Observations on the after-histories of men suffering from the effort syndrome. *Heart* 1926;12:121–42.
126. Wood P. Da Costa's syndrome or effort syndrome. *BMJ* 1941;1:767–72, 805–11, 845–51.
127. Howell JD. "Soldier's heart": the redefinition of heart disease and specialty formation in early 20th-century Great Britain. In: Bynum WF, Lawrence C, Nutton V, eds. *The emergence of modern cardiology.* London: Wellcome Institute for the History of Medicine, 1985:34–52. (Med Hist, suppl no 5).
128. Paul O. DaCosta's syndrome or neurocirculatory asthenia. *Br Heart J* 1987;58:306–15.
129. Mackenzie J. *Diseases of the heart.* London: Froude, 1908:56–8.
130. There is a large collection of Mackenzie's case records for the years 1908–18 at the Royal College of Physicians of London. During the years of the first world war, he was one of the few consultant physicians left in London and, therefore, extremely busy.

Chapter 2

The Second World War and the NHS – the Framework for the Development of Cardiology

Geoffrey Rivett

Cardiology has long been recognised as a substantial part of general medicine. A hundred years ago, William Osler, in his *Principles and practice of medicine*, devoted 100 pages out of 1150 to diseases of the heart and circulation.[1] Yet its organisation as a specialty is relatively recent.

Hospitals and specialists before the war

Even at the outbreak of war in 1939, it was only in large cities that general physicians and surgeons were supplemented by doctors practising in narrower specialties such as ophthalmology or thoracic surgery. Country areas depended largely on cottage hospitals staffed by local family doctors, with occasional visits from city based specialists. Furthermore, the distribution of the specialists was determined by the economics of private practice. To find a "pure" cardiologist anywhere was nearly impossible.

Special hospitals and specialised units

In the great voluntary and teaching hospitals, there was often a prejudice against specialising beyond general medicine or surgery. Young men, keen to make a name for themselves in a developing but restricted area, gravitated to the "special hospitals" which had developed in large numbers in the 19th century. In the provinces, where there was only one medical school per city, special and general hospitals developed a modus operandi early on; diseases of women or of the eye were usually managed by the special hospitals. However, in London, with its 12 medical schools, the special hospitals undertook no undergraduate teaching and remained entirely separate.[2]

It was inevitable that large hospitals would develop their own specialist services, but these units were often small. Later, during the second world war, the risk of air raids and the need for new forms of treatment led to the development of special units, often attached to a general hospital but situated in the countryside. Many specialist units for neurosurgery, plastic surgery, burns, spinal injuries, and thoracic surgery started in this way.

Planning for district hospitals

Viewed from a national perspective, the organisation of hospitals in the 1930s was somewhat chaotic. Much discussion focused on the lack of system in delivering health care. Some local authorities improved the organisation of the hospitals that they ran, and the voluntary (not for profit) sector also took tentative steps towards rationalisation. However, during the critical months preceding the outbreak of war in 1939, the government planned an emergency hospital service within which command and control would be possible. The country was divided into regions, and with the outbreak of war a regional system was imposed. Substantial sections of the London teaching hospitals were evacuated to the surrounding country, so that people needing care or were wounded in the blitz could be moved to safety. The exigencies of war had imposed a national structure and a managerial organisation on British hospitals.

Culture of nationalisation

The years of war and their aftermath saw a ferment of ideas - organisational and clinical. Cardiological services took their place within this broader framework, and the discipline of cardiology responded to the pharmaceutical and technological progress that was taking place. The war had accustomed the country to central organisation with great purposes in mind and to applying scientific methods to war aims. In 1945, the Labour government embarked on a massive programme of nationalisation, a small part of which was the takeover of voluntary and municipal hospitals. It would have been possible to create something of a national health service merely by coordinating the existing organisations and funding them centrally or through local authority channels. Early plans envisaged something along this line, with various coordinating committees to sort out the organisational mess of the prewar hospital services.

Visionaries within central government and the medical profession wanted rather more. They, and far sighted people such as Lord Dawson (a consultant physician at the London Hospital who had military experience[3]) saw the possibility of a health system that provided the commoner types of hospital care locally, supplemented by more specialist services at distant centres. A series of regional surveys began in 1942 and were published in 1945–6. These provided the foundation for detailed planning. The survey of London and the south east is a good example.[4] Based on existing services, natural centres of population were identified and hospital districts were then proposed. The ambition was to create a single hospital in each district that would provide specialist services for commonly encountered health problems that required hospital care.

In 1947, health service planners were promised guidance on the pattern of clinical and specialist services; this was published the following year as *The development of specialist services*.[5] It was the work of a group of eminent specialists, from London and the provinces, and the secretary was George Godber, who was later to become chief medical officer to central government. The report reflected the current consensus at consultant level – it was a successful essay on general principles but not a reliable guide on details. However, the Royal College of Physicians liked it enough to ask for reprints to send to their members. Specialised services such as cancer treatment, ophthalmology, orthopaedics, obstetrics, and ear nose and throat were considered in detail, but cardiology was barely discussed. Cardiology and cardiac surgery were not then generally recognised as separate fields of endeavour and did not attain this status until the 1950s and 1960s.

The NHS provided the first opportunity to develop specialist services away from large conurbations. The change could not be immediate, but would be progressive. There was a clear vision against which local ambitions could be judged. From the outset, it was understood that education and service were intertwined. The Goodenough report, published in 1944, considered how medical schools, clinical teaching, and research should be organised within the context of a national hospital policy.[6] Based largely on evidence from the medical schools, the report stressed the importance of general as opposed to specialist experience at undergraduate level and in the earlier stages of postgraduate education.

Speciality development

The differentiation of clinical medicine into specialities has been going on for at least two hundred years. Specialities such as ophthalmology were products of the 19th century; endocrinology began to emerge in the 1920s, and the 1930s saw the development of cancer and trauma care. Cardiology and cardiac surgery became identifiable specialties after the second world war.

Effect of the war

Civilian hospitals received a boost from the postwar discharge of energetic young doctors from the services, and sometimes this changed the pattern of hospital work substantially. For example, anaesthesia, which was crucial to developments in surgery and cardiology, had barely existed as a speciality before the war. The NHS recognised anaesthesia as a discipline from the outset, and the many military anaesthetists who were being demobilised were able to move into new posts. However, only a few doctors and a single hospital saw cardiology as the centre of their work. That hospital was the National Hospital for Diseases of the Heart, in Westmoreland Street.

The hospital survey of London and the south east, lacking a rubric for cardiology, classified the 47 beds at the National Hospital as "other."[4]

Cardiology – a regional service

Many general physicians in the large teaching hospitals had an interest in cardiology, but there were few specialist cardiological units where cardiac physicians saw only cardiac patients. One such was a unit was set up at the London Hospital. Although Goodenough heard evidence from the London Hospital, he focused on the needs of medical education and believed that these units inevitably created difficulties and might cause a lack of balance in the clinical experience of students. From the service viewpoint, *The development of specialist services* believed that cardiology should be part of general medicine. It considered it "undesirable that general medicine should be so rigidly subdivided that all cardiological (or neurological) work became concentrated in the hands of specialists working only in these subjects."[5] Cardiology would find a place at the proposed regional centre, which would provide less common services including thoracic surgery. The regional cardiology centre would not "need to be a large unit," but it would be recognised as the place for special investigation and treatment, for second opinions, and for undergraduate teaching and research. The physician in charge would need at least one whole time registrar.

Development of cardiology and cardiac surgery

The rapid development of the NHS in the aftermath of war coincided with an explosion in understanding of the heart and circulation. Electronics, measurement, and imaging underpinned this explosion. Within the teaching hospitals, cardiologists slowly replaced "physicians with an interest in cardiology." This was largely because the new techniques of investigation demanded more than a general physician, with all his other interests, could deliver. The concepts, the language, and the techniques were new and different.

Problems over location

While modern cardiology could develop comfortably within regional teaching hospitals, cardiac surgery had a different natural base. It developed through the thoracic surgeons who mainly worked with tuberculosis, infection, bronchiectasis, and cancer of the lung. Although cardiologists and thoracic surgeons needed each other, they seldom worked in the same place. Thoracic surgery was generally practised at rural tuberculosis sanatoriums such as Papworth, where general physicians, let alone cardiologists, were rarely found.

Cardiology in London

The National Heart Hospital, though committed to cardiology, had no surgical facility. However, the Brompton Hospital, which specialised in pulmonary rather than cardiac diseases, had a chest physician with an interest in cardiology, and in 1947 appointed Paul Wood as its first "pure" cardiologist. Wood rapidly built up an independent cardiology unit. The surgeons at the Brompton Hospital - Brock, Cleland and Tubbs - had a background in thoracic surgery, but they increasingly undertook cardiac work. Some members of the Brompton staff were also working at Guy's Hospital, and some of the London Chest Hospital staff were working at the Middlesex Hospital. The Hammersmith Hospital was also involved in cardiology and cardiac surgery from an early date, and The Hospital for Sick Children, Great Ormond Street had its watching brief.

Importance of collaboration

While clinical advances in the 19th century were generally the result of accurate description of maladies and their differentiation by clinical observation rather than by laboratory studies and clinical research, this was no longer the case by the middle of the 20th century. It became increasingly important for clinicians, as they moved into ever more specialised fields, to collaborate with those in other disciplines and to share expensive equipment in developing areas such as imaging or genetics. It was imperative for modern cardiology to develop in close relationship with cardiac surgery. Cardiological units without access to surgery began to wither, and undergraduate medical education in cardiology was also difficult. Cardiology exemplified the principles of human physiology, and was an important and useful topic in the student curriculum. To have cardiology in one hospital and cardiac surgery in another made no clinical sense. In Oxford in the 1950s, cardiology took place at the Radcliffe Infirmary and surgery at the Churchill Hospital. University College Hospital undertook thoracic but not cardiac surgery, and patients with rheumatic heart disease were moved to the Middlesex Hospital. Some teaching hospitals were lucky in the quality of their staff as they developed new services, but the clinical results at others were disastrous. In one London teaching hospital, the medical staff ensured that their first cardiac surgeons stopped operating. Clinical research and the improvement of services were fastest and easiest where cardiologists and surgeons worked in the same place - as at the Hammersmith Hospital, Guy's, and the Brompton in London, and, in the provinces, in Leeds. Little or no initial strategic thinking underpinned the planning and location of these new and important units. More often than not, their development depended on clinicians of energy and foresight, who often had or developed links with colleagues in the United States.

Early accommodation

Because of the shortage of acute hospital beds in the first decade of the NHS, the establishment of a new cardiothoracic unit often took place within accommodation previously used for treating patients with tuberculosis. For example, the London Chest Hospital had a country branch at Arlsey which was accommodated in huts developed for the wartime emergency hospital service. These huts were used for patients with tuberculosis who might require thoracoplasty. However, by 1958, senior registrars with little in the way of specialised equipment were undertaking closed mitral valvotomies alongside other chest surgery in these isolated units. Harefield and Papworth were also sanatoria that developed thoracic and cardiac surgical services of the highest quality.

Ideally, cardiology and cardiac surgery should not only have been closely related but also supported by the full panoply of other specialities such as immunology and renal medicine. However, the way specialties developed was constrained by the money, buildings, and personnel available.

NHS organisation and specialist services

The drive to develop the broad range of health services came partly from the management and partly from medical staff of the different disciplines. There was much to be done, and each speciality had to compete with others that were equally deserving. Managers, planners, and indeed the media could see woeful inadequacies in services – for example, for frail elderly people, people with psychiatric illness, and those with learning difficulties.

Geographical imbalance

A geographical imbalance was also evident. The volume and quality of specialist services in the south east and in major cities far outpaced those in the north and in less populated areas. More specialists were needed, particularly in the support services such as anaesthetics, radiology, pathology, and geriatrics. However, young doctors often aimed for the more "glamorous" fields of medicine, even though increasing the number of cardiologists was not a priority for the regional hospital boards.

Before the NHS, such specialist development as there was in municipal hospitals later administered by the regional hospital boards depended on the medical officer of health and the local council. In only a few places was there much encouragement to push back frontiers. However, at the Hammersmith Hospital, the London County Council had agreed to host the British Postgraduate Medical Federation to provide postgraduate training, particularly to graduates from the Empire. The Middlesex County Council was also prepared to see the Central Middlesex Hospital develop specialised units. The NHS potentially provided new and more substantial opportunities, if there was the desire to utilise them.

Teaching hospitals links with the Ministry of Health

The teaching hospitals were better placed. Before the war their specialist staff had given their time free to the hospital, and had substantial freedom in the conduct of their hospital practice. They retained this freedom even when salaried under the NHS. Much could be done without extra costs apparently falling on the board of governors and its endowments or charitable income. Even more to their advantage, the teaching hospitals were explicitly concerned with research and development, and with the coming of the NHS they benefited from direct links with the Ministry of Health. Close and often warm relationships were established between these hospitals and the small team of administrators and doctors in the ministry. The ministry team was usually bright, innovative, and interested in the hospitals' work, so that teaching and postgraduate hospitals had a good chance of bidding successfully for new resources to develop services.

London issues

In London, the more complex medicine was often undertaken in general teaching hospitals and in the postgraduate teaching hospitals. Both types of hospital had boards of governors who were directly responsible to the Ministry of Health. Postgraduate hospitals were often at the forefront in their respective specialities. Great Ormond Street and the Evelina Hospital at Guy's were extending the scope of paediatric care. Moorfields Eye Hospital provided the greatest mass of expertise on ophthalmology in the country. In the south, the Royal Marsden was pre-eminent in cancer care. The Brompton and the National Heart Hospital were cardiac centres of great expertise.

Clinicians often had one foot in a general teaching hospital and another in a specialist postgraduate centre that was relevant to their interests and where they met their peers. Nevertheless, the organisational separation of postgraduate from general teaching hospitals was strongly defended. Integration, when suggested, was seen as a threat to the unity of purpose of the single speciality postgraduate hospitals – the integration that the lion offered the lamb – even though separation increasingly meant isolation from other growing areas in medicine. In 1962, after national plans for hospital development were announced by Enoch Powell (the Minister of Health), Professor Sir George Pickering examined the problems of the 12 London teaching hospitals. Pickering, previously of St Mary's and at the time a successor of Osler at the Radcliffe Infirmary, Oxford, proposed that the postgraduate hospitals should associate at the least with each other, in two large multispecialty groups in Holborn and South Kensington.[7] The cardiological hospitals would be sited in South Kensington. It was a visionary proposal, but it foundered on the practicalities of money and the hospitals' desire for continued independence.[8] The postgraduate hospitals concerned with the heart remained, and continue to remain, outside the organisations that manage general hospitals.

Rationalisation and concentration

A second and substantial London problem was that the presence of 12 teaching hospitals as well as the postgraduate centres led to competition, duplication, and small units with small workloads. Some cardiac units had short waiting lists, probably due to awareness within the profession of their outcomes in relation to heart surgery. In 1979–80, the London Health Planning Consortium – established by the Department of Health and the four regional health authorities to rationalise health services in London across boundaries – commissioned a series of reports on technologically driven specialities. A working group, which included many people who were knowledgeable about health provision in London, reviewed cardiology and cardiac surgery. The specialist expertise in heart disease came from clinicians working outside the capital to avoid special pleading. In line with reports from the royal colleges suggesting minimum workloads for centres that investigated and operated on the heart, the London Health Planning Consortium group suggested that some units should amalgamate or close.[9][10] Little action was taken, but subsequent reports, such as that of Tomlinson,[11] followed a similar line, and some amalgamation ultimately took place. This planned concentration is quite unlike the situation in the United States, where cardiac services are much more widely dispersed.

Equity, cost, and quality

Cardiology, like renal medicine, was at the forefront of broader debates on quality and accessibility within the NHS. Equity has been an issue in British medicine since at least the 19th century, when hospitals began to be developed out of the old workhouses by boards of guardians. However, there is always a tension between the desire to provide good services and to make them widely accessible today, and the requirement for clinical research to ensure better services in the future. Sir Francis Avery Jones, an eminent gastroenterologist, pointed to the dilemma that inequality might be the price of progress.

Geographical equity

Nationally, there were problems of geographical distribution of services. In 1948, few places had a specialist cardiological service; London, Leeds, and the large metropolitan areas were at the cutting edge. While such expertise might attract patients from vast distances, the probability of people with comparable problems receiving care depended largely on how near they lived to a centre of excellence. Wales and the West Country were long without a cardiac surgical service, although a few patients travelled to the Brompton. One aim of the NHS was to provide equity of access, and it became apparent that specialist units were needed throughout the United Kingdom. Hence the development of cardiac surgical services in Bristol and Cardiff.

Increasing demand

Cost and equity are inter-related. To begin with, increasing access to cardiology and cardiac surgery did not seem to create a substantial financial problem. There was a limit to the number of people with congenital heart disease, and rheumatic heart disease was declining. These conditions did not generate a continually and rapidly increasing workload. However, once coronary artery surgery was established, matters were different. Britain was well behind the United States in recognising the potential of surgery, but did so just as the country was entering recession after the 1973 Yom Kippur war and the rise in price of oil.

As cardiac surgery entered the phase of rapid expansion, the money dried up. Adding to the problems was a political recognition that too little had been spent on mentally ill, mentally handicapped and elderly people. Money was needed to develop services for these groups, and it had to be found. In London, difficulties were compounded by the report of the Resource Allocation Working Party.[12] Since 1948 it had been recognised that in terms of the population served, substantially more money was spent in the south east of England than in most other parts of the country. That situation was now remedied to the detriment of acute services in London.

Rationing by waiting list

As the service needs became increasingly apparent, the sheer expense of cardiological care placed cardiologists and cardiac surgeons in the same position as the renal physicians, who for years had been unable to provide care for all who would benefit from renal replacement programmes. In a cash limited health service, there was no alternative to rationing. Queues developed for investigations such as catheterisation, which were potentially life saving, and these queues were followed by a second wait for surgery. In specialties where time can be of the essence in patient survival, this was, and is, clearly unsatisfactory.

Private sector

A small but flourishing private sector inevitably developed to provide earlier care to those who could pay. Initially based on private facilities in suitably equipped NHS hospitals, private hospitals were soon providing services, and in the 1990s a single speciality cardiological hospital opened in London. Britain was not alone in facing the problem of providing for rising demands, but the financial pattern of the NHS is almost unique. Other developed countries accommodated the demand, albeit at a substantial cost.

Issues of ethics and quality

Finally, there are issues of ethics and quality. From the outset, the severity of the problems faced by some patients invited rapid intervention, even when operative techniques were still primitive. By the late 1940s, surgeons such as Brock were operating on infants with severe congenital heart disease. The survival rate was low. Brock had to explain to the local coroner that without surgery the possibility of survival was slim, and that only by operating could surgical techniques be improved. In the 1950s, the operative mortality for those with pulmonary stenosis was high, yet some surgery had to go ahead – sometimes because patients were near to death, sometimes to try new and possibly better techniques. When the heart–lung machine came into widespread use in the 1960s, postoperative neurological complications were well known but little publicised. How different the fate of patients would have been had surgery been delayed until techniques had improved, and how "informed" consent for operation really was, are open to question. The doctors did their best by their lights, some with more humility than others.

The learning curve

By the 1970s, cardiologists were beginning to establish confidential case registers (for example, for pacemaker insertion) to enable them to assess their patients' outcomes. There was now wide recognition that the outcomes of patients undergoing cardiac surgery varied between units. The best results were usually to be found in those units with the higher workloads. Professional organisations issued guidelines about the level of work that was conducive to good results. Hospital planners sometimes took advantage of these guidelines in their planning and rationalising of services. By the 1990s the era of the brave surgeon venturing into uncharted territory had largely ended.

Shortages of money . . . and donor organs

Lack of funding restricted the provision of services, even when there could be little argument about clinical need. Furthermore, the effectiveness of cardiac transplantation shown in the 1980s resulted in new ethical problems. Transplant organs were in short supply, so clinicians were constrained not only by their budgets but also by the supply of organs. This forced them to decide who lived and who died. How far these decisions should be taken by ethical panels and how far by individual clinicians is not resolved. These ethical problems are now more open to public debate. The era of litigation and enquiries has arrived, and clinicians and managers are held accountable for results as never before.

Government has adopted a quality agenda and a framework of accountability for clinical results, some would say willing the end without providing the means. The landscape of the health services, public and private, has changed. Over the past 20 years systems of medical audit have been created and the belief has grown that organisations and hospitals share the responsibility of senior clinicians for the quality of care.

In conclusion

Within the same decade, modern technologically based cardiology and cardiac surgery developed, the second world war was fought, and the NHS began. The specialities and the organisational framework within which they operate interact. Society has changed, with a new emphasis on information, public involvement, ethics, and quality in health care. Continuing clinical development remains the most important factor shaping the demands on the healthcare system. Its costs increase, and the United Kingdom, which places great emphasis on equity, will rely on the NHS for such services for many years to come. Yet the ability of surgeons and physicians to improve the outcome of many patients depends on the money available. In an increasingly affluent and well informed society, clinical development drives the provision of private services as well. Avoiding a two-tier service seems impossible, not least because it is now easier than ever before to draw international comparisons of access and outcome.

References and notes

1. Osler W. *The principles and practice of medicine*. 3d ed. Edinburgh and London. Young J Pentland, 1898.
2. Ministry of Health. *Postgraduate medical education and the specialties. With special reference to the problem in London*. London: HMSO, 1962.
3. Ministry of Health. *Consultative Council on Medical and Allied Services. Interim report on the future provision of medical and allied services*. (Chairman Lord Dawson) London: HMSO, 1920. (Cmnd 693.)
4. Ministry of Health. *Hospital survey: the hospital services of London and the surrounding area*. London: HMSO, 1945.
5. Ministry of Health. *NHS: the development of specialist services*. London: Ministry of Health, 1948. (RHB(48)1.)
6. Ministry of Health, Department of Health for Scotland. *Report of the Inter-Departmental Committee on Medical Schools*. London: HMSO, 1944.
7. Ministry of Health. *Postgraduate medical education and the specialties. With special reference to the problem in London*. London: HMSO, 1962.
8. Rivett GC. *The development of the London hospital system, 1823–1982*. London: King's Fund, 1986.
9. Units for cardiac surgery. (Leader) *BMJ* 1979;2:2.
10. London Health Planning Consortium. *Report on cardiology and cardiac surgery*. London: DHSS, 1979.
11. Department of Health. *Report of the enquiry into London's health service, medical education, and research*. London: HMSO, 1992.
12. Department of Health and Social Security. *Sharing resources for health in England. Report of the Resource Allocation Working Party*. London: HMSO, 1976.

Chapter 3

The Training, Numbers, and Distribution of Cardiologists

Douglas Chamberlain

Until very recently, postgraduate medical training was poorly structured and based on the old apprenticeship system. This applied to specialist medicine as well as to general practice – and cardiology was no exception. Moreover, training was not well focused on future professional requirements. Well into the 1960s, most of those hoping to become specialists with an interest in heart disease looked for their apprenticeship within general medicine, although usually under the guidance of physicians who had a special interest in cardiology. Personal experience showed that in 1970 it was possible to be appointed as cardiologist to an important district general hospital having worked only in training posts designated as "general medicine" which offered broadly based experience. Accreditation did not exist. The supplementary training that could be obtained during research years together with overseas experience were often needed to bolster the inadequate provisions of an outmoded system.

Training within the NHS

Before the inception of the NHS in 1948, most hospital physicians were "honorary" – working part time and unpaid. This was not altruism; a hospital base was important for credibility in the private practice that could provide a generous income. The "honoraries" were absorbed into the new service and became salaried "consultants," but most retained their private practices so that few senior hospital appointments were full time. Most commonly, physicians and surgeons worked within the hospital service for nine notional half days or fewer. In London and the larger provincial cities, many had to divide this commitment between two or more hospitals. The time and influence within any one institution of some very great postwar British cardiologists was therefore limited, as, to a degree, was their potential impact on the training of junior staff.

The first training step

The organisation of the first training grade has remained broadly unchanged for nearly half a century. The consultants were then – as now – at the head of a pyramidal training structure, generally with two or more grades supporting them. In the United Kingdom, house physicians or house surgeons are the lowest hospital grade, equivalent to interns in some other countries. They became more numerous in 1953, when one year of hospital experience (six months spent in medicine and six in surgery) became compulsory after professional qualification by examination. These house officer posts are therefore designated as preregistration. Full entry onto the *Medical Register* is granted only after this period has been completed satisfactorily.

During the early postwar years, some teaching hospitals used relatively specialised services rather than more broadly based ones to provide early experience. Some even made the division between medicine and surgery unequal, with the emphasis reflecting the future aspirations of the trainee – subject always to the availability of posts. But even then, cardiology was too esoteric for preregistration house physicians. The objective of providing a general training with wide experience at house officer level is now closely regulated.

Membership

From the very start of organised progression within the hospital service, and long before structured training was available, those who wished to embark on a hospital career ladder faced a formidable obstacle – an entry examination for specialist training. For medical specialties this is a diploma of membership of one of the Royal Colleges of Physicians (of London, Edinburgh, or Glasgow (MRCP)). A diploma from the fourth institution in Dublin has tended to be regarded as less relevant to the United Kingdom. No equivalent entry examination exists elsewhere in Europe. The "membership" demands a broad and detailed knowledge of general medicine and has served to maintain high standards of knowledge and medical care. The examinations may not be taken for at least 18 months after qualification, and the first attempt is usually made after two or three years. Only a minority pass first time.

Thus, continued broad based training is required after a house physician appointment. This is generally provided at senior house officer grade, with appointments of one or two years' duration. Although these posts existed from the 1950s, they originally tended to be specialist orientated and designed for a service rather than an educational need. The emphasis changed through the 1980s and 1990s. Trainees now rotate through a variety of specialties in posts that provide time and opportunity for continuing broadly based postgraduate education.

Progression into the specialty

Entry to specialist postgraduate training in the United Kingdom has been at registrar grade. In all but the least popular specialties, training at this level is open only to those who hold the MRCP. Until 1997, registrar posts were at two levels – senior registrar and middle grade registrar (so called because historically a senior house officer post had sometimes been called "junior registrar"). These were separate appointments and entry into the first held no guarantee of further progression. Sometimes trainees stayed in one institution and sometimes they moved far afield for the necessary advancement. The two levels were frequently separated by a period in a research post outside the official training ladder. This could serve several purposes: it formed a buffer period that maintained employment while waiting for a senior registrar appointment, it could boost specialist training if the middle grade registrar appointment had not been fully dedicated to cardiology, and it provided trainees with an opportunity to work towards a doctorate of medicine (MD or DM). In the United Kingdom, the ordinary medical qualification is a bachelor of medicine (MB or BM). The doctorate is a higher degree attained as a result of a thesis that may be expected to have a content equivalent to at least three strong scientific papers. The competition for senior registrar posts in cardiology has usually been intense enough for an MD to be regarded as essential to success.

Some junior doctors with frustrated ambitions to become specialists did not stay long in hospital posts. General practice was not always regarded as a specialty in its own right. Until the 1970s it could be a depository for those who were failing to progress in their chosen field. Some of those who wished to become cardiologists finally settled as general practitioners or – because of a shortage of higher training opportunities – emigrated to where prospects were believed to be better.

The final stage

Once a senior registrar's post in cardiology had been achieved, consultant status could be expected in time. The final training appointment was for a four year period, but extensions were given regularly if the trainee had not been appointed to a consultant post by the end of the term. Senior registrars generally spent the first two years providing a service at a level of expertise little different from that expected of a consultant. Indeed, most consultants believed that service needs were adequately covered if a senior registrar was available. This was useful in an undermanned service. It could also provide a cloak for dubious practice by a very small but well publicised minority who drew salaries appropriate to longer hours of hospital duty than they provided, while allegedly giving too much attention to private practice. Senior registrars often spent a third year gaining experience overseas, often in the United States. In the final year, the emphasis was on further service provision (often in general medicine) or additional research . . . and on searching in earnest for a consultant position. But an ambition for a career in specialised hospital medicine led through a poorly charted pathway in which luck and opportunity were the major determinants of success.

"Elderly" junior doctors

Thus, until recently most consultant cardiologists in the United Kingdom had had a period of training that was longer, if less well organised, than that of colleagues in most other countries. Eleven years from qualification to consultant was by no means unusual, and for some the period was longer. Assuming qualification at 24 years of age, the arithmetic of training ensured that few attained their professional goal before 35 years of age. In the period after the second world war, when two years' national (military) service was mandatory for most young men (with three years an option for those keen to obtain a commission at officer rank) progression took even longer. Thus, until the early 1970s many appointments were made at ages 38 to 40 years. Indeed, in 1968, at the time of the Todd Report[1] - the first major effort to reform medical training in the United Kingdom - nearly 400 senior registrars were older than 35. For many newly appointed consultants there were relatively few years left when youthful enthusiasm remained a driving force.

The pattern of training

The only controls in the structure of training related to the types of post an aspiring cardiologist was expected to have filled and the de facto need to have achieved membership of a Royal College. Details were not specified. No requirements were laid down for the numbers of procedures undertaken nor for the skills that had to be learned, but some knowledge of research was expected by most appointment committees. Trainees would strive to have published a dozen or so papers and to have an MD by the time they were competing for a consultant post. Thus, the stimulus of competition and prolonged experience in the specialty tended to compensate for the inadequate organisation of the training programmes.

In most centres, clinical acumen and good standards of clinical practice were certainly learned from senior medical staff. But with some exceptions, investigatory skills, including those of catheterisation and later of echocardiography, were passed down within the training ranks with little direct consultant involvement. The old aphorism "see one, do one, teach one" was not entirely without foundation.

Two types of cardiologist evolved, and although the distinction was never officially recognised, all understood the labels "type A" and "type B." The former worked in the major cardiac centres with responsibilities restricted to the specialty. The latter were appointed to district hospitals and shared with colleagues from other disciplines the responsibility for general medicine. The pattern of training determined, to a degree, whether individuals applied for posts variously designated as "general medicine with an interest in cardiology," "cardiology with general medicine," or "cardiology." It was also possible to develop a specialty after appointment to a post, with or without the encouragement of employing authorities.

The distinction between type A and type B cardiologists became blurred and outdated through the 1970s and 1980s. A range of skills was still required, but this was seen to extend from the interventionalist cardiologist working in a major centres to the cardiovascular physician who was a true specialist but nevertheless undertook duties in general medicine by sharing responsibility for emergency admissions. How far the continuing care of non-cardiac patients remained the responsibility of cardiovascular physicians depended on local practice. It was (and remains) a necessity for some, because appointments in general internal medicine became increasingly uncommon. To meet this need the Specialist Advisory Committee in Cardiology laid down that one of the years at senior registrar grade had to be spent in general internal medicine in addition to a year in research. Thus, only two of the four years at the highest training grade were dedicated specifically to cardiology.

Introduction of formal training

The apprenticeship system was adequate for the needs of clinical cardiology when diagnosis depended principally on history and physical signs, and treatment was expectant or based on the use of a small number of effective drugs. But the introduction of invasive and electrical methods of treatment together with the explosive growth of new technology presented trainees with major new challenges. These challenges included the need to:

- acquire more detailed knowledge of congenital heart disease;
- understand the principles of caring for patients with acute coronary syndromes;
- acquire new skills in diagnosing and managing patients with arrhythmias (which included ever more complex methods of pacing);
- gain experience in cross sectional echocardiography with colour flow Doppler;
- become adept at cardiac and coronary catheterisation and angiography;
- have at least some insight into the principles and diagnostic value of nuclear cardiology and newer radiological imaging techniques;
- develop an interest in epidemiology, prevention, rehabilitation, and resuscitation.

Skills in interventional procedures played an important part for at least some trainees. Considerable experience was needed in percutaneous transluminal angioplasty, balloon dilatation of valvular obstruction, and electrophysiological methods of diagnosis and treatment. Random opportunistic training could no longer guarantee that newly appointed cardiologists would have the knowledge and skills needed in the new technological age. Two implications could not be avoided: strategies had to be developed to ensure that all necessary aspects of training were adequately covered, and some degree of subspecialisation was inevitable. The need for structured training rather than a purely experiential preparation was underlined by the reduction in the working hours of trainees – and therefore of clinical exposure – which followed recommendations and later regulations over the past decade. But change was on the way.

The Royal Colleges, through the joint colleges higher medical training committee and its specialist subcommittees, became increasingly active from the mid 1970s. In 1990, proposals for a new training programme in cardiology were published by a group representing the cardiology committee of the Royal College of Physicians of London and the British Cardiac Society.[2] Two years later these were followed by recommendations for paediatric cardiology that were generally compatible with the adult programme.[3]

The first proposals

Cardiology was considered to require longer training than other medical specialties – nine years from registration compared with the norm of seven. An initial period of three years in general internal medicine was still seen as essential, with the expectation that the MRCP would be gained during this time. Two blocks of three years in the registrar grade were envisaged. The advantages of two distinct posts were broader experience, flexibility, competitive interchange, and the opportunity for a break between the blocks to allow for a period of research. Accreditation would follow after five years of specialty training that might include a research year. The need for general medicine training late in the programme was still recognised, with the suggestion it should occupy one year of the second block. Interventionalist cardiologists might require an additional year, which could extend training to 11 years from qualification or 10 from registration, and more if additional research time were taken or MRCP was delayed. This proposal was published three years before the official report on specialist education (the Calman report), and influenced the future of training, at least in the United Kingdom.[4]

Meanwhile, the cardiology section of the European Union of Medical Specialists had made independent proposals for five years of specialty training as the European standard for hospital cardiologists. This was compatible with the five years for accreditation suggested independently for the United Kingdom. Subsequently, the newly created European Board for the Specialty of Cardiology, comprising representatives of the European Society of Cardiology and the cardiology section of the European Union of Medical Specialists issued guidelines for a six year training (including a common trunk of two years in general internal medicine).[5] The European board does not favour a qualifying examination, but does require an annual assessment by the head of the training programme. The widely applied requirements for training have enabled the board to create a diploma that allows those who have completed the programme (or an equivalent one) to be called "European cardiologist." This designation does not replace the need for accreditation at national level. Needs vary in different countries. For example cardiology in the United Kingdom is much more a hospital based specialty than is the case in many other parts of Europe.

New UK guidelines

The definitive guidelines on training were published in 1995.[6] The old terms of registrar and senior registrar were abolished, and the new designation of specialist registrar was introduced. Trainees are allotted a number, which is kept for the duration of their training. Matching of training to consultant opportunities is thereby controlled centrally. After a minimum of two years' postregistration general professional training in approved posts, higher medical training is provided in four phases. The first, lasting for one or two years, should be spent in a general hospital with at least 60 nights of resident unselected medical intake and continuing responsibility for the patients. It includes basic experience in cardiac catheterisation and pacing. The second phase of two or three years, with instruction in non-invasive and invasive techniques and contact with cardiac surgery, is provided in a specialist centre. In addition to these four years there may be a third phase of research for one year or more which can be undertaken at any time, or omitted if good quality research has been undertaken before entry. A final phase of formal training allows the development during a period equivalent to 12 months (not necessarily consecutively) of a sub-specialty interest within cardiology or alternatively further training in general internal medicine. As well as defining the broad structure of the programme, the guidelines set out the requirements for skill acquisition. During years one to five, defined numbers of non-invasive and invasive procedures must be undertaken (including 200 coronary angiograms and 500 echocardiograms) together with pacemaker implants and some participation in electrophysiology. Other detailed recommendations for the subspecialist year are given.

A system of annual assessments by an expert panel under the aegis of a postgraduate dean was introduced. Trainees have a nominated mentor, who can take an overview of their progress throughout and can offer them counselling and advice. Documentation includes a log book for records of laboratory procedures and a register of training and assessment. The register includes a curriculum vitae, a record of training, a register of general medical experience, and a detailed assessment sheet. After completing the six years, trainees are awarded a certificate of completion of specialist training and an appropriate entry is made in the national list of medical practitioners held by the General Medical Council. Cardiologists may have dual accreditation by adding general internal medicine, provided this path was followed in the final training year.

An editorial, published at the same time as the guidelines, summed up the development in terms that would have surprised most lay people (who might have expected this advance somewhat sooner). "For the first time in the history of British cardiology, trainees beginning their training have a curriculum laid out for them with an indication of the subject matter that they should learn and understand as well as a guide to the numbers of practical procedures they should aim to undertake to become proficient."[7]

Regulating numbers

One of the principle reasons why cardiology in the United Kingdom languished with too few posts was because specialist medicine under the NHS had neither the stimulus of a free insurance-led market nor effective central control. Expansion of the hospital service was determined at district or regional level (the NHS had three or four levels of control from central government down to hospital authorities). Expansion should have occurred in response to perceived need – and indeed it often did – but perception generally caught up with reality only after years of delay. As long as complex investigations and treatments were not needed for most patients with heart disease, their clinical needs had largely been met by general physicians. Then there came ever more successful surgery – first for acquired valvular disease and congenital anomalies and later for coronary disease – with all the accompanying diagnostic needs. Arrhythmias became better understood and more widely diagnosed, while treatments became more diverse, more successful . . . and more dangerous.

General physicians were slow to accept that they could no longer provide an acceptable service for most patients with heart disease. They had become used to supervising coronary care units after their introduction in the 1960s, and were happy to provide care within the NHS and privately – with the knowledge that tertiary referral could be made as necessary to the major cardiac units in teaching hospitals and specialist centres. But many patients who should have been referred from primary care to hospitals or from generalist physicians to tertiary care did not receive the specialist advice and therefore the effective new treatments that became available. Most physicians working in district hospitals did not understand the potential benefits, and needs were not recognised. Moreover, patients were not educated to have high expectations. Without the stimulus of demand there was no response from medical and non-medical administrators who determined what new posts should be created and in what specialty.

To be fair, the Department of Health had encouraged an increase in the number of cardiology posts within district hospitals during the late 1960s, but at local level it was rarely seen as a priority. The medical profession and the specialty itself carried as much responsibility for this as administrators and managers. By the time this view was corrected, financial constraints had tightened, and cardiology faced stiffer competition from other specialties that were also seriously under manned.

Pressure for change

Movement for change came primarily from two sources – from a joint cardiology committee of the Royal College of Physicians of London and the Royal College of Surgeons of England, and from the British Cardiac Society. Membership of these bodies inevitably overlapped; they represented the cardiologists and cardiothoracic surgeons who were most prominent in medical affairs nationally and who were most aware of the shortcomings of their respective specialties in relation to need, and in comparison with the progress being made in most of western Europe and the United States.

The joint cardiology committee published four reports between 1968 and 1992. The first noted that the rapid advances in medicine and surgery for heart disease had led to the need for units for diagnosis, treatment, and research and that these should be set up in general hospitals, preferably within the orbit of a university.[8] This recommendation may now seem self evident, but at the time few centres had adequate arrangements for interdisciplinary liaison, even if they had the facilities appropriate to the period. Four consultant cardiologists and four consultant cardiothoracic surgeons were recommended for populations of two to three million, although the authors accepted that such staffing levels "may appear lavish."

The second report (in 1980) noted that financial constraints and changes in priorities had limited the implementation of the modest proposals in the original report, and also addressed the implications of new developments, notably the advances in coronary surgery.[9] The latest figures available to the authors indicated that only 30 coronary bypass operations per million population were being conducted in the United Kingdom, one-sixth of the rate in South Australia. The report suggested that centres should be achieving 600 open heart operations per year to serve a population of approximately three million and that this would require the services of three consultant surgeons and six consultant cardiologists.

The initial emphasis on the need for cardiac centres was appropriate; growth had to begin centrally in order to provide adequate training opportunities for a more broadly based service. Although the 1980 report did include a note on the needs of hospitals outside major centres, it did not stress these until the later statements. By 1985, the need for effective local services in echocardiography, stress testing, ambulatory monitoring, emergency pacing, rehabilitation, and cardiac intensive care was well recognised.[10] The recommendation that each hospital should have at least one physician with special expertise and training in cardiology did meet with a response, partly because general physicians recognised that they could no longer claim to provide modern technological services. Nevertheless, the fourth and final report of the joint committee in 1992 [11] showed that there was still a large shortfall in local service provision. Nearly one in five district hospitals in England and Wales still had no physician with appropriate training. This deficiency was largely met over the next few years. But once a service is provided, the large unmet need is revealed by a torrent of referrals from general practitioners who become aware of new opportunities. This experience is familiar to every cardiologist appointed to a district hospital that previously had no cardiological service.

The British Cardiac Society in its own first report on district hospitals drew attention to the gross inequalities that existed in 1987 and stated that a full district service for a population of 250 000 required two physicians trained in the specialty.[12] By the time of the second British Cardiac Society report of 1994, an important shortfall remained.[13] Coronary artery surgery and percutaneous transluminal angioplasty had developed substantially and an increasing number of patients needed local assessment by exercise testing and other non-invasive tests. Moreover, the British Cardiac Society was encouraging appropriately trained district hospital cardiologists to participate in the invasive investigation of their patients in regional centres. The need was then considered to be one physician trained in cardiovascular medicine for every 100 000 population – a target that would still leave the United Kingdom well short of the provision considered appropriate in most western European countries. Yet the United Kingdom was still 155 positions short even of the earlier proposals.

Progress in times of stringency

Even if recommendations are widely agreed and accepted, implementation must always lag well behind intentions. Given the climate in which the proposals of the last three decades were made, progress has probably been as rapid as might have been expected. The United Kingdom's late start in the transition to specialist medicine has always been an important factor. Satisfactory growth in percentage terms has left a seemingly widening gap between need and provision – a perception that has substance at least in some geographical areas and specialties. Progress continues, but it is determined now by the pressure of contracts within the new purchaser-provider arrangements of the reformed NHS, restrained as it is by financial pressures that have now been devolved to local level with even less flexibility than previously.[14]

Counting the numbers

In 1978, the cardiology committee of the Royal College of Physicians of London discussed concern at the excess number of senior registrars in cardiology who had finished their training but had no immediate prospect of a consultant post. Concern was well founded. Many excellent physicians were unable to obtain posts when they completed their training. Some remained too long as "time expired" trainees, but many emigrated and have served the specialty well in other countries. Whilst their own ambitions were often satisfied, the loss to the country was considerable.

The apparent imbalance led to suggestions that the number of trainees should be reduced, but the facts were not sufficiently well established for recommendations to be made. Although the then Department of Health and Social Security attempted to maintain a balance, its information depended on returns from hospitals that usually included only posts funded through the NHS. But for at least a year or two, most trainees held temporary research appointments that were outside the official system. Moreover, many consultant and training appointments that related to cardiology were listed, for historical reasons, as general medical posts. Some practitioners thus designated, but who had a responsibility to the specialty, practised cardiology virtually all their professional time; but the variation between general and specialist medicine was wide. No firm criteria existed for defining posts or the training required to fill them. Thus, from the information collected through official sources there could be no prospect of predicting the vacancies that were likely to become available nor the true number of those aspiring to fill them. The cardiology committee was also well aware of the shortfall in facilities for the specialty in many parts of the country. The view prevailed that any reduction in the number of trainees would be inappropriate at least until accurate data became available.

The cardiology committee therefore decided to undertake a survey of staffing and projected vacancies that would be managed within the specialty by individuals who could make all relevant enquiries. The exercise was restricted to England and Wales and considered only consultant and senior registrar posts, taking as a criterion those who spent 40% or more of their working time in cardiology. Multiple techniques were used to obtain and cross-check the information. The survey proved very successful and became a biennial event under the joint aegis of the Royal College of Physicians and the British Cardiac Society. It eventually covered the whole of the United Kingdom and encompassed clinical and academic cardiologists, paediatric cardiologists, and trainees of all grades. Confidential information was gathered on expected retirement dates and was published in anonymous (aggregate) form. Information on technical facilities and staffing was also included as the enquiries became more ambitious.

In all, eight surveys were conducted and presented in seven publications from 1981 to 1994.[15–21] These provide a record of the specialty's progress over a critical decade. Not only did they supply the data needed for accurate planning, they also provided ammunition for those struggling to establish cardiology in districts where expertise and facilities were poor. The data did not suggest any need to reduce the number of trainees, and no mandatory reduction was made. By 1987, the Department of Health and Social Security was making determined efforts to match the number of trainees to consultant opportunities,[22] and the joint planning advisory committee was set up to achieve this. The biennial surveys channelled through the Royal College of Physicians provided data that eventually allowed most trainees to move into consultant posts without excessive delay. A major problem, however, remains – the maintenance of an appropriate balance between trainees for interventional and non-interventionist careers.[23]

Growth and geographical distribution

Table 1 shows the numbers of cardiologists and paediatric cardiologists in the United Kingdom from 1980, when the first reliable data were available, to 1992, when the last survey was conducted. No data are available for Northern Ireland in 1980, but the assumption has been made that the 1980 figures for Northern Ireland were the same as those in 1982. This will introduce little or no error. The original overall figure of 280 cardiologists in the United Kingdom increased by 51% to 423 over the 13 year period, with a greater percentage gain in England and Wales (60%) than in the other two countries. Expressed in terms of cardiologists per million population, this represents an increase from 5.0 to 7.6, but the figures mask considerable differences between and within the countries of the United Kingdom (table 2).

Northern Ireland has had by far the best provision throughout the whole period, and although it has enjoyed slightly less growth than England and Wales, it maintained more than twice the number of cardiologists pro rata compared with the rest of the United Kingdom. Within England and Wales, there has consistently been pronounced inequality of provision. In 1992, the range was from 4.8 per million population in East Anglia to 8.4 per million in south east Thames. All of these figures are put into perspective by comparing them with the provision in the United States, which even in 1967 had 51 cardiologists per million population in line with an authoritative recommendation a little later that 60 per million would be an

Table 1 Number of adult and paediatric cardiologists in the United Kingdom between 1980 and 1992

Year	Adult cardiology	Paediatric cardiology	Total
1980	248	32	280
1982	282	26	308
1984	289	41	330
1988	313	40	353
1990	339	48	387
1991	351	51	402
1992	373	50	423

The figures for 1986 were available only for England and Wales and have not been included.

Table 2 Change in the number of cardiologists between 1980 and 1992, expressed per million population

Year	England & Wales	Scotland	Northern Ireland
1980	4.5	7.4	11.4*
1992	7.2	8.2	17.7

* The figure for Northern Ireland represents 1982, not 1980.

appropriate number.[24] This ratio is now considered much too large, but no authoritative view on the ideal number has been forthcoming.[25]

Within the European Union, the figures in relation to population have been two to 10 times greater than for the United Kingdom. The other exceptions are Eire, whose figures are similar to our own, and Italy, where numbers approach those in the United States. It must be remembered, however, that some European countries have physicians who are designated as cardiologists yet have no hospital appointment. Their function is clearly different from that of cardiologists in the United Kingdom.

The 10 cardiologists per million population (one per 100 000) recommended in 1994 for district hospitals takes no account of the additional numbers needed in tertiary centres.[13] With increasing subspecialisation, we might anticipate a realistic total target of 15 per million, or approximately 850 in all for the United Kingdom. The current (1998) recommendation of the Royal College of Physicians is for one cardiovascular physician for every 80 000 population [26] which falls slightly short of that figure – it represents 12.5 per million. But certainly progress has been made, and this latest recommendation may well be met within three years if the present rate of expansion continues. Meanwhile, the provision of modern cardiac services in any area inevitably reflects wealth or dearth of local facilities. It is worth noting that in 1982, 55 health districts in England and Wales (average catchment area approximately 250 000 people each) were without a specialist cardiologist. The figure had fallen to 30 by 1992, but even then, 41 districts (total population 8.03 million) had fewer than seven half days of consultant time per week dedicated to cardiology. More recent figures are not available because no further surveys have been published.

Concluding words

This book underlines a fact that nobody would deny – that the United Kingdom has made major contributions throughout the second half of the 20th century to clinical cardiology, to the development and the appropriate integration of technological advances, and to research at all levels. This has been achieved in the face of serious deficiencies in manpower and resources. Furthermore, the apprenticeship method of training remained long after it could be justified by any modern precept. That there have nevertheless been achievements of which we can justifiably be proud is due, in no small measure, to the giants of the specialty – they led us, and taught us, and handed down traditions that we hope still survive. Opportunities, especially in training, are better now than they have ever been, and staffing is approaching reasonable levels. The present-day cardiologist is able to maintain excellence in the specialty; preferably with a little less effort but doubtless with equal enthusiasm.

The author wishes to acknowledge the kind help he received from Dr Gillian Ford CB, late of the Department of Health, Miss Lesley Haggar at the Royal College of Physicians of London, and Dr Roger Boyle from the British Cardiac Society.

References and notes

1. *Royal Commission on Medical Education 1965–8. Report.* London: HMSO. 1968.
2. Chamberlain D, Julian D, Sleight P, Sowton E. Proposals for a new training programme for cardiology. *Br Heart J* 1990;63:317–20.
3. Hunter S, Bull K, Dickinson D, Godman M, Keeton B, Radley-Smith R, et al. The future of paediatric cardiology in the United Kingdom. Report of a joint working party of the British Cardiac Society and the Royal College of Physicians of London. *Br Heart J* 1992;68:630–3.
4. *Hospital doctors; training for the future. The report of the working group on specialist medical training.* London: Department of Health 1993.
5. The Executive Committee of the European Board for the Specialty Cardiology. Recommendations of the European board for the specialty cardiology (EBSC) for education and training in basic cardiology in Europe. *Eur Heart J* 1996;17:996–1000.
6. Hall RJC, Boyle RM, Webb-Peploe M, Chamberlain DA, Parker DJ. Guidelines for specialist training in cardiology. *Br Heart J* 1995;73(suppl 1):1–24.
7. Boyle RM, Hall RJC. Training in cardiology: the future. *Br Heart J* 1995;4:302–3.
8. Report of the joint cardiology committee. A combined medical and surgical unit for cardiac surgery. *Br Heart J* 1968;30:864–8.
9. Second report of a Joint Cardiology Committee of the Royal College of Physicians of London and the Royal College of Surgeons of England on combined cardiac centres for investigation and treatment with a note on the requirements of cardiology in hospitals outside such a centre. *Br Heart J* 1980;43:211–9.
10. Third report of a Joint Cardiology Committee. Royal College of Physicians of London and the Royal College of Surgeons of England. Provision of services for the diagnosis and treatment of heart disease in England and Wales. *Br Heart J* 1985;53:477–82.
11. Fourth report of a Joint Cardiology Committee of the Royal College of Physicians of London and the Royal College of Surgeons of England. Provision of services for the diagnosis and treatment of heart disease. *Br Heart J* 1992;67:106–16.
12. Report of a working group of the British Cardiac Society. Cardiology in the district hospital. *Br Heart J* 1987;58:537–46.
13. A report of a working group of the BCS. Cardiology in the district hospital. *Br Heart J* 1994;72:303–8.
14. Department of Health and Social Security. *Working for patients.* London: HMSO 1989.
15. Chamberlain DA, Goodwin JF, Emanuel RW, Bailey LG. Career prospects in cardiology in England and Wales. Survey of 15 health regions. *Br Heart J* 1981;45:460–3.
16. Chamberlain D, Bailey L, Emanuel R, Oliver M. Staffing and facilities in cardiology in England and Wales July 1982. Second biennial survey. *Br Heart J* 1983;50:597–604.
17. Chamberlain D, Bailey L, Julian D. Staffing and facilities in cardiology in the United Kingdom 1984. Third biennial survey. *Br Heart J* 1986;55:311–20.
18. Chamberlain D, Bailey L, Sowton E, Ballantyne D, Boyle D McC, Oliver M. Staffing in cardiology in the United Kingdom 1988. Fifth biennial survey. *Br Heart J* 1989;62:482–7.
19. Chamberlain D, Pentecost B, Reval K, Stevens J, Boyle D McC, Cobbe S, et al. Staffing in cardiology in the United Kingdom 1990. Sixth biennial survey: with data on facilities in cardiology in England and Wales 1989. *Br Heart J* 1991;66:395–404.
20. The British Cardiac Society, the Cardiology Committee of the Royal College of Physicians, and the Trafford Centre for Medical Research, University of Sussex. Seventh survey of staffing in cardiology in the United Kingdom 1991. *Br Heart J* 1992;68:621–9.
21. Chamberlain D, Parker J, Balcon R, Webb-Peploe M, Cobbe S, Boyle D, et al. Eighth survey of staffing in cardiology in the United Kingdom 1992. *Br Heart J* 1994;71:492–500.
22. Department of Health. *Hospital medical staffing – achieving a balance. Plan for action.* London: Department of Health, 1987.
23. Chamberlain D, Webb-Peploe M, Hall R, Parker J. More winds of change: the provision of cardiological services in the United Kingdom. *Br Heart J* 1994;72:218–9.
24. Adams FH, Mendenhall RC. Evaluation of cardiology training and manpower requirements. DHEW publication 1974; No. (NIH) 74–623. (Quoted in American College of Cardiology and Health Resources Administration DHEW. Cardiology manpower (9th Bethesda Conference). *Am J Cardiol* 1976;37:941–83.
25. Beller GA, Vogel RA. Are we training too many cardiologists? *Circulation* 1997;96:372–8.
26. A report of the Royal College of Physicians. Consultant physicians working for patients. Part 1: A blueprint for effective hospital practice. *J R Coll Physicians London* 1998; 32 (suppl 1):S1–20.

Chapter 4

Societies, Journals, and Books

Arthur Hollman

Modern British cardiology had started well before the 20th century began in 1901. In the previous 20 years, Walter H Gaskell had elucidated the physiology of cardiac contraction, T Lauder Brunton had completed elegant work on the pharmacology of the heart, Augustus Waller had recorded the first human electrocardiogram, and Byrom Bramwell had written a comprehensive textbook on diseases of the heart. Even so, 1901 was, in fact, an important year because Dr James Mackenzie was writing his internationally acclaimed book, *The study of the pulse, arterial venous and hepatic, and the movements of the heart.* Mackenzie's work and his original views on cardiac disease attracted many physicians to his general practice in Burnley, Lancashire. They would meet on Sunday afternoons to see patients and discuss polygraph tracings, and Mackenzie suggested that a small club should be formed for meetings and discussion.[1] [2] This was the first time that an organised cardiac group had been considered, but with Mackenzie's move to London in 1907 the idea was dropped.

There were, however, a few formal occasions when physicians with an interest in heart disease could get together. One such was the first meeting of the Association of Physicians of Great Britain and Ireland in 1907. William Osler, the founder, invited Mackenzie to open a discussion on the heart. Another was a special meeting on electrocardiography organised in 1912 by the Royal Society of Medicine's section of medicine. Willem Einthoven of Leiden, inventor of the string galvanometer, was the guest speaker at that meeting.[3] Between 1908 and 1912, Mackenzie read four papers before various sections of the society, so there was a fair amount of interchange of information about the heart but still no separate organisation for heart disease.

The Cardiac Club

During the first world war, rates of cardiac disability among soldiers were very high. By 1918, even though many soldiers had the effort syndrome (soldier's heart) with normal hearts, 36 000 men had been discharged and were eligible for pensions.[4] But the inexperienced doctors on the pension boards made inaccurate diagnoses and assessments, and on the initiative and advice of Thomas Lewis, the Ministry of Pensions appointed consultants in every region to supervise and instruct the boards.[3] These consultants were general physicians with a special interest in heart disease. In 1921 and 1922, the ministry held conferences for them at which clinical problems as well as administrative matters were discussed. The conferences, which enabled cardiologists to meet for the first time as an organised group, were an important step towards the development of the specialty that was just beginning to be called cardiology.

The ministry conferences were so useful that on 21 February 1922 William E Hume wrote to John Cowan (the senior member) suggesting that they should get together at the next meeting of the Association of Physicians, to which, as hospital consultants, they naturally all belonged. Hume and Cowan were joined by Thomas F Cotton and Carey F Coombs as the "official accoucheurs," and the Cardiac Club was founded at Oxford on 22 April 1922 with Alexander G Gibson in the chair.[2] There were 15 members and Sir James Mackenzie was elected as an honorary member. The original members of the club deserve to be remembered as the pioneers of British cardiology.

THE CARDIAC CLUB

Original members

CF Coombs • TF Cotton • J Cowan • JG Emanuel • AG Gibson • TW Griffith • J Hay • Sir Thomas Horder • WE Hume • Sir Thomas Lewis • JE MacIlwaine • J Parkinson • WT Richie • HJ Starling • KD Wilkinson

Secretaries 1922–37

J Cowan • AG Gibson • J Crighton Bramwell • D Evan Bedford • J Maurice Campbell

Cardiac Club meetings

The club held its first meeting on 22 November 1922. Sir Thomas Lewis was in the chair, which was appropriate since the club had been born out of his initiative in getting the ministry to nominate cardiac consultants. Thereafter, the Cardiac Club always met on the day before the Association of Physicians meeting, in whichever city that meeting took place, and with the local member in the chair. At most of the meetings there were two set subjects with chosen speakers and informal discussions of short communications. The subjects discussed included: the heart in pneumonia and in influenza, the heart and athletics, heart disease in children, diseases of the pulmonary artery, heart block, angina pectoris, digitalis and quinidine.

In 1932, members were in a dilemma about Sir Thomas Lewis – he had been absent without explanation from more than two meetings, and according to rule two his membership had therefore ceased. However, the letters of the secretary, AG Gibson, make it clear that they hesitated to tell him this; he was, after all, a rather important person. Should they just stop sending him notices, or strike him off? The club's minutes (unpublished) reveal the solution they struck upon. A category of extraordinary membership was created and Sir Thomas Lewis was elected as the first member.

By 1936 the club had held 15 meetings and a further 19 members had been elected. It was then decided that with the increasing numbers of physicians interested in cardiology the club should expand into a larger and more representative society.

The British Cardiac Society

At a final special meeting of the club on 8 January 1937, members decided to create a new society. Several names were suggested – the Society of Cardiologists, the Heart Society, the Society for the Study of Cardiovascular Disease – but the name chosen was the Cardiac Society of Great Britain and Ireland, renamed the British Cardiac Society in 1946.[5]

Among the new rules was one stating that the society should have up to 60 ordinary, 25 associate, and 20 extraordinary members, and also honorary members. There were 69 members at the outset, and the first annual meeting was held in Edinburgh on 15 April 1937 with A Rae Gilchrist[6] in the chair. In 1940, the first lady members, Dr Janet Aitken[7] and Dr Doris Baker,[8] were elected. The society created the *British Heart Journal* in 1939, and after 1941 the "Proceedings of the Society" were always published in the journal and these are a very helpful archival source.

The onset of the second world war limited the society's activities, but the meetings continued and medical officers from the Commonwealth and North America were invited to attend. Usually there were 40 to 50 members present and 20 guests. The society advised the government on the medical examination of service recruits and on the rehabilitation of cardiac patients, and it had a joint committee with the British Paediatric Society on the care of children with rheumatic heart disease. As early as 1943 there was a discussion on cardiology in a coordinated medical service in anticipation of the National Health Service which began in 1948.

Soon after the end of the war in 1945, the society asked the Royal College of Physicians of London if it would appoint a cardiology committee. The committee was duly formed under the chairmanship of Sir Maurice Cassidy, and in 1947 it published its first report dealing with the training of specialists in cardiology and the practice and teaching of cardiology.

Cardiac surgery comes of age

The autumn of 1947 found the society closely involved with the meeting in London of the International Conference of Physicians, bravely arranged by Lord Moran despite the very difficult postwar conditions. At this meeting, cardiac surgery was discussed fully for the first time. Dr Alfred Blalock and Dr Helen Taussig of Johns Hopkins Hospital described their operation for tetralogy of Fallot, Professor Clarence Crafoord of Stockholm discussed coarctation of the aorta, and Mr Oswald Tubbs from St Bartholomew's Hospital spoke on patent ductus. In 1939, Tubbs had been among the first surgeons in the world to operate on a ductus (in fact an infected one), and by 1948 British cardiac surgery was at the forefront of progress. Thomas Holmes Sellors had undertaken the world's first pulmonary valvotomy in December 1947,[9] and Russell Brock carried out one of the earliest mitral valvotomies in 1948. It was therefore more than appropriate that the cardiac society should begin to elect surgical members. The first ones, elected in 1949, were Brock, Sellors, Tubbs, and Price Thomas.

The society enlarges

In 1952 the rules were changed to allow a total of 250 members, an increase of 105 since 1946. By 1962 only a few vacancies existed; there were now 30 surgical members, but still only five lady members. The rapid increase in membership reflected the development of the specialty. After 1947 it was necessary to have a second meeting each year, held in London in the autumn. The annual general meeting in the spring, held at the university city where the Association of Physicians was meeting, continued the practice of the Cardiac Club. The scientific programmes always contained discussions on particular subjects such as acute rheumatism and anticoagulants, but in 1952, for the first time, a whole day was given over to short communications.[5]

A very high standard was expected of speakers at scientific meetings, and this was indeed upheld by them. The rule that communications must be spoken and not read was strictly adhered to, and no speaker would dare to run over their allotted time of 10 or 15 minutes. Furthermore, members had to be referred to by their surnames only – titles were not allowed, even for the most senior members, and first names were entirely out of order.

In the discussion after a paper, questioners would often be called by name as soon as they raised their hand to speak. This surprised new members, but either the chairman or the secretary knew many of the audience by sight, and up to 1976 all sessions were plenary ones. Names of the questioners – and there might be several – were written on the blackboard, and although one honorary secretary tried to get out of this chore, the custom persisted until simultaneous sessions made it impractical.

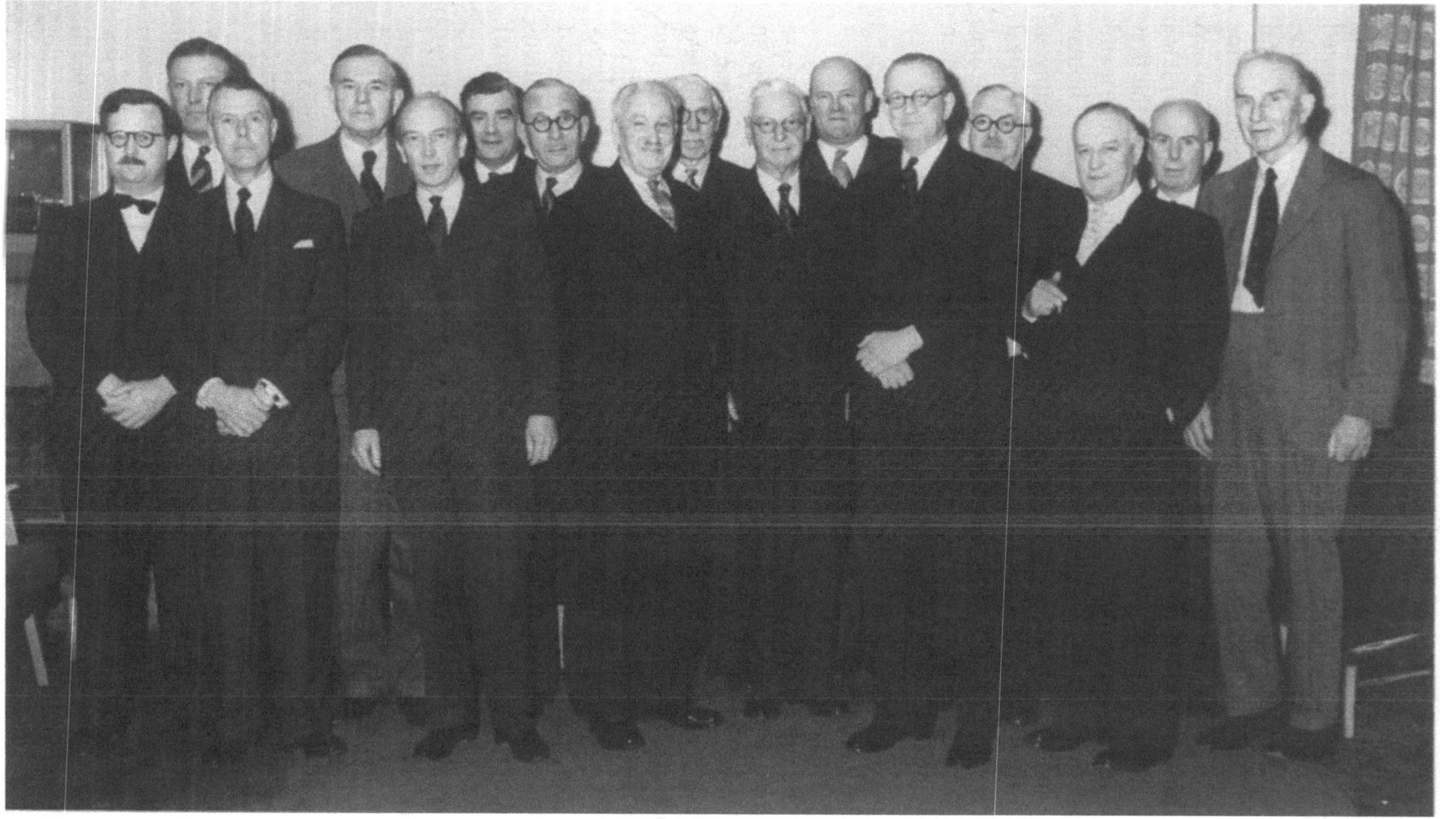

Figure 1 A group of senior members of the British Cardiac Society in 1958. Left to right: back row – GW Hayward, G Bourne, AM Jones, DE Bedford, AA Peel, AR Gilchrist, W Evans, W Phillips; front row – W Whitaker, KS Smith, PH Wood, JM Campbell, J Parkinson, JR Towers, JH Wright, SB Campbell (Reproduced with permission from *Br Heart J* 1962;24:688).

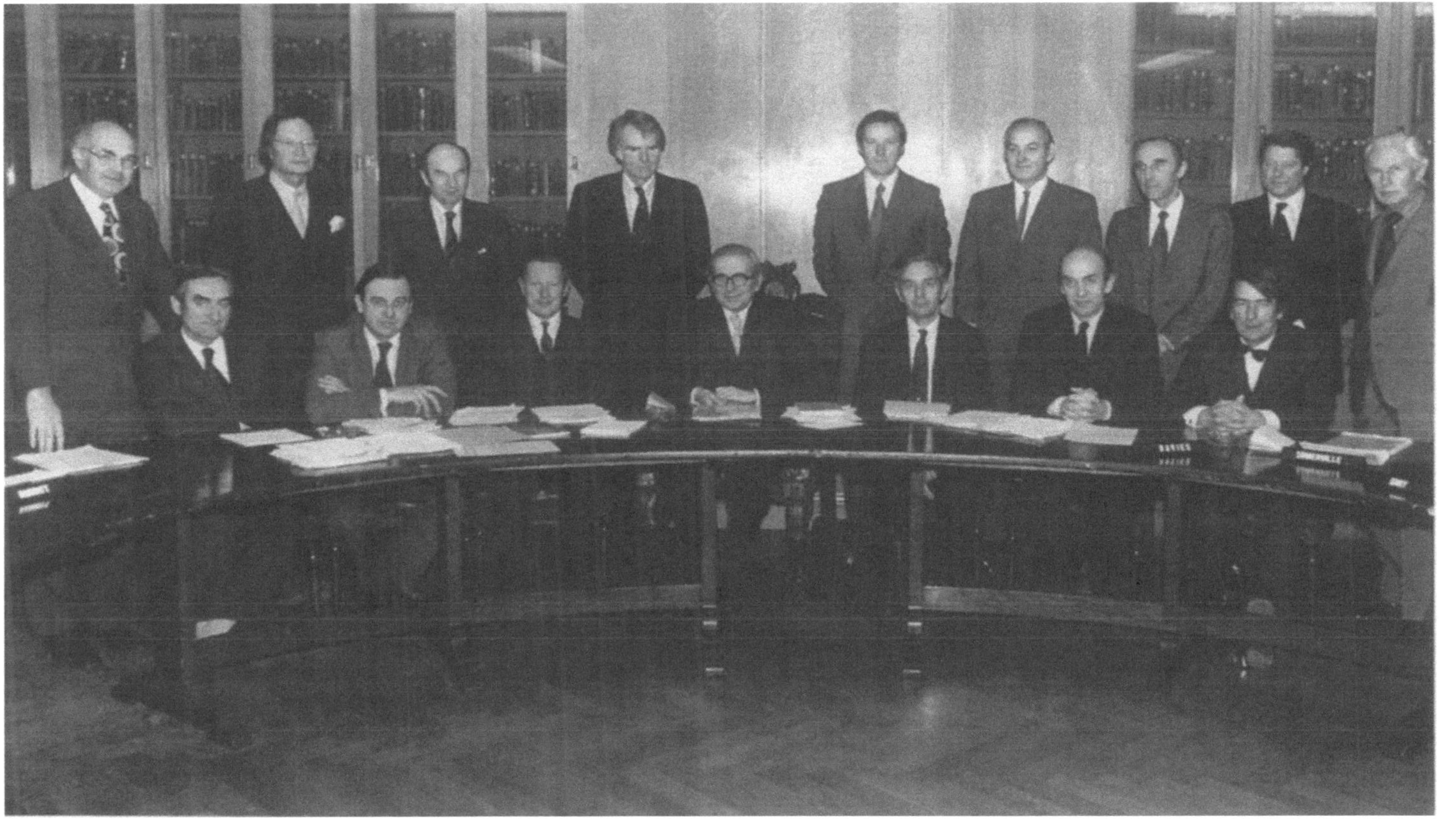

Figure 2 The council of the British Cardiac Society in 1975. Left to right: back row – LG Abrams, RM Marquis, DS Short, EG Wade, BL Pentecost, RJ Linden, JM Barber, G Howitt, W Somerville; front row – DW Barritt, GA Miller, A Hollman, JF Goodwin, MK Towers, LG Davies, IR Gray.

Named lectures

A valuable addition to meetings came in 1963 when the first Thomas Lewis Lecture was delivered. This lecture was founded by a generous donation from Dr Samuel Levine of Boston in recognition of the inspiration and friendship that he and other American physicians had gained while studying with Lewis. A further donation came from the Canadian born physician, Dr Tom Cotton, a close associate of Lewis. The lecture has been given every two years since its inception. In 1994, the society founded the Paul Wood Lecture in honour of Dr Paul Wood, the first director in 1949 of the Institute of Cardiology and an inspiring leader of British cardiology up to his death in 1962. The first lecture, delivered in 1995 by his former colleague Dr Jane Somerville, recounted Wood's career and achievements. In 1998, the society's president, Professor Ronald WF Campbell,[10] died in office at the age of 50, and this tragic event led to the establishment of a series of five lectures in his memory. The first Ronnie Campbell Lecture was given in 1999 by Professor A John Camm.

Three lectures associated with other groups were transferred to the society. The first was the St Cyres Lecture of the National Heart Hospital, established in 1926 by Viscountess St Cyres in memory of her husband. He had been a patient of Dr Strickland Goodall, a physician at the hospital. The bequest's purpose was for further investigation into diseases of the heart, and the stated subject of this annual lecture was, "Myocarditis in the widest possible sense, including every variety thereof, the term to cover all diseases of the myocardium." The National Heart Hospital's Keith Jefferson Lecture on cardiac imaging was founded in 1980 with a bequest from Dr Jefferson. He had been a distinguished radiologist at the hospital. Lastly, the Worshipful Society of Apothecaries of London asked the society to host its lecture and gold medal. These had been founded in 1936 by colleagues and patients in memory of Dr Strickland Goodall, a liveryman of the Apothecaries, who was said to be the first physician in London to practice exclusively in cardiology.

The society and international cardiology

The society has always played an important part in promoting international cardiology. In 1949, Evan Bedford represented the society at a meeting in Brussels when delegates from 14 countries met to inaugurate a European Society of Cardiology, and the first European Congress of Cardiology was held in London in 1952. Two years previously the first World Congress of Cardiology had been held in Paris, and several of the speakers were British. In 1970, the British Cardiac Society hosted the World Congress of Cardiology in London. Professor Jack Shillingford did a truly remarkable job in organising the whole congress with the assistance of his secretary and a small committee – it must have been one of the last big congresses to have been arranged without professional conference organisers. The president of the congress was Sir John McMichael. In 1976, Professor John

Goodwin was elected president of the International Society and Federation of Cardiology, the body that promotes the world congresses and which has now been renamed the World Heart Federation.

The need for representation at international meetings was the main reason for the decision to have a president of the society. It was natural for Sir John Parkinson to be elected to this post in 1952 because he had been the main inspiration of the society in its earlier days. He served for four years, as did his successors, but in 1985 the increasing complexity of the post required there to be a president elect for two years, who would then become president for a further two years. This arrangement allows the president elect sufficient time to learn the job before his term of office.

The international role of the society was strengthened after 1981 when there was a large increase in the number of corresponding members from abroad; by 1993 there were 255 members in that category. In addition, there were joint meetings with other European societies - with the Swedish society in Stockholm in 1975, the French society in Paris in 1977, the Finnish society in Helsinki in 1978, and the Czech society in Prague in 1981. However, the increasing strength and importance of the European Society of Cardiology made it less necessary to have intersociety meetings. This was well demonstrated by the large attendance from all European countries at the European society's first annual congress in Vienna in 1988 (these had previously been four yearly). Through their national societies, 47 countries are currently members of the European Society of Cardiology, giving a total membership of 27 000. The *European Heart Journal* is published by the society and is warmly supported by British cardiologists, two of whom have been its editors.

Organisation and offices

A succession of honorary secretaries, working from their own hospital departments or their private consulting rooms, organised the society in its earlier days. The first executive secretary, Miss EG North, was appointed in 1964, but she worked from the office of the honorary secretary at Hammersmith Hospital. By 1974 it was clear that the society required an office of its own, and this was set up at the Royal Society of Medicine, with Mrs Gay Read in charge. A medical precinct was established in 1986 next to the Royal College of Physicians, and in company with other medical bodies the society moved into St Andrews Place. However, the society outgrew even this accommodation, and in 1994, it acquired its very own home - an elegant spacious house at 9 Fitzroy Square, London. The house was designed by the famous Adams brothers in 1798, and its historical importance is indicated by the fact that English Heritage have given it a grade II* listing. Earlier occupants included the Royal physician and translator of Laennec, Sir John Forbes (1824–49), and a blue plaque on the building tells us that the noted chemist, Professor W Hofmann, lived there a few years later. There are two lecture rooms and a council room in addition to the offices of the staff and the journal *Heart*. Although the society's home is steeped in history, its organisation is up to date; it has its own web site at www.bcs.com

Society of Cardiological Technicians

The introduction of the electrocardiograph meant that physicians needed help to deal with technical problems and to record the increasingly large numbers of electrocardiograms required in hospital practice. But this requirement for technical help became much more important with the introduction of cardiac catheterisation, and a 1948 survey showed that an organisation to represent staff engaged in technical cardiology would be welcomed. The Society of Cardiological Technicians was founded in 1949. It had 149 members and Dr William Evans was its president. The society started a quarterly journal and established a library. In the next few years the first examinations for membership were held and an annual lecture in memory of Sir John Parkinson was created. In 1957, the society initiated its training courses for the society's examination, the syllabus for which was compiled jointly with the British Cardiac Society. The growth of the Society of Cardiological Technicians was reflected in the creation of branches throughout the United Kingdom and New Zealand, with affiliated societies in South Africa and Australia. In 1968, with the support of the Department of Education and Science, an ordinary and then a higher national certificate in medical physics and physiological measurement were introduced. The Society of Cardiological Technicians had over 700 members by 1999.

Annual scientific meetings started in 1949 and grew steadily in importance. The society mounted its first exhibition of equipment in 1960. There was continuing emphasis on education and qualifications, as evidenced by the introduction in 1991 of a specialist course developed jointly with the British Pacing and Electrophysiology Group and the inauguration of a BSc degree in clinical science at the University of Belfast in 1994. The importance of cardiac technology was emphasised in 1995 when the society's name was changed to the Society of Cardiovascular Science and Technology and its members were designated cardiac clinical scientific officers.

British Cardiac Society Meetings

As mentioned previously, the society had a spring meeting at a university city and, after 1947 an autumn meeting in London. Until 1976 all the sessions were plenary ones, and although this gave a welcome sense of unity to the meetings, the system could not continue. The numbers attending were too large, and it was increasingly difficult to cater for the needs of members specialising in, say, paediatric cardiology. Simultaneous sessions were therefore introduced in 1977. However, attendance at the meetings was restricted to members and their guests until as late as 1984 when the numbers attending increased from the usual 400–50 to nearly 700. This was also the year when posters were first introduced. 1985 saw the first three day meeting. Members were finding it difficult to attend two meetings a year as well as meetings overseas, and the idea of having a single annual meeting was proposed. The first such annual conference was held over four days in Torquay in 1990. Four lecture theatres were required, and the 1600 delegates included 300 nurses. Harrogate and London were subsequent venues, but the continuing growth of cardiology has meant that since 1995, Glasgow and Manchester have been chosen as the only ideal large conference centres. At Glasgow in 1998 there were 2114 delegates using six lecture theatres, and at Manchester in 1999 there were 2470 delegates.

The increasingly important part played by the nursing profession was recognised by the society when a nurses' educational programme was started at the meeting in 1987, and "nurses' day" as it came to be called had over 500 delegates in 1999. The Association of British Cardiac Nurses was founded in 1995.

A very important development at the meetings occurred in 1978 when, in collaboration with the Society of Cardiological Technicians, the first commercial exhibition of equipment was held. That year, 60 companies had stands occupying $500m^2$. The commercial exhibition has become very popular with delegates, and the society has derived a very satisfactory income from it. At Glasgow in 1998, over $3000m^2$ of stand space was sold to 127 companies.

Affiliated groups

The invention of new technology such as cardiac pacing and the development of academic departments funded by the British Heart Foundation were the two main reasons for the formation of specialist groups within mainstream cardiology. The people working in specialised areas naturally wanted to meet with each other and exchange views. The first group – physicians interested in heart muscle metabolism – was soon followed by a paediatric cardiology group. Nine specialist groups are currently affiliated to the society (see below), and each has a seat on the council of the society.

Affiliated specialist groups

- British Pacing and Electrophysiology Group
- British Cardiovascular Intervention Society
- British Nuclear Cardiology Society
- British Society of Echocardiography
- British Paediatric Cardiac Association
- British Society for Cardiovascular Research
- British Association for Cardiac Rehabilitation
- Association of British Cardiac Nurses
- Society for Cardiological Science and Technology

Other British cardiology organisations

In addition to the national society, local organisations for physicians and other hospital doctors who had a special interest in heart disease have been founded.

Newcastle Cardiac Club

Sir William Hume[11] founded this club at Newcastle upon Tyne in 1949, and its 12 members included radiologists and surgeons. The club met three times a year at members' homes on a Saturday evening. A paper on a selected topic was followed by supper provided by the host and then short presentations of interesting case histories illustrated by radiographs and electrocardiograms. The last and 125th meeting of the Newcastle Cardiac Club was held in 1994. It was hosted by Hewan Dewar, then 80, the only surviving original member.[12] Other cities such as Edinburgh and Glasgow also had clubs, and local medical societies provided the venue for meetings of cardiologists in Manchester and Liverpool.

Hugh's Club

Travelling clubs are popular with various specialty groups within medicine. In 1963, Dr Hugh Fleming of Cambridge founded a club for cardiology, which came to be called Hugh's Club. Its aim was "to enable people who were on friendly terms to meet regularly and to have frank discussions of all aspects of their work in cardiology."[13] The first members were HA Fleming, LG Davies, AM Johnson, C McKendrick, PR Fleming, and A Hollman. The club met twice a year and was active until 1978.

The London Cardiological Club

This club started around 1948 and had a well defined membership – it was open only to consultant cardiologists in private practice. The secretary for many years was Dr Charles Baker of Guy's Hospital. Initially, the club met at members' homes after dinner and discussed a topic presented by a member. When, in 1960, a newer member showed slides with his paper Evan Bedford objected that this was out of keeping with a domiciliary gathering! Like the Newcastle club, the London club eventually had to meet at members' hospitals, or at Durrants Hotel, and so the proceedings became more formal. During the 1960s there was concern that physicians engaged in full time academic work were excluded from membership; as a result, Professors John McMichael and John Goodwin were elected. The club gradually lost impetus and stopped meeting in 1985.

The Junior Cardiac Club

The expansion of cardiology after 1948 meant that many young doctors were eager to join the specialty, but they were not eligible to join either the British Cardiac Society or the London Cardiological Club. They badly needed a forum, and on the initiative of Walter Somerville the Junior Cardiac Club was founded in 1948. Its members were registrars or junior consultants, and they had to leave when they had the honour of becoming a full member of the British Cardiac Society.[13] Although the club met in London, initially at the Middlesex Hospital and later at other hospitals, its membership came from Cambridge and other centres too. Two or three papers would be discussed vigorously, and the dinner beforehand was also valuable for exchange of ideas. The club flourished. In the 1980s, it was having monthly meetings at several hospitals in London with attendances of between 50 and 70. Usually three research papers were given, accompanied by the kind of frank discussion that was acceptable among friends but unheard of at the British Cardiac Society. The club also had annual meetings abroad and a highly competitive research prize, judged by a panel of members and distinguished consultants, and sponsored by the firm of Rorer. Another innovative idea was a "short case" meeting where errors could be presented and discussed - sometimes with a brisk exchange of views. This was an effective and early introduction to audit. Many of the members of the club felt that it was their most important membership, both academically and socially. The Junior Cardiac Club is now over 50 years old - a fine testimony to its founder and to its value among the younger members of the profession.

Interhospital meetings

Much less interchange took place between the cardiac departments in London hospitals; there should have probably been more. In 1958, Dr Wallace Brigden said that the few units doing open heart surgery should have joint meetings, but his advice was ignored. However, in 1963, Walter Somerville of the Middlesex initiated a useful monthly meeting between the cardiac departments of the Middlesex Hospital and University College Hospital. The meeting was extended to include St Mary's Hospital and the Royal Free Hospital, and continued until 1980.

Journals and books

Journals

Throughout the last half of the 19th century, and especially towards its end, there was a surge of interest in the clinical features, investigation, and treatment of diseases of the cardiovascular system and also, importantly, in animal physiology and pharmacology. Naturally this led to a big increase in publications, and by writing a textbook an author could confine the subject matter to his own field of interest. Examples of these textbooks are: AE Sansom's *Manual of the physical diagnosis of diseases of the heart including the use of the sphygmograph and cardiograph* (1881), B Bramwell's *Diseases of the heart and thoracic aorta* (1884), and WH Broadbent's *The Pulse* (1890). However, when it came to publishing articles in the periodical press there was little specialist identity, except when an author published all his papers in one volume, as did Lauder Brunton with his 1906 *Collected papers on circulation and respiration*. The early research workers had to place their articles in a wide variety of journals. Physiologists such as JA MacWilliam, WH Gaskell, and AD Waller were able to publish in the *Journal of Physiology* or the *Proceedings of the Royal Society of London*, but it was not so easy for clinicians to find a home for their work. For example, the work of Dr James Mackenzie, the leading clinical investigator in heart disease around the turn of the century, appeared in the *Lancet*, the *British Medical Journal*, eight local British journals, and also in three German and three American journals.

Heart

Dr Thomas Lewis of University College Hospital London, whose distinguished career in elucidating cardiac irregularities started in 1908, also had an important role in medical publishing. After 1907, when Mackenzie moved to London, he and Lewis eagerly shared their joint interest in arrhythmias. Lewis had already written 10 papers on cardiac topics, and it was obvious to both of them that an English language journal specialising in cardiovascular problems was needed. They would have know about the French journal *Archives des Maladies du Coeur et des Vaisseaux et du Sang* founded in 1907. By January 1909, Mackenzie had taken the crucial step of finding a publisher – Shaw and Sons of Fetter Lane, London. In March 1909, Mackenzie invited Lewis to be the editor of the new journal. Although Lewis was only 26 and had no editorial experience, he was soon hard at work in getting six physicians to help select papers and 44 more to be collaborators – what we would now call the assistant editors and the advisory board. Twenty-two of the collaborators were from the United States, and included men like Harvey Cushing and Alexis Carrel who later became so well known. It would be fascinating to learn how Lewis and Mackenzie knew of these men. Perhaps William Osler, now at Oxford, helped them.

Progress on the new publication was swift. According to Lewis, "One of the chief reasons for accelerating publication was that several articles were ready." The four papers of part 1, volume 1 went to press on 9 June and the first issue came out on 1 July 1909, a momentous day for British cardiology.[14] The prefatory note was written by the Cambridge physiologist, Walter H Gaskell, whose work on the rhythmical contraction of heart muscle was much admired by Lewis. Indeed it is instructive to note that the early pioneers of clinical cardiology were eager to discuss problems with physiologists. Mackenzie was a keen visitor to Ernest Henry Starling's laboratory at University College London. In his editorial note, Lewis wrote, "The Journal

HEART.

A JOURNAL FOR THE STUDY OF THE CIRCULATION.

EDITED BY

THOMAS LEWIS, M.D.,

AIDED IN THE SELECTION OF PAPERS BY

Dr. W. H. Gaskell.

Prof. A. R. Cushny (London).
Dr. Leonard Hill (London).
Dr. J. Mackenzie (London).
Prof. A. W. Hewlett (Ann Arbor).
Prof. G. N. Stewart (Cleveland).

WITH THE COLLABORATION OF

Prof. J. G. Adami (Montreal).
Sir T. Clifford Allbutt (Cambridge).
Prof. W. M. Bayliss (London).
Dr. C. Bolton (London).
Prof. J. R. Bradford (London).
Dr. W. Langdon Brown (London).
Sir Lauder Brunton, Bt. (London).
Dr. W. J. Calvert (Dallas).
Prof. A. J. Carlson (Chicago).
Dr. Alexis Carrel (New York).
Dr. A. E. Cohn (New York).
Dr. C. M. Cooper (San Francisco).
Dr. John Cowan (Glasgow).
Prof. George W. Crile (Cleveland).
Prof. Harvey Cushing (Baltimore).
Dr. George Dock (New Orleans).
Prof. W. Einthoven (Leyden).
Prof. J. Erlanger (Madison).
Dr. A. G. Gibson (Oxford).
Dr. G. A. Gibson (Edinburgh).
Dr. A. M. Gossage (London).
Prof. F. Gotch (Oxford).
Prof. T. Wardrop Griffith (Leeds).
Prof. Ch. C. Guthrie (St. Louis).
Dr. J. Hay (Liverpool).
Prof. Y. Henderson (New Haven).
Dr. W. P. Herringham (London).
Dr. A. D. Hirschfelder (Baltimore).
Prof. Ch. F. Hoover (Cleveland).
Prof. Wm. H. Howell (Baltimore).
Prof. T. C. Janeway (New York).
Prof. A. Keith (London).
Prof. J. A. MacWilliam (Aberdeen).
Dr. S. J. Meltzer (New York).
Prof. Joseph L. Miller (Chicago).
Sir R. Douglas Powell, Bt. (London).
Dr. W. T. Ritchie (Edinburgh).
Prof. Torald Sollmann (Cleveland).
Prof. E. H. Starling (London).
Prof. Graham Steell (Manchester).
Prof. W. S. Thayer (Baltimore).
Prof. A. D. Waller (London).
Prof. G. S. Woodhead (Cambridge).
Sir Almroth E. Wright (London).

VOL. I.
1909-1910

London:
Shaw & Sons, Fetter Lane, Fleet Street, E.C.

1910

Figure 3 The title page of the first volume of *Heart* 1909–10.

affirms a single object, the progress of knowledge of the mechanism by which the blood circulates in health and disease . . . (and) the mechanism by which it distributes the constant stream of blood, bathing and feeding the tissues of the body." The journal was called *HEART. A journal for the study of the circulation.*

Heart continued until 1933 when Lewis changed its title to *Clinical Science, incorporating Heart.* This reflected two things. First, about half of the total of 326 papers had come from his own department and, second, he had given up work on the heart, as emphasised by the title of his Department of Clinical Research. The full run of *Heart* comprised 16 volumes. Although each one contained four issues, Lewis brought them out at irregular intervals when there was enough material available, so that occasionally the issues were only one or two months apart. Looking back it is surprising to find the considerable length of the papers; those by Lewis and his co-workers ranged from 6 pages to 76 pages with an average of 30 pages (about 9000 words). Of the other contributors to *Heart*, about a quarter came from the United States until 1926 when the *American Heart Journal* was founded.[3]

During the 1930s British cardiology became an active specialty, as shown by the increasing membership of the Cardiac Club and the work of its members. John Parkinson was a pioneer of cardiac radiology, D Evan Bedford[15] emphasised the entity of left ventricular failure, Carey Coombs[16] wrote a good book on rheumatic heart disease, and Crighton Bramwell[17] gave the Lumleian Lectures on the arterial pulse. But now, as was the case before *Heart* was founded, papers went into the *Quarterly Journal of Medicine* and the weekly journals. The formation in 1937 of the Cardiac Society of Great Britain and Ireland, the successor to the Cardiac Club, gave impetus to the creation of a new journal – one that belonged to the society. The *British Heart Journal* was founded in 1939 with the British Medical Association as the publisher. Sir Thomas Lewis wrote a spirited foreword enjoining contributors to "bow loyally to editorial decision." He added, "The success of the new journal will depend upon the quality . . . of the matter which it publishes. Originality of observation and of view will be the touchstone of quality. The best contributors will submit . . . only sound and original matter . . . they will judge their own text impartially thinking of the standard of work accomplished and not of personal interest."[14] The *British Heart Journal* served the society very well under a succession of able and devoted editors (see box, p. 67), all of whom had busy professional lives.

The war and its aftermath, with paper in short supply, curtailed the size of the journal. In its first 10 years the average volume had 267 pages, but by 1954 this had risen to 478 pages. In 1961, the frequency of publication increased from four to six numbers per year, and in 1972, with volume 34, the 1334 pages were spread over 12 numbers.

The *British Heart Journal*, perhaps unique among cardiac journals, had cumulative indexes, and thanks to the work of Dr Sheila Howarth these were prepared for volumes 1–17 in 1955 and from 18–29 in 1967. Another

Editors of the British Heart Journal

1937–47	edited jointly by Maurice Campbell[18] and Evan Bedford[15]
1947–58	Maurice Campbell
1958–61	K Shirley Smith
1961–81	Walter Somerville
1981–92	Dennis M Krikler
1992–99	Michael J Davies
1999 to date	Roger J Hall

valuable feature has been the publication of the Proceedings of the British Cardiac Society, containing abstracts of the papers given at their scientific meetings. The British Medical Association (BMJ Publishing Group) did well financially from publishing the journal, and due to the initiative of Walter Somerville it agreed to share the profits with the society.

In the late 1950s increasing numbers of papers dealing with research rather than clinical aspects were submitted, and this research was greatly promoted by the foundation of professorial chairs by the British Heart Foundation. The society responded by establishing a journal called *Cardiovascular Research.* The first volume appeared in 1966 under the editorship of Professor JP Shillingford. There was one volume per year containing about 700 pages. Subsequent editors were Professors RJ Linden, PJ Sleight, and DJ Hearse, and by 1992 the volume had 740 pages. In 1995 (volume 30), control of the journal was transferred to the European Society of Cardiology. After 1997 there were four volumes per year, each of 600 pages published in three numbers – a nearly fourfold increase on the early years.

By 1994 it was clear that for any specialist journal to survive it had to adapt to changes in the needs of readers, subscribers, and authors in the increasingly international world of cardiology. It was thought that there would be fewer journals with a clearer division between national and supranational ones. Much of work published in the *British Heart Journal* in the previous decade had come from the United Kingdom, though since 1992 submissions from mainland Europe had risen substantially. Even so the time seemed right to underline a commitment to be an international journal, and to emphasise this the journal was renamed *Heart.*

The newly named journal continued to use the volume numbers of its predecessor, and the first volume of *Heart* was number 75. When the *British Heart Journal* was started many titles were considered including even *De motu cordis*! Campbell was then in favour of the title *Heart* and although Sir Thomas Lewis rather reluctantly agreed to its use, the permission of the publishers was not obtained. Campbell persisted and asked Shaw and Sons if he might approach them again in the future, but his foresight was not rewarded until 58 years later.

To emphasise and enhance its new image *Heart* created an international advisory board with 39 members, almost the same number as Lewis had recruited way back in 1909. Three associate editors help Professor Roger Hall with the hard, day to day grind in the office. Another new departure was the decision to have four assistant editors, representing general cardiology, electrophysiology, paediatric cardiology, and surgery. A full text web site at www.heartjnl.com is now available for the journal.

The end of the century was signalled by volume 82 of *Heart*. It comprised over 700 pages and included contributions from 32 countries in every continent.

British Journal of Cardiology

The *British Journal of Cardiology* is the official organ of the Primary Care Cardiovascular Society. It was started in 1993 with the objective of providing a link between hospital cardiology and primary care. It is sent free of charge to cardiologists and to interested general practitioners and is also available on subscription. Articles are subject to peer review. It is edited by K Fox, P Poole-Wilson, and H Purcell and has a circulation of 19 000.

Books

Monographs 1900–50

The first British book on heart disease in this century was James Mackenzie's outstanding monograph, *The study of the pulse arterial venous and hepatic and of the movements of the heart*. Published in 1902, it comprised 319 pages and 332 illustrations of recordings made by the author on smoked paper with his modified Dudgeon sphygmograph (which he called the clinical polygraph). The monograph was based on Mackenzie's intensive investigations and was greatly admired by those working on cardiac topics in Europe and America and Britain. It is one of the classic cardiac texts of the century.

But it was Mackenzie's next book that made him famous, because it reached a much wider audience. *Diseases of the Heart* was published in 1908, went to a fourth edition in 1925, and was translated into four European languages. His other books were: *Symptoms and their interpretation* (1909, 4th edition 1920); *Principles of diagnosis and treatment of heart affections* (1916, 3rd edition 1926); *Future of medicine* (1919); *Heart disease and pregnancy* (1921); *Angina pectoris* (1923), and *The basis of vital activity* (1926).

The next British monograph after those of Mackenzie was that of Dr Thomas Lewis. Like Mackenzie, Lewis distilled his own personal work (largely on the newly invented electrocardiograph) into *The mechanism of the heart beat* (1911), but he also included many references to other workers. This is also a classic text, and was hailed in America as the bible of electrocardiography. The very fine third edition of 1925, now named *The*

THE

STUDY OF THE PULSE

ARTERIAL, VENOUS, AND HEPATIC

AND OF THE

MOVEMENTS OF THE HEART

BY

JAMES MACKENZIE, M.D. (EDIN.)

BURNLEY

EDINBURGH AND LONDON

YOUNG J. PENTLAND

1902

Figure 4 The title page of James Mackenzie's epoch making monograph of 1902.

Other important early monographs

- *Diseases of the arteries including angina pectoris* by Sir Thomas Clifford Allbutt (1915)
- *Hyperpiesia and hyperpiesis* by Charles Bolton (1922)
- *Rheumatic heart disease* by Carey Franklin Coombs (1924)
- *The action and uses in medicine of digitalis and its allies.* by Arthur Robertson Cushny (1924)
- *Heart disease and pregnancy* by J Crighton Bramwell and Edith A Longson (1938)
- *Congenital heart disease* by James W Brown (1939)

mechanism and graphic registration of the heart beat, comprised 529 pages, 400 figures, and 1003 references and was a tremendous enterprise for a single author. Other important early monographs are shown in the box. The successful series, *Recent advances in cardiology*, was edited by Curtis Bain and Terence East and started in 1929.

Textbooks

Then there were the textbooks of cardiology. *Diseases of the heart. Described for practitioners and students* by Sir Thomas Lewis in 1933 enhanced the reputation of British cardiology. It was translated into six European languages, over 11 000 copies were sold in America, and it went to a fourth edition in 1946. Other early textbooks were: *Diseases of the heart* by Dr Frederick W Price (1930) and *Principles and practice of cardiology* by JC Bramwell and John T King (1942).

1950–2000

Dividing the century into half has greater significance than might appear because it was in 1950 that a textbook was published which heralded a new era of cardiology. This book was *Diseases of the heart and circulation* by Paul Hamilton Wood. It had 589 pages and 343 good illustrations, and it introduced the reader to the new information obtained by cardiac catheterisation and linked this with the clinical examination of the patient. It was more than a conventional textbook because Wood gave first hand evidence in the text, just as if he were writing a scientific paper. The book gave Paul Wood and British cardiology a worldwide reputation, and he wrote a larger second edition in 1957. It was followed in 1964 by William Evans's *Diseases of the heart and arteries* (761 pages, 643 figures) and in 1971 by Samuel Oram's *Heart disease* (920 pages, 560 figures).

These three books marked another significant change because they were the last of the large single author textbooks. When Wood was writing his third edition, he told J Willis Hurst of Atlanta Georgia of the considerable strain that this involved, and Hurst conceived the idea of producing his very successful multi-author book *Heart*. Wood's third edition had to be completed after his premature death by other authors under the editorship of Walter Somerville. But continuity of British authorship was established in 1989 with the 1630 page *Diseases of the Heart* edited by DG Julian, J Camm, KM Fox, RJC Hall, and P Poole-Wilson, which went to a second edition in 1996.

The number of cardiology books by British authors has increased appreciably in the past 30 years and it would be difficult, even if it were desirable, to name all of them. The topics covered include: teaching books for undergraduates, cardiovascular physiology, hypertension, pathology of the heart, cardiac radiology, cardiac catheterisation, difficult cardiology, beta blockers in clinical practice, surgery of congenital heart disease, heart disease in infants and children, left ventricular hypertrophy, cardiac problems in the adolescent and young adult, clinical trials in cardiology, epidemiology of coronary heart disease, cardiac arrhythmias, and heart disease in pregnancy.

History of British cardiology

From the inception of the *British Heart Journal* in 1939 until 1991, full obituary notices of the leading figures in British cardiology were published in the journal. This useful historical source no longer exists; the historian will have to rely on the entries in *Munk's Roll* of the Royal College of Physicians of London and on articles in various journals such as the *Journal of Medical Biography*. An account of the life and work of Paul Wood was written by Jane Somerville and published in *Heart*.[19] In addition there are biographies of two famous men. A good personal account of Sir James Mackenzie was written by R Macnair Wilson in 1926 and Alex Mair produced the definitive biography in 1973.[20] The biography of Sir Thomas Lewis by Arthur Hollman was published in 1997.[3]

Personal recollections of people and events are invaluable, and luckily two good accounts have been published. "Some notes on the Cardiac Club," written by John Cowan and others in 1939 gives details of the membership and of the subjects discussed at their meetings.[2] "The British Cardiac Society and the Cardiac Club: 1922–61" written by Maurice Campbell is a long, well illustrated article with very full references.[5]

It is appropriate to mention here the two books on the general history of cardiology written by British cardiologists. *The story of heart disease* by Terence East is the published account of his Fitzpatrick Lectures given before the Royal College of Physicians of London in 1956 and 1957.[21] *A short history of cardiology* by Peter R Fleming is an excellent account of cardiology from 1680 to 1970.[22]

The Evan Bedford Library of Cardiology

Individual members of the society have built up their own libraries of important books. The outstanding collector was Evan Bedford, who, for nearly 50 years, systematically sought and acquired books on heart disease and created a very fine and unique library which he generously donated to the Royal College of Physicians of London in 1977. His splendid gift of over 1000 volumes was as great as any benefaction that the College had received in the past two centuries and he enhanced it by writing notes on many of the books. The Evan Bedford Library of Cardiology and its catalogue are recognised worldwide, and a book will often be identified as "Bedford number. . . ."

In conclusion

The British Cardiac Society has developed through this century from a small informal group that met at the house of Dr James Mackenzie in 1905 to an association with over 1000 members, large annual meetings, and nine affiliated specialist organisations. Books and journals, highly acclaimed in the first decade, have remained excellent. International cooperation, which began on a personal basis, continues to grow, and, in addition, there are now European congresses at which the British Cardiac Society and its members play an important part.

Notes and references

1. Hay J. A lecture on James Mackenzie and his message. *BMJ* 1930;1:1033–6.
2. Cowan J and others. Some notes on the Cardiac Club. *Br Heart J* 1939;1:97–104.
3. Hollman A. *Sir Thomas Lewis. Pioneer cardiologist and clinical scientist.* London: Springer Verlag, 1997.
4. Lewis T. *The soldier's heart and the effort syndrome.* London: Shaw and Sons, 1918.
5. Campbell M. The British Cardiac Society and the Cardiac Club:1922–61. *Br Heart J* 1962;24:673–95.
6. Alexander Rae Gilchrist (1899–1995) was a dominant figure in Scottish medicine and cardiology for many years. He was on the staff of the Edinburgh Royal Infirmary, noted for his work on heart block and anticoagulants He was twice president of the Royal College of Physicians of Edinburgh.
7. Janet Kerr Aitken (1886–1982) had a special interest in juvenile rheumatism and was a consultant physician at the Elizabeth Garrett Anderson Hospital, London.
8. Doris Manning Baker (1895–1971) established a rheumatism supervisory clinic, wrote on left infra-mammary pain and was a physician at the South London Hospital for Women.
9. Hollman A ,Treasure T. Pulmonary valvotomy 50 years ago. *Lancet* 1998;352:1956.
10. Ronald WF Campbell (1944–98) was the British Heart Foundation professor of cardiology at Newcastle upon Tyne from 1986 until his untimely death in 1998. A world authority on cardiac electrophysiology and arrhythmias. President of the British Cardiac Society 1997–8.
11. Sir William Hume (1880–1960) was a physician at Newcastle upon Tyne and was the pioneer of cardiology in north east England, taking his first electrocardiogam in 1912. He was an RAMC colonel in world war one and stated that "soldier's heart" was not caused by neurasthenia. He helped to found the Cardiac Club.
12. Dewar H. *The story of cardiology in Newcastle.* Durham: Durham Academic Press,1998.
13. Fleming H A. *Papworth Cardiac Unit 1957–1967.* Cambridge: Papworth Hospital, 1996.
14. Hollman A. *Heart* and the *British Heart Journal. Heart* 1996;75:3–5.
15. Davis Evan Bedford (1898–1978) was on the staff of the Middlesex Hospital and National Heart Hospital. He was a research fellow at the London Hospital under John Parkinson, and they wrote

a pioneering paper on the electrocardiogram in cardiac infarction. In collaboration with his surgical colleague Sir Thomas Homes Sellors, a large and notably successful series of patients with atrial septal defect were operated on under hypothermia at the Middlesex. He was known at the Middlesex as "the old top". This nickname came from his comment while playing billiards, "Give it a bit of the old top," meaning top spin on the ball. Bedford did much for the British Cardiac Society. He was co-editor when the journal was founded and its president in 1960–4. The Evan Bedford Library of Cardiology is referred to in the text.

16. Carey Franklin Coombs (1879–1932) found a typical diastolic murmur in children with acute rheumatic fever at the Bristol Children's Hospital between 1905 and 1907. This became known as the Carey Coombs murmur. His detailed study of 700 patients over a period of 15 years formed the basis of his 1924 monograph on rheumatic heart disease. He had been encouraged to study the condition by FJ Poynton.
17. John Crighton Bramwell (1889–1976) was on the staff of the Manchester Royal Infirmary, where he carried out important cardiological research – for example, using the cathode ray oscillograph to record heart sounds in 1934. He was appointed professor of cardiology in 1946, the first such post in Britain.
18. John Maurice Hardman Campbell (1891–1973) started his career in cardiology as a junior under John Parkinson at the National Heart Hospital. He joined the staff in 1931 and later gave the St Cyre's lecture. He was the cardiologist at Guy's Hospital when, in 1946, he talked to RC Brock about the possibility of surgery for mitral stenosis. He later said, "Probably he, and certainly not I, did not realise how this talk would change our lives." Starting in 1947, they collaborated in pioneer work on the surgical treatment of congenital heart disease and mitral stenosis. Maurice Campbell gave tremendous service to the British Cardiac Society; he served for 10 years at its first secretary and was president from 1956–60. He was editor of the *British Heart Journal* for 20 years.
19. Somerville J. The master's legacy: the first Paul Wood lecture. *Heart* 1998;80:612–9.
20. Mair A. *Sir James Mackenzie, MD 1853–1925, general practitioner.* Edinburgh: Churchill Livingstone, 1973.
21. Terence East (1894–1967) was a consultant cardiologist at King's College Hospital, London. He co-founded, with CW Bain, the series *Recent advances in cardiology*, first published in 1929.
22. Fleming PR. *A short history of cardiology.* Amsterdam-Atlanta: Editions Rodopi, 1997.

Chapter 5

The British Heart Foundation

Desmond Julian and Brian Pentecost

In the 1950s, large sums were being raised for cardiological research in other parts of the English speaking world but very little in the United Kingdom, which was still in the grip of post war austerity. John McMichael observed in 1961 that the Medical Research Council probably did not spend more than £50 000 a year on research into heart and vascular disease. Two organisations were keen to foster cardiological research - the Chest and Heart Association and the British Cardiac Society - but who was to take the lead? The former had initially been created as the National Association for the Prevention of Tuberculosis - an organisation committed to combating tuberculosis, but it changed its name in 1959 so that it could encompass both pulmonary and cardiac diseases. As a mark of its new role, it planned to launch a campaign to raise £1 million for heart research.

Founding committee

From the Cardiac Society came the impetus to create a British Heart Foundation. In 1958, Maurice Campbell, then president of the society, wrote to members suggesting that either a new association should be created to raise money for research or that there should be some cooperation with the National Association for the Prevention of Tuberculosis, as it then was. After protracted discussions, a founding committee was set up. The British Cardiac Society representatives on the committee were Campbell, Paul Wood, Evan Bedford, and William Evans. The latter had been particularly inspired by what he had seen in Australia, where £2 million had been raised in a single day. The committee was later expanded to include additional members of the Cardiac Society as well as representatives from the Royal Colleges of Physicians of London and Edinburgh, the Royal College of Surgeons of England, the Royal College of Physicians and Surgeons of Glasgow, and the Royal Postgraduate Medical School.

In 1960, plans were made for the creation of the Council of the Foundation, which was to include a substantial proportion of lay members. In the same year, the Duke of Edinburgh agreed to become patron and Field Marshal the Earl Alexander of Tunis to be president. Delicate but successful negotiations were undertaken with the Chest and Heart Association, which resulted in Dr Harley Williams (from the Association) being appointed as secretary to both charities for a period of 3 years.

Statement of purpose

The British Heart Foundation (BHF) was officially incorporated on July 28, 1961. In the agreement with the Chest and Heart Association (CHA), it was stated that:

> ... the Foundation was established (*inter alia*) to raise funds by public appeal or otherwise for the following purposes:
>
> - The primary purpose being to undertake and promote medical and scientific research relating to diseases of the heart and circulation and subjects related thereto and to promote postgraduate medical training in cardiology
> - The secondary objective being to promote through the Association, so long as the Association retains the status of a charity, the welfare and rehabilitation of patients who have suffered from heart disease, and health education in subjects relating to the heart and circulation.

This separation of functions was clear at this time and remained almost unchanged for 25 years. The foundation throughout its existence has seen the support of research as its main purpose, and it is only since the mid 1980s that it has taken a more active role in public education and promoting rehabilitation.

Fundraising

The founding committee decided that the British Heart Foundation would launch a major fundraising campaign and nominated an appeals committee of prominent and influential individuals. The target set for the appeal was £5 million.

Leslie Lazell, chairman of the Beecham Group, chaired the appeals committee, with William Evans and Lord (Horace) Evans as vice-chairmen. The latter was well known as a physician to the Queen, and was friendly with many leading industrialists and businessmen. Among those who joined the committee were the governor of the Bank of England, Lord Cobbold and the proprietor of the *Times* newspaper, Gavin Astor. After one year's work, the committee had received promises of nearly £1 million, although much of this sum was in the form of covenants, payable over a 7 year period.

Public appeal

It was then decided to launch a public appeal. On 11 June 1963, a high profile press conference was held at the headquarters of the Royal Society. Speeches were delivered by Field Marshal Earl Alexander, Lord Evans, Sir

John McMichael, and Mr Lazell, who said "the foundation will need £500 000 a year to finance research on an adequate scale." In spite of personally signed letters to 12 000 companies and mailings to 500 000 householders, only about £350 000 was raised in the first year.

This disappointing start did not discourage a relatively small band of enthusiasts, led by Brigadier Ereld Cardiff, who was initially the director of appeals, and, from 1966, the foundation's first director general. Although a few glamorous gala events were held with leading show business personalities such Arthur Askey, Peter Sellers, and Eric Morecambe attending, these did not raise much money and it was realised that a more diversified approach was required. Thus, local committees were set up, grouped according to their geographical regions, and over the years these committees have played a major role in fundraising. Regional committees have helped to support national schemes such as "National Slim," "Jump Rope" in schools, and many other local events – and, just as importantly, became the link between the British Heart Foundation and the general public. Successful fundraising charities must be responsive to the public mood and require a point of contact where the charity can explain its actions and elicit support. In recent years British Heart Foundation researchers have been encouraged to make contact with local supporters and, where appropriate, to hold open days so that supporters can see for themselves what their efforts provide.

National and international events

The British Heart Foundation also organises a programme of national events. One outstanding and continuing success has been the London to Brighton Bike Ride held every June. By 1998 there were 27 000 registered cyclists taking part, raising £1.84 million for the charity. For the more adventurous there are opportunities to cycle in Jordan, Israel, and Vietnam, even to walk the Great Wall of China! Between 1994 and 1998, a total of £1.5 million was raised through these international events. Back home again "Walkabout UK," which encourages walking as a healthy pastime, has raised nearly £1 million since 1993. Participation as a selected charity in the London marathon has also resulted in substantial income.

Legacies, shops, and investments

The biggest single component of fundraising has proved to be legacies. Starting modestly with £2500 in 1963, they increased very rapidly during the property boom of the 1980s, rising from £3 million in 1982 to £7.7 million in 1988. By 1999, this figure had risen to £26.4 million, constituting 46% of the total income of the foundation. However, the proportion of total income from this source has fallen, as other forms of fundraising have become more successful.

In 1988, the decision was made to start charity shops. Their distinctive red and white fascia has become a recognised feature of many high streets and the total of shops now stands at nearly 400. British Heart Foundation Shops is a successful commercial enterprise and a highly professional organisation.

The foundation's portfolio of investments, from which it now derives a substantial income, has grown very considerably over the years. The greater proportion of the investments, though, could be classed as liabilities, as the money has already been pledged to fund the activities of the British Heart Foundation chairs and to pay for research projects.

Governance

The chief executive of the foundation since 1966 has been designated the Director General, whose job it is to oversee all its activities. The organisational skills of the military have been highly valued. Brigadier Ereld Cardiff was succeeded in 1976 by Brigadier Christopher Thursby-Pelham, and Major-General Leslie Busk took over in 1990. Directors now exist in the areas of finance, communications, fundraising, shops, and medicine. They, together with the director general, answer to the executive committee, itself appointed by Council.

The medical department

The medical department is responsible for advising on the disposal of the foundation's funds on medical research, education, and the welfare of cardiac patients. The chief executive of this department is the Medical Director, a position that was held by Professor Jack Shillingford from 1981–6 and by Desmond Julian from 1986–93. He was succeeded by Brian Pentecost, who retired in 1999 and was replaced by Sir Charles George.

Research

Research has always been the prime concern of the foundation. Project grants, which provide support for staff and materials for up to three years, account for more than half of the money spent on research. The average value of a British Heart Foundation project grant in 1999 was approximately £100 000. Programme grants provide longer term support. These normally last for five years, and may be renewable.

Fellowships and exchanges

The fellowships committee oversees the foundation's investment in the future of British cardiovascular research. Junior research fellowships (for one or two years) and PhD studentships provide an introduction to research, while intermediate research fellowships (for three to four years) give more prolonged support for those who have become established as independent researchers. Senior research fellowships (for five years or longer) are awarded to outstanding research workers thought likely to achieve senior academic status in the next few years. An early feature was the creation of British/American exchange fellowships in 1967; many of the successful candidates have become leaders in their respective fields. Exchanges with other countries followed, especially with the Netherlands.

Basic scientists have fewer career opportunities than clinicians and so the British Heart Foundation instituted a system of basic scientist lectureships/senior lectureships. Two or three are awarded each year.

Professorial chairs

Early in the history of the British Heart Foundation a decision was made to create a professorship. As a result of a donation by Lord Marks of Marks and Spencer, the Simon Marks chair was endowed at the Institute of Cardiology in London. The first occupant was Peter Harris. The decision to fund further chairs was stimulated by the reluctance of young cardiologists to enter academic cardiology because of the lack of a career structure and the attractions of clinical practice. The research funds committee decided that the creation of academic departments was a priority, and over the next 20 years it helped to create an additional 13 academic departments of cardiology or cardiac surgery (see box, p. 79). In each case, an endowment was provided by the foundation, but this was usually accompanied by local fundraising together with an undertaking by the host university to contribute towards accommodation, running expenses, and future financial support. The long term financial implications of creating new departments became formidable when it was decided that, at a minimum, a professor, senior lecturer, lecturer, technician, and secretary should staff a university department of cardiology.

By the mid 1980s it became evident that the foundation could no longer donate the very large sums that were required to fund such positions in perpetuity. It was decided to create no more departmental chairs, but that personal chairs would still be granted to outstanding researchers. These represented a commitment to an individual rather than to an academic department and, in most cases, it was anticipated that the chairholder would progress to an established senior position in their university. There are now 28 British Heart Foundation chairs in a range of clinical and basic scientific disciplines from molecular genetics to cardiac surgery.

Education

From the outset, postgraduate medical education was seen as an important function of the foundation. Over the years, this has taken many forms. Symposia and workshops on specific topics of current interest have catered

British Heart Foundation endowed chairs

Institute of Cardiology, London (1965) – Peter Harris then Philip Poole-Wilson

Birmingham (1971) – Melville Arnott then William Littler

Glasgow (Medical Cardiology) (1973) – Veitch Lawrie then Stuart Cobbe

Leeds (1973) – Ronald Linden then Stephen Ball

Oxford (1973) – Peter Sleight then Hugh Watkins

Newcastle upon Tyne (1974) – Desmond Julian then Ronnie Campbell

Glasgow (Cardiac Surgery) (1974) – Philip Caves then David Wheatley

Institute of Child Health, London (1975) – Fergus Macartney then John Fabre

Royal Postgraduate Medical School, London (1976) – Jack Shillingford, Attilio Maseri, then Dorian Haskard

Edinburgh (1978) – Michael Oliver then Keith Fox

Cardiff (1980) – Andrew Henderson then Michael Frenneaux

Royal Postgraduate Medical School (Surgery) (1983) – Kenneth Taylor

St George's Hospital, London (1986) – John Camm

National Heart and Lung Institute, London (Surgery) (1986) – Magdi Yacoub

for research workers. A wider audience has been reached by lectures in postgraduate medical centres throughout the country, and general practitioners have been made aware of recent advances by monthly *Factfiles* on cardiological topics.

Educating the public

At first the BHF did not see a major role for itself in public education. There were two reasons – the original agreement that the Chest and Heart Association would be doing this and some uncertainty over what it was appropriate to tell the public. In some areas, however, the BHF has played an important role in providing advice. This applied particularly to the treatment of cardiac arrest and in providing practical information for those with pacemakers and those at risk from infective endocarditis. Starting in 1969, the BHF published a series of booklets entitled *Heart Research Series* pamphlets, which provided articles on subjects such as congenital heart disease, angina, and cardiac catheterisation. These were intended for patients and their families.

In 1977, the then Director General reported that "the policy remains to avoid proselytising amongst the general public until there is much more agreement generally about the origins and causes of cardiovascular disease," and this approach was reconfirmed the next year. In 1979, it was stated in the Director General's report to Council, in reply to requests for advice on prevention on heart disease from the public, that "only smoking had been generally agreed to be harmful . . . For the time being we do not wish to suggest any changes in lifestyle. For general bodily health we recommend moderate exercise and avoidance of obesity."

Coronary Prevention Group

In 1980, the BHF came under attack from the *British Medical Journal* for not doing enough about public education and prevention. Sir Ronald Bodley Scott, then chairman of council, replied, pointing out that the foundation had been set up specifically to fund research. Nonetheless, there were many critical voices around and, as a consequence, some prominent medical and lay personalities set up the Coronary Prevention Group, which took a very active approach to the correction of risk factors. The foundation was most unhappy about the use of the word "prevention," and in 1981 it stated formally that "It was therefore probably misleading to talk about 'prevention' of a heart attack but more accurate to substitute the words "increase" or "decrease" the risk."

Leaflets for patients

Attitudes change with time. As new information accumulated over the succeeding years, the BHF became much more active in public education and now provides advice on many topics including those relating to lifestyle. Leaflets in the *BHF Heart Information Series* give patients and their families information on a wide range of clinical questions. Several highly successful videos have been made by the BHF dealing with subjects as diverse as basic life support and heart surgery. In an attempt further to explain its activities to the public, videos have been made that attempt to describe in an easily understood way, much of the Foundation's research. In particular, increasing efforts are made to ensure that the message of healthy lifestyle reaches the young. An additional source of information on cardiological topics is the recently formed department of medical information, which provides both telephone and written replies to approximately 12 000 enquiries each year.

The foundation has deliberately avoided political action or lobbying, but it has supported organisations such as Action on Smoking and Health (ASH) and the National Heart Forum that are concerned with turning scientific evidence on the prevention of coronary disease into policy.

Cardiac care

A cardiac care committee was formed in 1970 with the purpose of providing "life-saving equipment" for hospital and ambulances. This was popular with local fundraisers, but it posed two problems. Firstly, its very attractiveness might divert money that would otherwise go to fund research. Secondly, it might, in effect, subsidise the NHS. It was, therefore, decided to impose quite strict limits on funding for this purpose.

Defibrillators in ambulances

The success of defibrillators in the treatment of cardiac arrest and the finding that ambulance personnel could be trained to use them led to a great expansion in the activities of the cardiac care committee. The Department of Health had, at first, been antagonistic to the provision of defibrillators, and many ambulance services were reluctant to provide the appropriate training, but the foundation led the way in encouraging this development from the mid 1980s. Eventually, the Department acknowledged the success of the programme ... but not before the Foundation and its local supporters had equipped most of the ambulances in the country! Defibrillators were also given to general practitioners in country districts who could reach patients with heart attacks more quickly than could ambulances.

More recently still, the concept of *First responder defibrillation* was at the centre of a further British Heart Foundation initiative to increase the availability of defibrillation within the community. External automated defibrillators are supplied to organisations willing to provide the appropriate level of training, re-training, and maintenance of professional standards among their membership, like St John Ambulance and other voluntary organisations.

The philosophy of most of the British Heart Foundation's activity in the cardiac care field has been one of innovation; to explore the benefits of a particular therapeutic strategy which, if successful, might be adopted by government rather than to simply provide substitute funding for the NHS.

Heartstart UK

Aware of the fact that the chances of successful resuscitation from ventricular fibrillation outside hospital were increased by effective basic life support, the Foundation, together with colleagues in St John's and St Andrew's Ambulance, the Red Cross, the Royal Life Saving Society, and the ambulance services formed *Heartstart UK* in 1991. Its purpose was to establish community based training programmes in basic life support of which there are now more than 300 throughout the United Kingdom.

Cardiac rehabilitation (see also Chapter 18)

Cardiac rehabilitation had been deliberately excluded from the British Heart Foundation activities under the original agreement with the Chest and Heart Association. By the mid 1980s, it had become apparent that the Chest and Heart Association did not have the resources to meet the public demand and it was decided that the British Heart Foundation and the association should jointly undertake a "pump priming" exercise to help create rehabilitation centres in hospitals which wished to have them. This arrangement continued for three years – until the Chest and Heart Association changed its focus to stroke and its name to the Stroke Association. The British Heart Foundation has continued its support until the present time. Between 1989 and 1996 the number of cardiac rehabilitation centres increased from 91 to nearly 300. Similarly, the British Heart Foundation took over the role of encouraging the development of patient support groups run for and by patients. There are currently more than 200 of these groups affiliated to the foundation.

British Heart Foundation nurses

The most recent major initiative has been the British Heart Foundation nurses whose role is to bridge the gap in care between hospital and the community for heart patients. In the case of patients with coronary disease, for whom the scheme was designed, the role of the nurse is to ensure that the benefits of rehabilitation and secondary prevention are not lost. The scheme is therefore a natural sequel to the interest of the foundation in rehabilitation as foreseen by our founders.

In conclusion

At the end of the century, the British Heart Foundation remains the main source of funds for cardiovascular research in the United Kingdom. In recent years, however, it has been substantially increasing its involvement in public and professional education and in stimulating improvements in the prevention and management of heart disease.

Acknowledgement

The authors wish to acknowledge their debt to the information contained in *Fighting heart disease; the history of the British Heart Foundation 1961–88* by David N Matthews.

Chapter 6

PART I • The National Heart Hospital: The First of its Kind

Mark E Silverman

London hospitals prior to special hospitals

In early 19th century London, there were two basic types of institutionalized medical care: workhouse infirmaries for the sick pauper and general "voluntary" hospitals for the sick poor.[1–3] Patients who could afford to avoid the contagion and uncertain benefit of hospitals paid for their treatment at home. The voluntary hospitals, mostly supported by public donations, were governed by a lay committee of good standing in the community who selected both the patients who could be admitted to the hospital as well as the physicians who would provide their care. Although unpaid, these "honorary" physicians – often referred to as "the great men" – received enormous benefits: the satisfaction of doing charitable work, an association with a prestigious hospital which greatly enhanced their reputation and private practice, and lucrative referrals from their students and the Board of Governors.[1] An appointment to the staff of a voluntary hospital was, therefore, highly sought after, and the number of physicians desiring a position greatly exceeded the limited number of spaces.[4] Competition was fierce, sometimes politically unfair, and jealousies inevitable. The honorary physicians preferred not to share their rewards and would successfully oppose expansion of their numbers or the creation of a new specialty area.[1] The junior physicians, who often provided the day-to-day care, found the bottleneck frustrating and their opportunities restricted. The reluctance of the entrenched medical staff to allow a new specialty to develop prevented research and hindered the younger physicians from learning a new technique that might enhance their practice.

The British Medical Journal in June 1889 commented: "*. . . How many men are there waiting outside the hospitals, doing dreary drudgery at the dispensaries; or, who, having at length been received within the coveted circle, are exhausting their best efforts in the outpatients' department, waiting anxiously for promotion and relief from the thraldom of seniors! What these men, and many more who are not aspirants to the general hospitals, want* *is opportunity for independent work. And they want it while they are young, with energies unimpaired, still burning with the fresh spirit of original research.*" [5]

The rise of special hospitals

The "Special Hospitals", as they were called, sprang up mostly in the early and mid-19th century, either because a physician felt that his career as an honorary physician was thwarted or there was an unmet need not covered by the general hospitals, such as obstetrics, eye, consumption, fever, or sick children. New instruments, such as the laryngoscope, stethoscope and ophthalmoscope, requiring special expertise in their use, inevitably led to specialization and the increasingly affluent population was able to pay specialists for this type of care. The specialty "hospital building" often required no more than a small home and physicians could raise funds fairly easily by campaigns appealing to grateful patients or the charitable public. [1,2] For example, an appeal from the National Hospital for Diseases of the Heart and Paralysis for funds included the following:

"*Heart Disease and Paralysis! To the Wealthy these diseases are most distressing, but what are their sufferings compared with the poor man or woman working for their living with the constant care of a paralyzed husband, wife, or child.*

"*The National Hospital for Diseases of the Heart and Paralysis was established in 1857. Medical Statistics clearly prove the increasing prevalence of this class of disease, whilst the benefits conferred by this Hospital are evidenced by the fact that whereas in 1857 only 435 patients were prescribed for, in 1874 no less than 6045 attended.*"[6]

By 1891, 160 of these special hospitals had been established in England and Wales. Some of these hospitals, such as the ones for fever, sick children, eye and neurologic disease, were greatly respected. Many of the others were looked upon with hostility by established physicians. "The British Medical Journal in 1889 stated: "*Those who by good fortune or merit - the two qualifications are not always united - have achieved hospital rank are apt to lament the multiplication of special hospitals. To some extent they themselves are responsible for this evil - if evil it be. Enjoying what approaches to a monopoly they should not be surprised if young men seek independent outlay.*"[5]

Special hospitals gain recognition

The honorary physicians also looked down contemptuously upon specialists, sniffing that they did not have the broad range of knowledge and ability to provide comprehensive medical care. Nevertheless, the special hospitals, started and controlled by renegade physicians, some reputable and some not, would often lead the way in developing that field. Eventually, the general hospitals would be forced to start their own specialty areas, and voluntary consultants would willingly attend at both the general and the special hospital. In that way, the special hospitals eventually gained recognition and prestige. In 1923, the respected Sir Sydney Russell-Wells summarized how far the change in attitude had come. "*Medicine is so vast a subject, and has grown so greatly both in extent and complexity, that specialization is inevitable. It is no longer a question whether specialties are desirable or not, but rather how they can best be learnt, taught, and practised . . . so far as the sick poor are concerned, I have no doubt that they are adequately, skillfully, and humanely treated both in our general and special hospitals . . . In a general hospital a specialty is only a small part of a great whole; in a special hospital it is the be all and end all of the institution. The staff consists of a team of specialists, each urging the others on to increased efforts, each contributing his own quota, each influencing and modifying the views of all. An atmosphere is created which makes for growth.*"[7]

The origins of the National Heart Hospital

A "Hospital for Diseases of the Heart", apparently the first in the world to be designated solely for patients with heart conditions, was founded by Dr. Eldridge Spratt in 1857 "*to afford relief to the poor suffering from diseases of the heart.*"[6] The original hospital was a small house with a waiting room, consulting room, and two bedrooms with 8 beds at 67 Margaret Street in London. Dr. Spratt was a licentiate of the Faculty of Physicians and Surgeons of Glasgow and had written treatises on mange in dogs as communicated to man and on diseases of the heart. He was the sole physician as well as its treasurer, secretary, and fund-raiser for a number of years. The fund-raising went poorly and the name of the hospital was changed several times, apparently in an attempt to elicit sympathy and generate revenues. In 1871, it became known as "*The National Hospital for the special treatment of Paralysis, Epilepsy, Nervousness, and the Primary Stages of Insanity and other diseases arising from affections of the Heart*", an apparent deliberate confusion with the hospital at Queen Square.

The Dr. Eldridge Spratt melodrama

The first two decades of the hospital were fraught with perils worthy of a melodrama. Dr. Spratt, as amusingly described by Robert Whitney in 1957, was an irascible, duplicitous, and dictatorial person who repeatedly manipulated the fortunes of the hospital for his own advantage.[8] Debts were unpaid for years, and lay committee members invariably resigned quickly upon learning the truth about the hospital or the character and dealings of its founder. In 1868, the newest secretary, Captain Portlock Dodson, a man of integrity and determination, helped to pay off its debts from his own pocket thereby maintaining the solvency of the operation during an acute period of recurring financial crises. The hospital moved to 85 Newman Street in 1869 and in December 1872 they again appealed for funds stating that the house, "*which had afforded relief to nearly seven thousand poor people*", would close unless funds were immediately forthcoming. The appeal ended by saying, "*They would ask all who spend a Merry Christmas and look forward to a Happy New Year to think of their afflictions of paralysis and epilepsy, unable to enjoy mirth, and hardly daring to hope for the New Year. Shall they ask in vain at this season of "goodwill towards men?*" A suggestion for a "National Subscription" of 5 shillings a year from 4000 subscribers was urged.[6]

Because of increasing complaints about its legitimacy, the hospital was investigated by The Lancet in 1872 who reported that it was a very modest house with a small waiting room and consulting room with only two of the fifteen available beds occupied. The Lancet commented, "*Started as a so-called hospital for diseases of the heart, the institution in question appears now to be ashamed of its name, and to appeal for support to the public by the taking title of "National", which, coupled with the words 'epilepsy and paralysis', has a direct tendency to mislead and create confusion, since the well-known hospital in Queen-square has for years been called the 'National Hospital for the Paralysed and the Epileptic'. The absurdity of attributing these diseases or the 'primary stages of insanity' to heart disease is sufficiently patent.*"

The Earl of Glasgow was persuaded to become its treasurer and a new and more responsible medical committee was formed. By 1874, the debt had been considerably reduced and the hospital was able to move to finer quarters on Soho Square, the former home of the Linnean Society. In 1875, Dr. Spratt was forced to resign because of "peculation" (embezzlement) related to setting out his own collection boxes for donations and not turning the money over to the treasurer. In addition, he was secretly using the hospital pharmacy for his private patients. His name was struck from the hospital registry. Always resourceful and vengeful, he returned with a van at night and removed a considerable amount of the contents of the hospital, including furniture, instruments, pictures, an organ, and even some lead from the roof. Pratt then submitted a bill for £855 for expenses incurred in founding the hospital.[8] This could not be substantiated, and he was not reimbursed. Later, he attempted to establish a new Hospital for Diseases of the Heart. This venture apparently never got off the ground. After continuing to plague the operations of his former hospital for many years, Dr. Spratt died in 1902. Despite the havoc that he caused, he was fondly remembered at the 80th anniversary of the hospital by Whitney as "*a Physician of skill and foresight and very definitely a medical pioneer. His conviction that diseases of the heart merited special study and treatment stamps him as being very much in advance of his time.*"[8]

The National Heart Hospital gains sound footing and respect

By 1880, the name of the hospital had been shortened to the "National Hospital for Diseases of the Heart and Paralysis" with 22 beds, four physicians, a resident house surgeon, 3 nurses, and 3 servants. The previous year the records show that 87 in-patients, who stayed an average of 57 days, and 8886 out patients were treated. Problems occurred related to the matron and the professionalism and reputation of several of the physicians. The hospital continued to struggle until a sound financial footing was established under the leaderships of the Earl of Glasgow (1875–1881) and Colonel Roberson-Aikman (1881–1890) with royal patronage by the Duke of Albany and then the Duke of Cambridge.[9] By the end of the 19th century, the hospital was functioning smoothly with a resident medical officer, regular out-patient sessions, a busy in-patient operation, and an improved financial condition, aided by a £4000 donation from the Pickard estate in 1894. Several physicians of reputation, including Sydney Russell-Wells (later Vice-Chancellor of London University) joined the staff. In 1897, the hospital contained 25 beds and cared for 141 admissions and 10,079 out-patients.

In 1908, the hospital name was "*Hospital for Diseases of the Heart*" and the number of out-patients had risen to 21,578 with an average inpatient stay of 52 days. In 1910, a pathology department and an x-ray unit were purchased about the same time, both housed in a new iron shed on the property. The first electrocardiographic machine, a Bock-Thoma model, was purchased in 1911. Because there was no space available for the bulky equipment, it was kept for two years in South Kensington in the physiologic laboratory of A.D. Waller. Patients needing an electrocardiogram had to be sent by cab to the South Kensington laboratory. Waller, who had been the first to record electrical activity from the human heart using a capillary electrometer in 1887, became a consulting physician, adding to the prestige of the hospital.

By 1912, the hospital's operations had been revised by sound businessmen and had an endowment fund of £2,188 and a building fund of £10,400. With the increased number of patients, the hospital was declared unsuitable by the King Edward's Fund.[9] Under the guidance and inspiration of Dr. Russell Wells, Sir James Harrison, and Captain Whitney, and despite great misgivings and opposition by some of the committee, considerable funds were raised and the hospital moved to Westmoreland Street in January 1914. There was space for 42 beds and each bed in the new building was wired for transmission of an electrocardiogram. Soon thereafter, the hospital volunteered to become the center for examining World War I recruits with possible heart disease.[8, 10] Before long, hundreds of recruits were arriving unannounced for an extensive examination which required the professional staff to work from morning until midnight. This led to a 1918 report in the British Medical Journal entitled, "Ten Thousand Recruits with Doubtful Heart Conditions."[11] This evaluation was continued following the war for disabled soldiers with heart disease, and by 1926 the hospital had evaluated a total of 60,000 servicemen, an immense service at no charge to the country.

With the introduction of the electrocardiogram and the influence of James Mackenzie, Thomas Lewis, and others, cardiology had become a highly respected discipline and the reputation of the hospital grew. Much of its success and prestige can be attributed to the joint appointments held by the physicians at the leading undergraduate hospitals.[10] Well-known consultants, such as Frederick Price, the editor of "The Textbook of Medicine", J. Strickland Goodall, John Parkinson (London Hospital), B.T. Parsons-Smith, and Thomas Cotton joined the staff between 1914 and 1924. In the 1930s, Maurice Campbell (Guy's Hospital) and Paul Wood (Hammersmith Hospital) were added. William Evans (London Hospital) [12], Evan Bedford (Middlesex Hospital), Graham Hayward (Bart's Hospital), and Wallace Brigden (London Hospital) came in the 1940s. These physicians were regarded as the elite cardiologists in London who greatly influenced the practice of cardiology locally as well as internationally through their publications, teaching, and organizations.

The Second World War period

In 1938, as warning signs of war became increasingly apparent, a decision was made to find an alternative hospital outside London which would be safer for the care of hospitalized patients. After careful deliberation, Maids Moreton Hall, a $8\frac{1}{2}$-acre site in Buckinghamshire was purchased for £3500. A benefactor left £3000 in his will because of the kind reception that he had received only at the National Heart Hospital at the time of an unannounced visit to "look around". The building was quickly modified in time to transfer patients beginning in August 1939 and was completed September 3rd at the time that war with Germany was announced.[13] Sir Charles Hambro, Chairman of the Board and also a Director of a railway company, arranged for several railway carriages to be transferred to the grounds for administrative offices. The in-patients were transferred to the Maids Moreton site, where they were treated by the local general practitioners, supervised weekly by B.T. Parsons-Smith and resident medical officers first appointed in 1945 beginning with Aubrey Leatham and then Lawson McDonald. The out-patient clinic continued to function at the Westmoreland site with John Parkinson and Thomas Cotton working with seven Clinical Assistants, caring for an average of 100 follow-up and 16 new patients twice weekly despite air raids and the effects of a bomb and parachute land mine. Teaching, in the form of lectures, twice yearly courses, and in-patient demonstrations, was maintained throughout the war. In 1946, the hospital was designated as a postgraduate teaching hospital under the National Health Service Act with the title of the National Heart Hospital prior to its official association with the Institute of Cardiology.

The National Heart Hospital and Institute of Cardiology

At the conclusion of the war, the hospital reopened for in-patients. Because the number of beds was limited (47), the Buckinghamshire branch was kept as a place to transfer patients needing longer hospitalization. The Institute of Cardiology, which had been planned during the war, was inaugurated in 1947 with Paul Wood as its director.[14] The "National" in the title of the hospital, although used for years, became official in 1948 as a Statutory Instrument of the Government.

At the time of its centenary in 1957, a dinner celebration was held and a history was published by Robert Whitney, the long standing secretary and its historian who had been at the hospital for forty-five years.[13] A poem, written by Whitney, introduces his monograph:

1857–1957
Festival time!
Let the bells chime!
Such an occasion is really sublime
(for added importance I'll say it in rhyme)
It should be told in letters of gold
The National Heart is
ONE HUNDRED YEARS OLD!
Our founder was Spratt
We cannot help that
(A very queer fish and a very bad hat:
His endeavors thereafter to kill us fell flat)
So rejoice with one voice
Let the wide world be told
The National Heart is
ONE HUNDRED YEARS OLD!

He concluded the monograph by saying: *"To be a member of its Consultant Medical and Surgical Staff is a distinction which is rightly prized by any eminent member of either branch of that great profession and the standard set by those now associated with the Hospital will very surely be maintained by those who come after them in the future."*

Cardiac catheterization and cardiovascular surgery

At all times, space remained a severe limitation.[14, 15] Additional adjoining space on Westmoreland Street was purchased in the 1920s and 1930s which allowed the out-patient clinic to increase in size and scope. On 6 April 1948, the first cardiac catheterization was performed successfully by Paul Wood, assisted by Walter Somerville and John Norman, on a patient with an atrial septal defect. In the 1950s, expansion of a limited nature was made possible through the purchase and leasing of property on Wimpole Street, directly behind the hospital.

Cardiac surgery was highly desired for years but not possible until 1962 when a new building with two operating theatres was constructed. Holmes-Sellors (Middlesex Hospital), the first surgeon, was appointed in 1957 and Donald Ross (Guys Hospital) in 1963. Subsequently, Keith Ross, Magdi Yacoub, and John Parker (as Senior Registrar) joined the staff. Pioneering cardiac surgery procedures, including the use of homograft aortic valves (1962), the correction of pulmonary atresia (1966), the pulmonary autograft (Ross procedure,1967), and the world's second cardiac transplantation performed by Donald Ross in 1968 enhanced the international reputation of the National Heart Hospital as an active surgical and research program. In 1973, an eight bed children's unit was added bringing the total number of beds to 88.

Closure and rebirth of the Heart Hospital

In 1989, the hospital on Westmoreland Street closed when the National Heart Hospital with its Institute of Cardiology fused with the Brompton Hospital, London Chest Hospital, and the Institute of Diseases of the Chest and moved to the Brompton site. The old heart hospital on Westmoreland Street remained vacant, slowly deteriorating and becoming an eyesore to the community. A group of eight cardiologists and cardiovascular surgeons, known as G-8, maintained optimism that one day the hospital might be restored. Eventually, Gleneagles Ltd, a component of Parkway Group Healthcare, provided funding from a Singapore private hospital group for a private heart hospital. The old building was demolished, except for the central facade which was maintained as a treasured link to the past. On October 19, 1998, a £30 million new complex, equipped with the latest advances in cardiology, was opened as the first acute single specialty unit in the private sector in the UK. Now called "The Heart Hospital", the facility includes 95 beds, four operating theatres, three cardiac catheter laboratories, a paediatric unit, out-patient facilities, and day care. The new building connects by a glazed garden to four adjacent houses on the Wimpole Street side which provide a lecture theatre, telemedicine facilities.

Acknowledgements

The following are greatly appreciated for their review of the chapter and helpful suggestions: Raphael Balcon, Wallace Brigden, RJ Denney, Fiona Hammond-Green, Arthur Hollman, Aubrey Leatham, Geoffrey Rivett, Keith Ross, and Donald Ross. The archives of the London Metropolitan Archives and the University of London were invaluable.

References

1. Abel-Smith B. *The hospitals: 1800–1948*. London: Heinemann, 1964,
2. Rivett G. T*he development of the London hospital system 1823–1982*. London: King Edwards Hospital Fund., 1986, Oxford Press, pp 24–50.
3. Evans AD, Howard LGR. *The romance of the british voluntary hospital movement*. London: Hutchison & Co, pp 124–182.
4. Stevens R. *Medical practice in modern England. The impact of specialization and state medicine*. London: Yale University Press, 1966.
5. Editorial. The metropolitan hospitals, general and special. *Brit Med J* 1889;1:1412.
6. Metropolitan Archives. *Hospital records project (H25)* (A/FWA/C/D11/1 and 2).
7. Russell-Wells R. *The aim and use of special hospitals*. J. Laryng 1923;38:173–178.
8. Whitney R. *The place of hearts: being a history of the National Heart Hospital, London and Buckingham, 1857–1937*. London: New Goswell Printing Co., undated.
9. London Metropolitan Archives. *King Edwards Hospital Fund for London*. Box 9 (A/KE/253/1–9).
10. Campbell M. the National Heart Hospital (1857–1957). *Brit Heart J* 1958;20:137–139.
11. Wells SR. Ten thousand recruits with doubtful heart conditions. *Brit Med J* 1918;1:556–559, 2:248–251.
12. Evans, William. William Evans (1895–1988) was a greatly loved and highly respected physician, teacher, and writer. Born in an isolated farmhouse in Wales, where he also retired and eventually died 92 years later, he graduated from the London Hospital Medical College in 1925 and was appointed house physician to John Parkinson at the London Hospital in 1927. In 1944, he became consultant to the National Heart Hospital and in 1948 he succeeded Parkinson as physician in charge of the cardiac department at the London Hospital. Known as "Willie", he was a portly man with a charming and quaint manner whose humanity, integrity, and wit inspired great loyalty and deep affection from his many colleagues and friends. As a clinician, he was regarded as an astute observer with great common sense. He was a master of the doctor-patient relationship who believed that "the patient should never be worse for seeing the doctor". Evans was a memorable teacher and lecturer, often quoted for his impressive and dogmatic statements which were long remembered though sometimes counter to prevailing opinion. His writing and research were influential, especially in the area of electrocardiography, familial cardiomyopathy, and cardiac radiology. He contributed over 100 article and 5 books on cardiology as well as an autobiography "Journey to Harley Street" and was the first, with Clifford Albutt, to use controls in drug trials.
13. Whitney R. *The place of hearts* (part two): 1938–1957. Published privately.
14. University of London. The Institute of Cardiology, 1963.
15. University of London. The Institute of Cardiology. *Progress Report* 1954–1958.

Chapter 6

PART II • The Institute of Cardiology and the National Heart and Lung Institute

Mark E Silverman and Aubrey Leatham

After the second world war, there was an immediate necessity for specialty training.[1] Advances in medicine, partly as a result of the war, had stimulated an opportunity for specialists who could perform the new laboratory and diagnostic procedures and take care of patients with more complicated disorders who were likely to be admitted to hospital. With the introduction of the National Health Service in 1948, the government had assumed control over all the teaching hospitals and nearly all the district hospitals. There was both a great need and an opportunity to upgrade the level of hospital practice outside London.[2][3]

Formation of special institutes for postgraduate education

Before the second world war, the Chelmsford committee had recommended that the British Postgraduate Medical School at Hammersmith provide postgraduate training at the special hospitals, whose staff consisted mainly of the leaders in their specialty at the London undergraduate teaching hospitals. The special hospitals, however, declined the invitation. In 1944, a report by the Goodenough interdepartmental committee on medical education stressed the importance of postwar training of specialists and education for those whose training had been interrupted by the war.[4][5]

Francis Fraser, who had left Hammersmith Hospital during the war to serve as director general of the Emergency Medical Service, was appointed the first director of the redesigned British Postgraduate Medical Federation in 1945.[6] This would serve as an umbrella federal organisation of the University of London in charge of postgraduate education, including the programme at Hammersmith Hospital.[5] The school at Hammersmith was renamed the British (later Royal) Postgraduate Medical School of London. Fraser felt that postgraduate education in specialty areas could be best accomplished through newly created Institutes for education and research attached to the leading special hospitals. He stated:

> The aim is to provide opportunities for research and higher education in each of the major clinical specialties, with staffs appointed to advance knowledge not only in the clinical field but also in the sciences upon which the practice of each is based. Each institute should be the centre in London of thought and practice to which the specialists will look for help and above all for inspiration.[1]

Requirements

To qualify, the institute had to meet the following requirements:

- Provide postgraduate education of academic standard;
- Accept postgraduate students only;
- Provide lecture rooms, a library, refectory, a student common room, and laboratory space;
- Develop new methods for the study of patients and their diseases;
- Perform research.

Fraser pointed out in 1948:

> Clearly it will take some time to provide at each institute the laboratory accommodation and equipment, the libraries and museums, that are required, but until this is done the institutes cannot fulfil their main purpose; for teaching must always be dull, uninspired, and lacking in the essential element of excitement unless there is an atmosphere of investigation and progress. This is especially necessary in advanced or postgraduate education.[1]

The bait for the hospitals was strong. The special hospitals would receive grants to provide repair from the war damage and upgrade their facility and staff, be designated as a "teaching hospital" responsible to the Ministry of Health rather than to a regional board, and they were promised further maintenance and development support.[7] When the institute reached a certain standard, it would be approved by the University of London and recognised as a federated institute of the British Postgraduate Medical Federation. In this manner, the Institute of Cardiology, based at the National Heart Hospital, became a reality in 1947 as one of the second group to be selected to be a constituent of the federation.[5][8]

National Heart Hospital

Postgraduate education at the National Heart Hospital dates from 1874 when "medical men on presentation of their cards were admitted free to witness the practice of the hospital." Students were allowed to come, upon payment of a fee. A medical school – with Dr P Hammill as the first dean, teaching in the outpatient clinic, and courses in cardiology – started in 1919.[8][9] In 1927, the Viscountess St Cyres endowed a lectureship, the

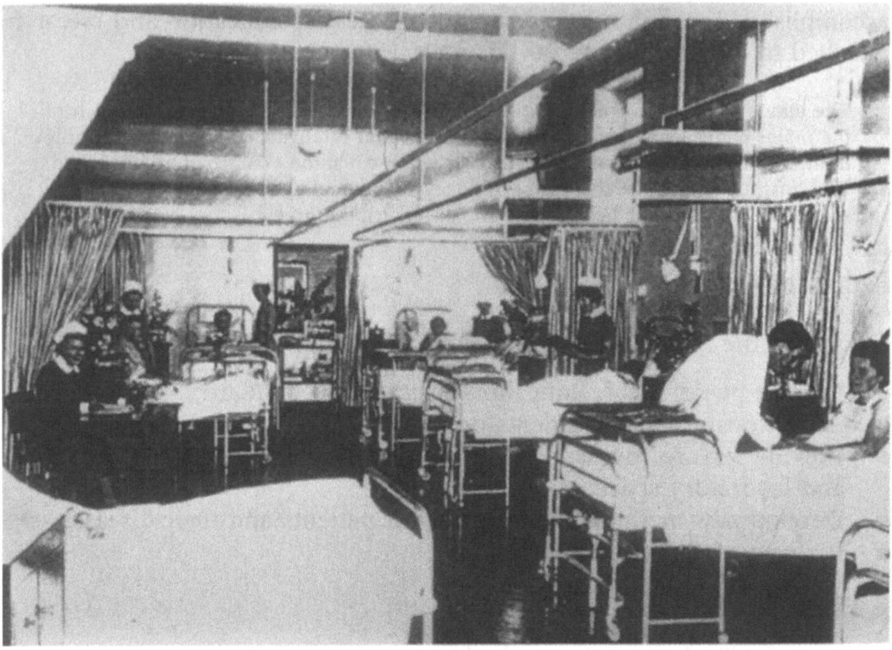

Figure 1 John Parkinson Ward, the National Heart Hospital circa 1963.

St Cyres Lecture. The St Cyres lecturers have included internationally famous speakers such as Karel Wenckebach, Thomas Lewis, Paul Dudley White, Samuel Levine, and Lewis Dexter, and many distinguished cardiologists from Britain, and the lecture is now presented by the British Cardiac Society.[8][9] John Parkinson established the principle that election to the honorary staff of the hospital should come from the leaders in cardiology at the undergraduate teaching hospitals. In 1946, before its official association with the Institute of Cardiology, the hospital was designated as a postgraduate teaching hospital under the *National Health Service Act*, with the title of The National Heart Hospital (figures 1 and 2).

Institute of Cardiology

Paul Wood, who had been a resident medical officer at the National Heart Hospital in 1933 and on the consulting staff since 1937, was the obvious choice by Francis Fraser to be the first director of the institute.[6][10] The original consultants were John Parkinson, BT Parsons-Smith, Thomas Cotton, Maurice Campbell, Evan Bedford, and later William Evans. Paul Wood and the other honorary consultants were appointed lecturers. The members of the honorary staff met monthly as an academic board. At its

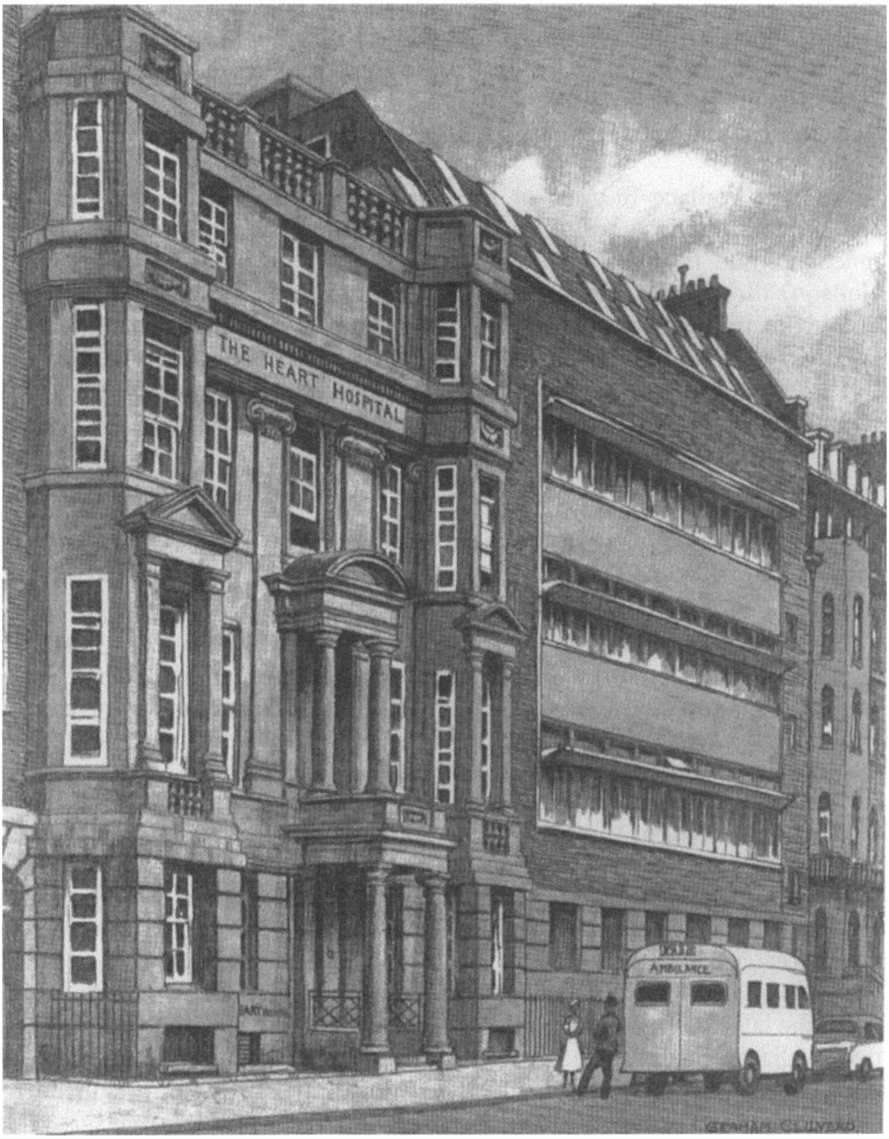

Figure 2 Engraving of National Heart Hospital.

first meeting, on 4 March 1947, John Parkinson was elected as chairman and Paul Wood as dean. The institute, consisting initially of two small administrative rooms, a lecture space created from the waiting hall for outpatients, three small research rooms, a library containing several journals and leading cardiac textbooks, and a basement room for a museum and storage, had to be wedged into the already cramped National Heart Hospital. Teaching was accomplished at the outpatient sessions (with each consultant spending a half day each week) and through regular lectures.

In 1949, Wallace Brigden of the London Hospital was appointed as a consulting physician and Reginald Hudson, whose background was in pharmacology and bacteriology, became the director of pathology.[11] Under Hudson's direction, a fine museum of pathology and a stereographic photographic technique was developed and important studies on the conduction system and aortic homograft were conducted. In 1965 and 1970, Hudson published an authoritative text on cardiac pathology. It was the first major textbook devoted to this subject and comprised 3300 pages.

The academic unit

An academic unit, with Paul Wood as a part time director, was formed in 1949, at which time Graham Hayward from St Bartholomew's Hospital succeeded Wood as dean of the institute.[10] Acquisition of space at 47 Wimpole Street in 1949 and 35 Wimpole Street in 1951 allowed the institute to establish additional research laboratories, a photographic department, a cardiac catheterisation laboratory, a small library, common rooms for students and registrars, a pathology museum, combined board room and lecture room, and administrative offices.[11]

By 1951, the institute had met the requirements to be recognised as a federated institute of the British Postgraduate Medical Federation. Aubrey Leatham, who was appointed as the first full time assistant director and lecturer under Paul Wood, started a phonocardiographic laboratory to establish a scientific basis for auscultation. At that time, there were two senior registrars and four registrars in advanced training for one to two years and a small number of selected postgraduate students.

By the late 1950s, the hospital medical staff consisted of six cardiologists, two cardiac surgeons, three anaesthetists, three radiologists, three pathologists, and a clinical physiologist. The educational programmes included courses of instruction of 2 to 11 weeks duration several times a year, attendance at outpatient clinics and ward rounds, interpretation of electrocardiograms, and special lectures and demonstrations.[13] Over the next four years, despite unmet plans for expansion, the institute thrived by imaginative use of its limited space. Research in congenital and rheumatic heart disease, cardiomyopathy, ischaemic heart disease, lipids, clotting, pulmonary hypertension, arrhythmias, and heart failure resulted in 77 publications.[13]

Despite the lack of surgical theatres, Mr T Holmes Sellors was appointed consultant surgeon and lecturer in 1957, followed later by Mr Donald Ross.[10] The postgraduate teaching programme expanded with the addition of competitive honorary assistant registrars. Up to four a year came from around the world for up to 12 months training. Short- and long-term courses and special instruction was given for consultants, general practitioners, candidates for membership of the Royal College of Physicians, and senior registrars.

International reputation

The reputation of the Institute of Cardiology had now become worldwide and large numbers of candidates applied to attend the courses and for year-long registrar positions. In particular, the postgraduate students were excited to witness the bedside analysis of the history and examination and correlation with the chest *x* ray, electrocardiogram, and haemodynamics, as taught by the charismatic Paul Wood. His ability to link together the clinical data and incorporate the cardiac catheterisation findings brought a new approach and understanding to rheumatic and congenital heart disease, and led to many published reports.[14] The consultants, especially Paul Wood, were invited to speak internationally.[13] A symposium entitled, "Current problems in relation to congenital heart disease" was held in October 1957, and was published in the *British Heart Journal*. A progress report to the British Postgraduate Medical Federation in 1958 applauded the accomplishments of the institute but deplored the lack of space, saying, "It will not be possible for the Institute to develop satisfactorily until more research laboratories are available and space can be provided for a new pathology department and a new biochemistry department."[13] By that time, expansion had been planned and was to be completed by 1959; frustratingly, however, the rebuilding of the south block was not finished until 1963.

Nevertheless, progress continued between 1958 and 1963.[10][15] A special research fund was started and grants were obtained from Imperial Chemical Industries to support a research assistant working in atherosclerosis. A genetics and expanded respiratory laboratory was developed, and the pathology department was enlarged. A new outpatient department and lecture theatre (later named the Paul Wood Theatre) were finished by autumn 1961. The same year, after a professional visit by Wood to see the Emperor of Abyssinia, a Haile Selassie lectureship was inaugurated to honour an outstanding worker in cardiac research, and the National Institutes of Health in Bethesda awarded a grant to finance two American fellows to come to the institute annually to train. This programme would lead to important Anglo-American interactions. In 1961, Wallace Brigden succeeded Graham Hayward as dean.

Deans of the Institutes

Institute of Cardiology

Dr Paul Wood 1947–50
Dr Graham Hayward 1950–61
Dr Wallace Brigden 1961–62
Dr Aubrey Leatham 1962–69
Dr Simon Rees 1969–72

Cardiothoracic Institute

Dr Joe Smart 1972–73
Professor Lynne Reid 1973–75
Dr Raphael Balcon 1975–79
Dr Eddie Keal 1979–84
Professor Margaret Turner-Warwick 1984–87

National Heart and Lung Institute

Dr Malcolm Green 1987–90
Professor Tim Clark 1990–97
Head of Division: Professor Philip Poole-Wilson 1997

Initiation of cardiac surgery

Cardiac surgery was finally initiated and pioneering work was done by Donald Ross and others, particularly in relation to homografts and surgery for congenital heart disease. Important work was also published on rheumatic heart disease, the natural history and diagnosis of congenital heart disease, phonocardiography and auscultation, cardiac pacemakers, genetically determined heart disease, and myocardial metabolism. Key figures of this period included Paul Wood, Wallace Brigden, Aubrey Leatham, Maurice Campbell, Graham Hayward, Peter Kerley, Keith Jefferson, Edgar Sowton, Lawson McDonald, Richard Emanuel, Jane Somerville, and Reginald Hudson.[10][15]

Formation of the National Heart and Lung Institute

The institute suffered a devastating blow with the sudden death of Paul Wood aged 54 in July 1962.[14] Wallace Brigden succeeded Wood as director and Aubrey Leatham then moved into the position of dean for the next seven years.[16] With a bequest from the Simon Marks Foundation honouring Evan Bedford, Peter Harris was appointed to the first chair of cardiology supported by the British Heart Foundation in 1964. A department of myocardial metabolism, under the direction of Peter Harris, was established in a house in Wimpole Street, purchased through gifts related to the pioneering surgery of Donald Ross. The institute was instrumental in persuading the two royal colleges to form a joint cardiology committee to make recommendations on the appropriate size and staffing of cardiac medical and surgical centres to achieve optimal patient outcome.[15]

The expansion in surgery continued, led by Donald Ross and later Magdi Yacoub. An innovative development was the replacement of the diseased aortic valve by the patient's own pulmonary valve with insertion of a homograft in the pulmonic position. Nearly all the leading cardiac surgeons in the United Kingdom, as well as many cardiologists throughout the world, were trained at the National Heart Hospital and its Institute of Cardiology. Later, a successful department of paediatric cardiology was started by Jane Somerville. Important advances in artificial pacing were made by Edgar Sowton and Tony Rickards.

Move to Brompton and amalgamation

The cancellation of the proposed expansion of the National Heart Hospital dashed hopes for further development of teaching and research at the Westmoreland Street site. In 1968, Aubrey Leatham as dean at the National Heart Hospital and John Batten at the Brompton Hospital approached John McMichael, director of the Postgraduate Medical Federation, suggesting that the National Heart Hospital and the Institute of Cardiology be combined with the Brompton Hospital and the Institute for Diseases of the Chest to form a single institution.[16] This would be built on a large site south of the Brompton Hospital and called the National Heart and Chest Hospital. Since the Brompton Hospital had become a leader in cardiac surgery, a move to that site made sense to some, but it angered others. A decision to proceed with this fusion was formalised in 1971, but it was not finally completed until 1988. The new hospital was named Royal Brompton Hospital, unfortunately obliterating any reference to its origin and previous cardiological associations. It was officially opened by the Queen in 1990.

At the time of the 21st anniversary of the Institute of the Diseases of the Chest in October 1970, JG (Guy) Scadding, the first dean, commenting on the merger said:

> We must welcome such changes. If in 40 years' time, someone is able to review the history of the world-famous Cardio-Respiratory Centre at South Kensington, or whatever it is eventually called, tracing it back to the amalgamation of the Hospitals for Diseases of the Chest and the National Heart Hospital and of the Institutes of

> Diseases of the Chest and Cardiology, our Founders and we could be cognisant of it, should feel well satisfied with the results of the fusion of our traditions and our histories.[17]

National Heart and Lung Institute

The fusion of the two specialties began in 1973 when the Cardiothoracic Institute was established under a common committee of management, academic board, and dean. The two institutes had moved to a site in Chelsea adjoining the site of the new hospital in April 1988, and its name was changed to the National Heart and Lung Institute (NHLI). The new institute, which was the largest academic centre for heart and lung disease in Europe, consisted of 15 departments, including cardiac medicine, respiratory medicine, cardiothoracic surgery, immunology, microbiology, experimental pathology and pharmacology, together with library and museum facilities. The centre was responsible for all aspects of the medical and surgical care of children and adults with heart disease, and its objectives were as follows:

- To increase knowledge of the causes of heart and lung disease as the basis for their prevention
- To increase understanding of the basic mechanisms of heart and lung disease at the cellular and molecular level to improve treatment
- To evaluate the effects of intervention – both medical and surgical, in hospital and in the community – to define optimal management of these important diseases.

The success of the heart and lung institute can be seen in the many developments that have taken place over the last 16 years. In 1984, the assets of the Midhurst Medical Research Institute, including staff, equipment, and investments valued at £6.5 million, were transferred to the institute. In the same year, a chair in clinical pharmacology was established, with Professor Peter Barnes as the first incumbent. In 1988, a close association with the Wynn Institute of Metabolic Research (formerly the Cavendish Clinic) was formalised with Professor Michael Oliver as director. The Wynn Institute brought expertise in the early detection and prevention of coronary artery disease. In the same year, Professor Philip Poole-Wilson succeeded Peter Harris as the Simon Marks British Heart Foundation professor of cardiology. In 1994, he became the first Englishman to become President of the European Society of Cardiology. Poole-Wilson, Andrew Coats, the current Viscount Royston BHF Chair in Cardiology, and others developed their research interest in congestive heart failure, which has led to many publications in this area. Over the years, the institute became increasingly self-funded with little more than 25% of its annual budget contributed by government sources. It has also developed an extensive partnership with industry and is now capable of exploring almost all areas of cardiovascular disease and treatment.

Undergraduate education at the National Heart and Lung Institute, undertaken in collaboration with Charing Cross and Westminister Hospitals, dates back to 1985. A teaching auditorium, named the Paul Wood Lecture Theatre opened 1989, and many postgraduate courses attracting an international audience have subsequently been held there.

Further rationalisation

In 1992, the Tomlinson report recommended integration of medical institutions with multifaculty colleges of the university, and in 1995 the National Heart and Lung Institute became a component of Imperial College of Science, Technology and Medicine. The institute is now one of nine divisions of the medical school and has activities on each of the campuses.

Conclusion

The vision of Sir Frances Fraser to attach postgraduate institutes for education and research at the special hospitals has proved to be prescient. From its origin as the Institute of Cardiology at the National Heart Hospital to its fusion as the National Heart and Lung Institute at the Royal Brompton Hospital, the institute has been a major force in the growth and worldwide recognition of British cardiology in the last half of the 20th century.

Acknowledgments

Our appreciation is expressed to Irene Oddi, Wallace Brigden, and Peter Harris for their review.

References

1. Fraser F. The training of specialists. *BMJ* 1948;1:135–8.
2. Rivett G. *From cradle to grave: fifty years of the National Health Service.* London: King's Fund, 1998.
3. Stevens R. *Medical practice in modern England: the impact of specialization and state medicine.* London: Yale University Press, 1966.
4. Great Britain, Ministry of Health and Department of Health for Scotland. *Report of the interdepartmental committee on medical schools.* London: HMSO, 1944.
5. Fraser F. *The British Postgraduate Medical Federation: the first fifteen years.* London: The Athlone Press, 1967.
6. Obituary of Sir Francis Fraser. *Br Heart J* 1965;27:449–51.
7. Rivett G. *The development of the London hospital system 1823–1982.* London: King Edwards Fund for London, 1986.
8. Campbell M. The National Heart Hospital (1857–1957). *Br Heart J* 1958;20:137–9.
9. Whitney R. *The place of hearts: being a history of the National Heart Hospital, London and Buckingham, 1857–1937.* London: New Goswell Printing Co, undated.
10. University of London. *The Institute of Cardiology handbook, 1963.* London: University of London, 1963.
11. Olsen EGJ. Reginald E.B. Hudson. *Clin Cardiol* 1987;10:277–78.
12. University of London. Institute of Cardiology. *Inspectors report, 1954.* London: University of London, 1954. (Appendix A.C. & C.C.1.)

13. University of London. Institute of Cardiology. *Progress report, 1954–58.* London: University of London, 1958.
14. Silverman ME. "To die in one's prime." The story of Paul Wood. *Am J Cardiol* 2000;85:75–87.
15. University of London. Institute of Cardiology. *Progress report, 1957–62.* London: University of London, 1962.
16. Silverman ME. Aubrey Leatham: twentieth century pioneer in auscultation. *Clin Cardiol* 1999;22:155–7.
17. Scadding JG. *The institutes of diseases of the chest 1946–1972: a personal history.* Library for the National Heart and Lung Institute.

Chapter 7

The Hammersmith Hospital and the Royal Postgraduate Medical School

Mark E Silverman, Arthur Hollman,
and Dennis M Krikler

In 1918, Sir William Osler, regius professor at Oxford, said, "The profession must get over its infantile fears of government finances, and must start to think about postgraduate education on an imperial scale." Osler and others proposed that a hospital be used solely for the purpose of postgraduate education.[1]

Foundation

In 1921, the Athlone committee was appointed by the Ministry of Health "to investigate the needs of medical practitioners and other graduates for further education in London." The committee recognised the lack of organised postgraduate education and recommended selecting a well financed, centrally located school attached to a hospital with 400 or more beds. Furthermore, the committee stipulated that the hospital should not be associated with an undergraduate medical school, which would divide the teaching effort. By 1925, it was clear that none of the acceptable London hospitals or schools was suitable or willing to divest itself of its undergraduate school in order to undertake the new educational venture, and building a new facility was deemed impractical. Thus, in 1930, the Hammersmith Hospital was chosen as the site and the British Postgraduate Medical School of the University of London was born.[2][3]

The postgraduate school and hospital were officially opened in 1935 by King George V. He expressed his hope that they "would play an imperial role in the winning and dissemination of medical knowledge, in the relief of suffering among my peoples in this country and overseas, and in enabling the doctors of all lands to come together in a task where all must be allies and helpers." This royal blessing set the tone that the Hammersmith would become an international centre, not just a London centre, for educating physicians and investigating disease.

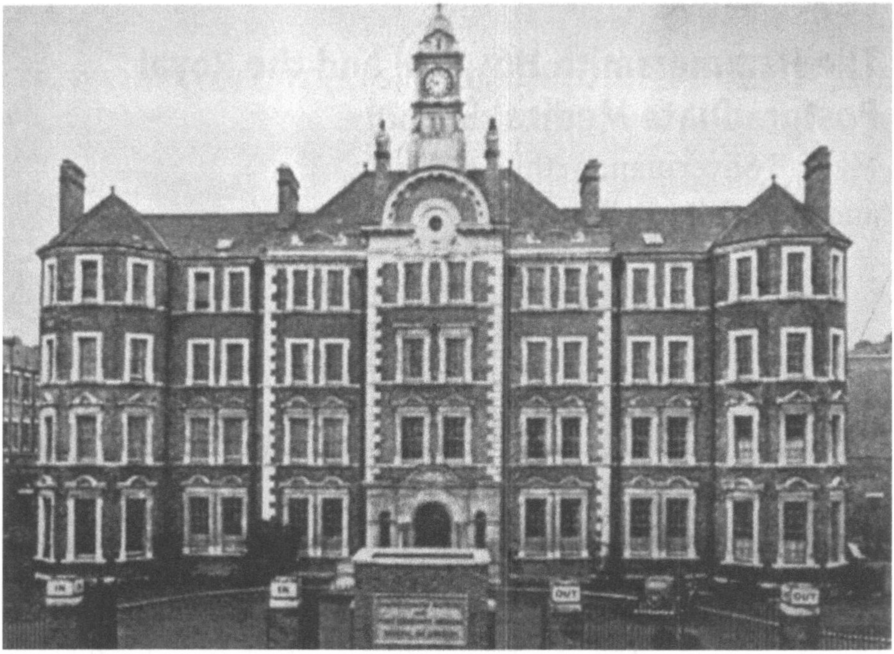

Figure 1 The Royal Postgraduate Medical School.

The new facility had four clinical departments - medicine, surgery, obstetrics and gynaecology, and pathology - each under the direction of a professor, with a reader, four assistants, and a few part-time specialist consultants.[2] Francis Fraser was appointed the first professor of medicine in 1934; an inspired choice for the future of training and research in Britain. Fraser had worked at the Rockefeller Institute in New York under the influence of Abraham Flexner and William Welch. They had been successful in developing the Germanic concept and structure, whereby the professor was an outstanding clinician-investigator-teacher who passed on his knowledge to postgraduate students from around the world.[4]

Voluntary hospitals and research

At that time, all teaching hospitals in England were voluntary - supported mostly by philanthropy and public donations - and their consultants had honorary appointments. These hospital consultants were part-time, donating their services conscientiously to attend a hospital ward twice a week and to see outpatients. Within this system, there was little opportunity or laboratory space available for organised research and, at best, a junior might spend a year on a project before entering private practice. Facilities for some clinical research did develop in London after 1920 with the foundation of five chairs of medicine and the establishment under Sir

Thomas Lewis of a department of clinical research at University College Hospital. However, most of the clinical practice at the voluntary hospitals continued as it had since Victorian times - each consultant had his own teaching firm and there was no coordinated medical practice within the hospital.

The Hammersmith model

Francis Fraser was determined to create at Hammersmith a department of medicine that was based on the Rockefeller model and consisted of full time physicians paid by the university to do research and teach. His initial selections included Robert Aitken as reader and Paul Wood, JG (Guy) Scadding, Peter Sharpey-Schafer, and CH Stuart Harris as first assistants. All were under 30 years of age. Each was given responsibility for 30 general medical beds, an outpatient clinic, and the opportunity to pursue his own academic interests.

The striking feature of medicine at the Hammersmith working under Fraser was freedom of expression. The deference paid to senior consultants elsewhere was replaced by an encouragement to challenge and argue openly at bedside rounds and at Wednesday morning staff rounds. The teaching was of the highest calibre. It was carried out at joint weekly bedside rounds, short courses, and at lectures, and spilled over into the lunch and tea sessions in front of the postgraduate students. Daily pathology conferences in the autopsy room, attended by many of the seniors in the department, were an essential learning opportunity. The cramped quarters, in which all were forced to share and interact, seemed to provide rich soil for productive research. Papers presented at national meetings were rehearsed before a critical department meeting - a terrifying experience, which might mean a total revision but ensured a polished final performance.

Cardiac catheterisation

In 1939, John McMichael from Edinburgh succeeded Aitken as reader in medicine.[5] Then, when Francis Fraser left in 1939 to direct the Emergency Medical Service, McMichael became the head of the department of medicine. While in Edinburgh, John McMichael had made a thorough study of the cardiac output in heart failure using the acetyline method of Grollman. At Hammersmith with Peter Sharpey-Schafer he tried to use this method to study cardiac output after venesection, but found the sequential changes difficult to assess. They were therefore immediately attracted by the paper on right heart catheterisation in 1941 by Cournand and Ranges.[6] McMichael and Sharpey-Schafer undertook their first cardiac catheterisation on 24 November 1942, initiating a series of important studies on the physiology and pharmacological response of the normal and diseased heart and circulation, especially in the area of heart failure, which was first published in 1944.[7] Their work not only shed new light on the heart and circulation but also helped to establish cardiac catheterisation as a safe technique for studying the heart, bringing great prestige to the medical school and the Hammersmith Hospital. By the end of 1943, they had performed 135 catheterisations without incident.

Sharpey-Schafer at the Hammersmith (and after 1952 at St Thomas's Hospital) became interested in the peripheral circulation, realising that there was more to the circulation than the heart and arteries. He accomplished important studies on venous tone, postural effects, the Valsalva manoeuvre, and reflexes related to the development of syncope.[8–11] His two Oliver-Sharpey Lectures on venous tone in 1961 gave a fine account of the subject.

The Second World War

In 1939, the hospital was designated a casualty centre of 400 beds. Many of the staff left for military service or were transferred elsewhere. Despite the difficulties and some bomb damage, training and research continued apace throughout the war under the direction of McMichael. Seventy two courses were held, and these were attended by 3700 officers from the Allied Forces. The training was directed towards the war effort, and important research in crush injuries, renal failure, jaundice, and shock was carried on as a natural consequence of the types of patients referred at that time. The research would lead to pioneering investigation through the use of liver biopsy and cardiac catheterisation. This type of invasive research was bold and controversial and was carried through in the face of criticism outside the hospital. Using plethysmography on a volunteer donating blood, they were able to show for the first time that the low blood pressure accompanying fainting was due to vasodilatation in muscle – not to a low cardiac output.[12] Investigation of the action of intravenous digoxin was a world first.[13][14] Other studies led to an appreciation of the concept of high and low output heart failure. Sheila Howarth, McMichael's house officer, joined the team, and, in 1946, they demonstrated the haemodynamic features of congenital heart disease.[15]

The Postgraduate Medical School of London

After the second world war, Francis Fraser left Hammersmith to become the first director of the British Postgraduate Medical Foundation of the University of London. The school at Hammersmith was renamed the Postgraduate Medical School of London.[3] In 1946, John McMichael was appointed to succeed Fraser as professor of medicine, a post he would retain until 1966.[5] In 1950, McMichael published a monograph – *The pharmacology of the failing human heart* – which reviewed his studies on heart failure and offered a revised definition of the disorder.[16] This signalled the end of his cardiac work.

Severe hypertension became an important area of investigation, and in 1950 an outpatient clinic was established to follow patients with this problem. A series of investigations, including auscultatory findings, the retinal vessels, and the mechanism of antihypertensive drugs, undertaken by J Barlow, CT Dollery, P Kincaid-Smith et al., led to a new understanding of the problem and its treatment. A department of clinical pharmacology was established under the direction of CT (later Sir Colin) Dollery.

After Peter Sharpey-Schafer moved to St Thomas's Hospital in 1948 and Paul Wood went to the Brompton and National Heart Hospitals in 1949, John Goodwin took charge of clinical cardiology. Under Goodwin's direction, Hammersmith Hospital became known internationally as a centre for the investigation of cardiomyopathy with a special interest in the study of hypertrophic cardiomyopathy. In 1974, Goodwin provided a classification of the various types of cardiomyopathy that became adopted world wide.[17] Goodwin was coeditor of *Progress in cardiology* from 1973–88.

Robert Steiner, who became director of radiology in 1950, was interested in cardiac catheterisation and played an essential role in introducing coronary arteriography in 1970.[18] John B West and Dollery (see chapter 12) capitalised on the availability of the MRC's cyclotron unit with an elegant radioisotope study of regional pulmonary blood flow in patients with mitral stenosis. In 1962, Celia Oakley joined the staff. She had a strong interest in cardiomyopathy, valvular heart disease, and infective endocarditis. Later, she was awarded a personal chair in clinical cardiology.

Cardiac surgery

Cardiac surgery began at Hammersmith in 1948, with operations for coarctation, patent ductus, the Blalock–Taussig shunt, and closed mitral valvotomy. In 1953, Denis Melrose pioneered the development of a heart–lung machine at Hammersmith. It became a custom to place a specimen rose plucked from the garden that morning on the machine to bring good luck. Three years later Bentall, Melrose, and colleagues were the first to publish a report on experimental potassium citrate arrest. WP Cleland, who performed the first open heart surgery on mitral and aortic stenosis and congenital heart disease at Hammersmith, recalls those days:

> Melrose was a physiologist and became involved in elective cardiac arrest with potassium citrate and with the development of a heart lung machine designed to take over the function of both heart and lung and permit unhurried intracardiac surgery ... About 1950 Bentall and I became involved with Melrose and others with the Melrose rotating disc heart lung oxygenator. Experimental operations were originally carried out in the laboratories of the department of surgery at the PGMS. But soon a full blown team assembled every Saturday morning at the Royal Veterinary College at Camden Town where our open heart procedures were performed. With this information we were prepared to start clinical operations. In 1953 six patients were selected, each of whom was considered to be unlikely to survive unaided for six months. The lesions were varied – aortic stenosis, mitral valve disease, etc. Of these six patients (all adults) all survived the immediate operation but five of the six

> succumbed in the postoperative period. The one survivor lived on for several years. This was not good enough and the exercise was brought to a halt. At this time Kirklin and Lillehei in the USA were both doing open-heart operations with good results and Melrose and I spent three months commuting between the Mayo Clinic with Kirklin and Minneapolis with Lillehei. It immediately became apparent that both these teams were operating mainly on children with congenital heart disease, but children who were not in imminent danger of death. But, apart from the selection of patients, the big lesson we learnt was the importance of meticulous postoperative care and especially the management of blood and fluid balance. With this information further practice enabled us to restart a clinical programme in 1957. This time the results were encouraging enough for us to continue steadily and in the following 10 years our team operated on 1200 patients. We were much helped in launching this drive by Dr. Richard Bonham Carter, cardiologist at the Children's Hospital in Great Ormond Street. He promised to send us up to 50 youngsters with serious congenital abnormalities but all with right sided heart lesions (VSD and ASD and pulmonary stenosis). No questions would be asked about the progress of the group until all 50 had been operated upon. Fortunately at the end of this period our operative mortality was recorded at 10% for this group. (personal communication)

In 1968, Cleland, Bentall, Melrose, Goodwin, Oakley, and Hollman published their decade of experience gained in the 1200 open heart operations at Hammersmith from 1957–67.[19] Cleland and Bentall, in 1958, were the first in the world to perform a ventricular myomectomy on a patient with hypertrophic cardiomyopathy. The Hammersmith surgical team - including Bentall, Cleland, and Hollman - travelled to Russia in 1959 to perform open heart surgery and introduce their techniques so that a Russian surgical programme could be started. They operated on four of 40 desperately ill children, and also performed two closed mitral valvotomies. The surgical procedures went well to their great relief. Goodwin started a joint consultation clinic at the Hammersmith between the cardiologist and cardiac surgeon, and this became a model for other centres.

Further research

John P Shillingford established an academic unit in 1956 located in a new three storey addition, the Collier Building. His investigative work included blood flow and the use of dye dilution techniques to make serial cardiac output measurements during pregnancy and in congenital heart disease.[20] He organised an early coronary care unit and was the first to use continuous monitoring and magnetic tape recording of physiological data.[21] Shillingford was the first holder, in 1976, of the Sir John McMichael chair of cardiovascular medicine established by the British Heart Foundation.

In 1973, Dennis Krikler was appointed. He established an arrhythmia service and electrophysiological investigative unit and initiated a course in arrhythmia and electrophysiology called "European cardiology." Krikler pioneered the use of intravenous verapamil for arrhythmias. Attilio Maseri from Pisa became the holder of the McMichael chair in 1980. Maseri and his staff investigated the dynamic factors that modulate coronary blood flow in angina and infarction and the mechanisms of anginal pain. Together with Goodwin, he initiated a highly praised annual meeting, European and American Cardiology at the Hammersmith, which attracted opinion leaders from around the world. An international diploma course in cardiology, subsequently adopted by London University, was also started. In 1981, a clinical research unit on the third floor of the Collier Building was developed for molecular biology and genetic studies in coronary disease together with laboratories for angiography and non-invasive cardiac studies. After Maseri left in 1992 to take a chair in Rome, the McMichael chair became vacant and was eventually filled by a physician interested in rheumatic diseases. After Goodwin's retirement in 1985, Roger Hall moved from Cardiff to take up the chair in clinical cardiology. Later, the cardiology service was amalgamated with that of the Charing Cross Hospital, and, in 1998, became a unit of the Imperial College School of Science, Technology and Medicine.

Acknowledgements

The authors are grateful to the following for their review and constructive comments: Sir Christopher Booth, WP Cleland, John Goodwin, Attilo Maseri.

References and notes

1. Osler W. The hospital unit in university work. *Lancet* 1911;I:211–49.
2. Newman C. A brief history of the postgraduate medical school. *Med Hist* 1966;10:285–8.
3. Fraser F. *The British postgraduate medical federation: the first fifteen years.* London: Athlone Press, 1967.
4. Fraser F. Obituary. *Br Heart J* 1965;27:339–51.
5. Dollery C. Sir John McMichael. *Biographical memoirs of the Royal Society.* London: Royal Society of Medicine, 1995:283–96.
6. Cournand A, Ranges HA. Catheterization of the right auricle in man. *Proc Soc Exp Biol Med* 1941;46:462–66.
7. McMichael J, Sharpey-Schafer EP. Cardiac output in man by a direct Fick method. *Br Heart J* 1944;6:33–40.
8. Edward Peter Sharpey-Schafer (1908–63), was the grandson of the famous physiologist Sir Edward Sharpey-Schafer who supervised his education. He trained at University College Hospital where he was houseman to Wilfrid Trotter and to Sir Thomas Lewis, and then went to the National Heart Hospital. In 1936 he was selected by Professor Francis Fraser to join his academic department of medicine at the Postgraduate Medical School. Initially he specialised in endocrinology, but after 1939 his interest turned to cardiac investigation. With John McMichael, he was a pioneer of cardiac catheterisation in Britain. In 1948, he was appointed professor of medicine at St Thomas's Hospital where he developed his research interest in venous tone summarised in his fine Oliver-Sharpey Lectures in 1961. He had a flair for an imaginative approach to research and as a scientist he sought the elegant and decisive experiment, well shown in his study of the pattern of blood pressure response to the Valsalva manoeuvre in heart failure. Other research included work on syncope and the use of the tilt table to study haemodynamics. At St Thomas's he fostered an environment that attracted and inspired others who became leaders in their fields, and he gave priority to the prosecution and encouragement of research. Sharpey-Schafer married Dr Sheila Howarth his former colleague at the Hammersmith, and they had two daughters. He had many interests outside medicine, and was a keen naturalist and a fine photographer, especially of native orchids. His early death at age 55 removed a creative mind that had contributed importantly to the understanding of cardiac physiology.
9. McMichael J. Edward Peter Sharpey-Schafer. *Br Heart J* 1964;26:430–2.
10. Sharpey-Schafer EP. Venous tone. *BMJ* 1961;2:1589–95.

11. Sharpey-Schafer EP. Effects of Valsalva's manaeuvre on the normal and failing circulation. *BMJ* 1955;1:693–5.
12. Barcroft H, Edholm OG, McMichael J, Sharpey-Schafer EP. Post-haemorrhagic fainting: study by cardiac output and forearm flow. *Lancet* 1944;i:489–91.
13. McMichael J, Sharpey-Schafer EP. The action of intravenous digoxin in man. *Q J Med* 1944;13:123–35.
14. Cournand A. Cardiac catheterization. *Acta Med Scand* 1975;suppl: 579.
15. Howarth S, McMichael J, Sharpey-Schafer EP. Cardiac catheterisation in cases of patent interauricular septum, primary pulmonary hypertension, Fallot's tetralogy and pulmonary stenosis. *Br Heart J* 1947;9:292–6.
16. McMichael J. *The pharmacology of the failing human heart.* Oxford: Blackwell Scientific Publishing, 1950.
17. Goodwin J. Prospects and predictions for the cardiomyopathies. *Circulation* 1974;50:210–9.
18. Steiner RE, Hollman A. Radiological contrast studies of the left heart. *Br J Radiol* 1962;35:540–53.
19. Cleland WP, Bentall HH, Melrose DG, Goodwin JF, Oakley CM, Hollman A. A decade of open heart surgery. *Lancet* 1968;i:191–8.
20. Taylor SH, Shillingford JP. Clinical applications of Coomassie blue. *Br Heart J* 1959;21:497–504.
21. Shillingford JP. The organisation of an intensive care unit for patients following acute myocardial infarction. *Br Heart J* 1965;27:305–6.

Chapter 8

Bedside Diagnosis

Aubrey Leatham

The skills of bedside diagnosis peaked in the middle of the 20th century following the earlier pioneering work of Dr James Mackenzie. He emphasised the importance of symptoms and careful history taking and was sceptical about many of the beliefs current at that time, which were based on empirical ideas without scientific proof.[1] While working as a general practitioner in Burnley, Mackenzie had used primitive external jugular recordings to make remarkably accurate observations on the venous pulse. He noticed the disappearance of the "a" wave with pulsus irregularis, and attributed this to paralysis of the atrium.[2] Later, in 1909, Thomas Lewis showed by means of electrocardiography that this finding resulted from atrial fibrillation. Before the advent of the electrocardiogram, Lewis, Hay in Liverpool, and others used the venous and radial pulse to skilfully analyse arrhythmias. Optimal bedside use of the venous pulse had to await proof that the wave form in the right atrium was identical to the deep venous pulse and the logical application of physical signs at the bedside practised by Paul Wood. Wood's skills were beautifully demonstrated in his film, *The jugular venous pulse*, which was made in 1957. No clinical cardiologist would question Wood's statement: "It is hard to conceive of any physical sign that is more informative."

Principles of examination

In view of the recent decline in interest in physical diagnosis and the rapid recourse to expensive investigations, it is worth restating some of the principles of examination used first by Thomas Lewis and then by cardiologists in the 1950s and 1960s. Reclining the patient at an angle of 40° brings the top of the normal venous pulse about 3 cm above the sternal angle where its waveform can be studied (best on the right side). The easiest way of differentiating the venous from the carotid pulse is the knowledge that the dominant venous wave is inward ("y descent"), caused by opening of the tricuspid valve, contrasting with the earlier outward movement of the carotid pulse, timed by palpating the other side of the neck. Giant "a" waves, from a powerful right atrial contraction, are seen to precede the palpated carotid upstroke and indicate conditions such as tricuspid stenosis, right ventricular hypertrophy, or nodal rhythm. A pansystolic venous wave that can be obliterated by gentle pressure indicates tricuspid regurgitation from transmission of the right ventricular pressure pulse to the right atrium and neck. A normal venous pressure in an ambulant patient who is not taking diuretics excludes right heart failure and is an invaluable physical sign in a patient presenting with an undetermined cause of swollen ankles.

The most characteristic arterial pulse is the sharp "water-hammer" pulse of aortic regurgitation, best felt at the periphery as described in the previous century by Corrigan. Lesser degrees of arterial sharpness indicate a diagnosis of increased stroke volume from high output states or mitral regurgitation. A sharp pulse is also an important feature of hypertrophic cardiomyopathy (asymmetric hypertrophy of Teare).

Aortic stenosis

Accurate diagnosis of aortic stenosis became more important in the 1960s because of the availability of surgical treatment and the increased number of elderly patients with a calcified aortic valve. Thus, careful palpation of the carotid pulse became increasingly important. Except where there is a small carotid pulse that is difficult to analyse, a slow rise is diagnostic of aortic stenosis. This is a particularly useful sign in elderly people (who normally have quite a sharp pulse because of rigid vessels) and can be used to differentiate valvular aortic stenosis from left ventricular obstructive cardiomyopathy. For changes of rhythm, the carotid pulse is more useful than the radial one, but auscultation is infinitely superior to both – a lesson that seems to have been largely neglected nowadays with the widespread availability of electrocardiography.

Palpation of the heart was practised by Mackenzie, who recognised the difference between the left ventricle at the apex and the right ventricle in the parasternal area. However, advances in cardiac surgery for congenital heart disease and the need for accurate diagnosis in the Paul Wood era increased the amount of information sought from palpation. Inclining the patient to the left to analyse the beat of the left ventricle was found very useful for diagnosing a hypertrophied or a hyperkinetic left ventricle; these procedures were then applied to the right ventricle in the parasternal area. The hyperkinetic impulse of the overloaded right ventricle in atrial septal defect proved to be a valuable physical sign in the absence of systolic expansion of the left atrium from mitral regurgitation pushing the right ventricle forwards.

Development of the phonocardiogram

The most important advances in bedside diagnosis were made in auscultation. The enormous improvements in amplifying and recording

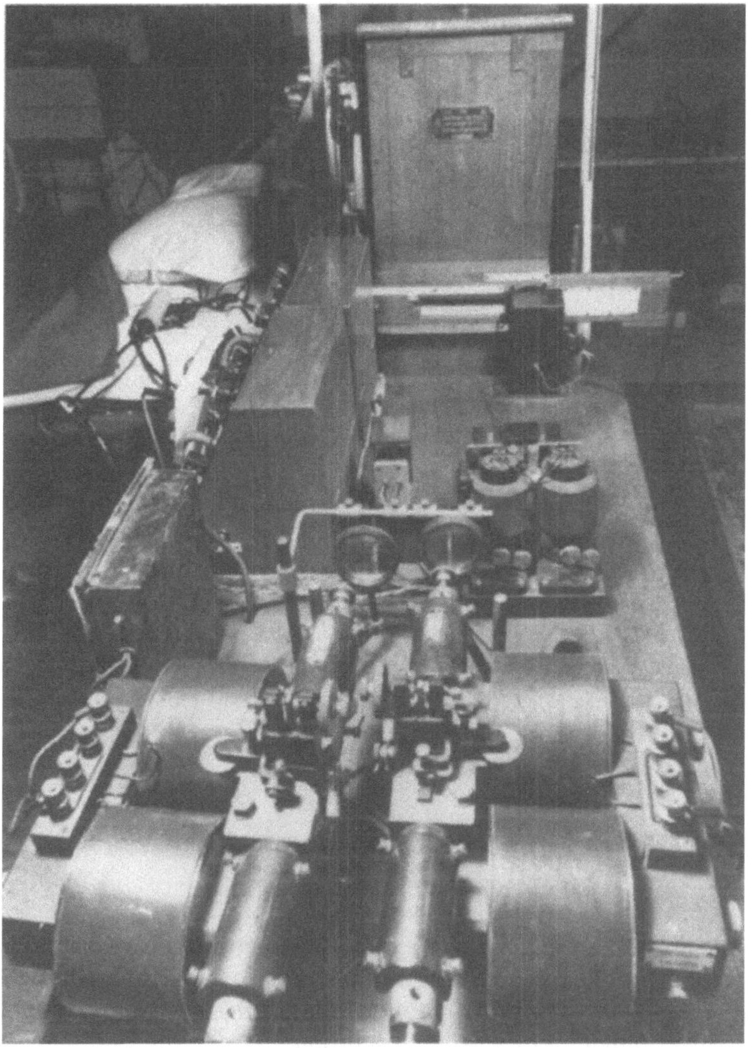

Figure 1 High definition phonocardiographic equipment, used in our laboratory in the 1950s, consisting of two Cambridge string and two mirror galvanometers (Reproduced, with permission, from Leatham A. *Auscultation of the heart and phonocardiography* London: Churchill Livingstone, 1975 and reference [4]).

techniques achieved in the 1950s permitted the recording of accurate phonocardiograms with several simultaneous channels to identify the timing of heart sounds and murmurs (figures 1–3).[3] For the first time, objective evidence of the auscultatory findings was possible.[4]

In 1946, using a telephone earpiece harnessed to a string galvanometer, I undertook primitive experiments on recording heart sounds. These had made it clear that recordings without filtration were dominated by low frequency oscillations bearing no resemblance to auscultation. The human hearing mechanism filters these low frequencies while passing on the higher

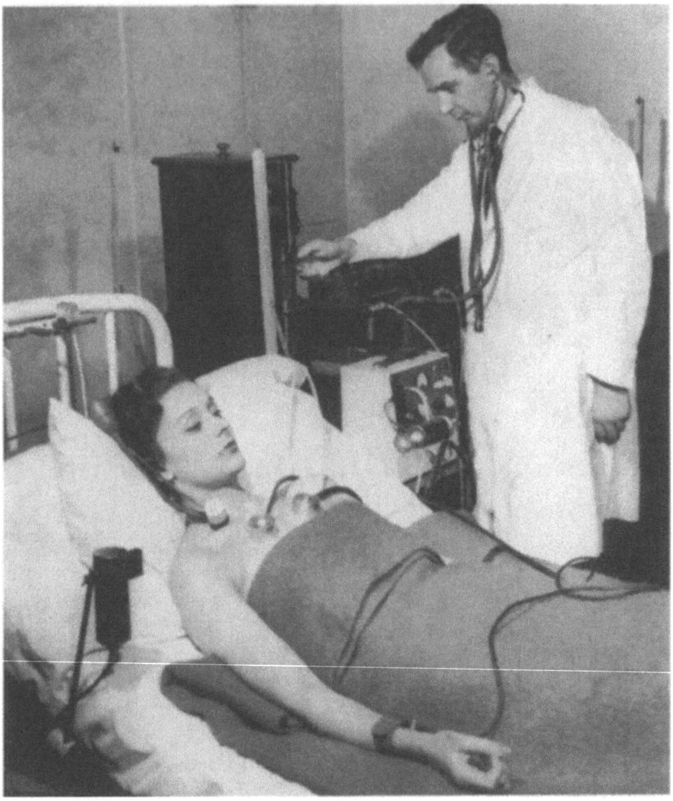

Figure 2 Recording the phonocardiogram, using several microphones.

frequencies. William Evans, aware of my interest in this area, appointed me the first Sherbrooke research fellow in the cardiac department of the London Hospital. He was attempting phonocardiography by using a double fibre string galvanometer, but was having problems with the dominance of low frequencies in his recordings.

Lewis's scepticism

Rappaport and Sprague in 1941 had shown that considerable filtration of low frequencies was required for the phonocardiogram to resemble auscultation. This seemed to be the first step if the graphic recordings were to clarify and improve auscultation – which at that time was largely discarded as a scientific diagnostic method, especially by Sir Thomas Lewis. The influential Lewis had stated that the murmur of mitral stenosis must be recognised by memorising its characteristics, rather like the bark of a dog, and he and other senior physicians completely disregarded systolic murmurs. I was impressed by the American physiologist, Wiggers, who had shown asynchrony between left and right ventricular pressure pulses, and

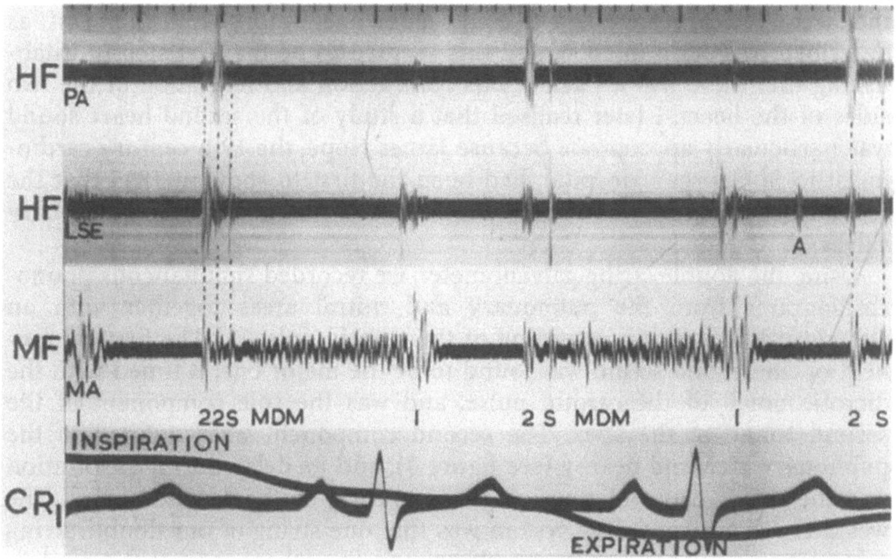

Figure 3 Tracings taken with the National Heart Hospital phonocardiograph showing the value of simultaneous recordings from different areas in a patient with mitral stenosis. In the expiratory phase of respiration the snap (S) might have been P2. In inspiration, however, the sequence of A2, a loud P2 (maximal in the pulmonary area), and a soft opening snap can be easily recognised. High frequency (HF) recordings from the pulmonary area (PA) and lower left sternal edge (LSE) and a medium frequency recording from the mitral area (MA) to show the mitral diastolic murmur (MDM). Nowadays, identification of sounds would have been achieved, perhaps more scientifically but not more clearly, by echophonocardiography. (Reproduced with permission from Leatham A. *Auscultation of the heart and phonocardiography* New York: Churchill Livingstone, 1975 and reference [4]).

by Wolferth and Margolies, who in 1935 had identified the two components of the second heart sound in bundle branch block by using a simultaneous carotid pulse. Their findings reversed Lewis's erroneous electrocardiographic interpretation of which bundle branch was affected.

Dock had popularised the hypothesis that the opening and closing of valves was the major cause of heart sounds. It seemed to me that filtration of the low frequencies not only resembled auscultation, but should also show whether high frequency transients synchronised with valve movement. If this were the cause of the sounds, it would make identification of the components of sounds relatively easy.[4] Fortunately, I was not aware that I would have to wait for 30 years for echocardiography to prove this correct.

Studies on identifying components of the second heart sound

After Bernstein in the physiology department of the London Hospital made amplifiers with suitable filters, Malcolm Towers and I started our work on the second heart sound. We could hear inspiratory splitting, just as described by Potain in 1866, and this seemed to be the first step in establishing that there was asynchronous contraction and relaxation of the two sides of the heart. I later realised that a study of the second heart sound was particularly appropriate because James Hope, the 19th century cardiologist to St George's Hospital, had been the first to show in 1835 that the second heart sound was related to closure of the aortic and pulmonary valves.

Using the double string galvanometer, we recorded simultaneous phonocardiograms from the pulmonary and mitral areas together with an electrocardiogram or a recording of the carotid pulse.[3] The first component of the second sound was found to be the major one; it timed with the dicrotic notch of the carotid pulse, and was the sole component of the second sound at the apex. The second component was confined to the pulmonary area and nearby (see figure 3), and its delay during inspiration was the major cause of physiological splitting of the second sound. The weakness of our recording system was that one string of our double string galvanometer tended to wrap itself around the other whenever it made a big deflection; this meant numerous trips to Cambridge in a 1934 "baby" Austin to visit an old technician who alone was able to unwrap the strings.

Elsewhere in Europe, particularly in Sweden and Germany, the Mannheimer system (comprising one microphone and several simultaneous channels with different frequency ranges) was being developed, but nothing important was discovered with this technique. Luisada in Chicago was using low frequency phonocardiograms, bearing no relation to auscultation, and multiple timing channels with variable delays.

At the London Hospital, cardiac radiology under Parkinson was making major advances. Each outpatient had to wait until the end of the afternoon for the fluoroscopy session. Parkinson's time in the *x* ray dark room would last for about an hour, during which time there was discerning and entertaining comment. With the help of the radiological findings described by Parkinson, Papp, and Bedford in 1939, it became possible to diagnose atrial septal defect. Barber, Magidson, and Wood had described the auscultatory signs as we were looking at the peculiar second heart sound. It was Bill Dicks, our technician and collaborator at the London Hospital, who said triumphantly, looking at the moving shadow of the string rather than at the finished graph, that the "split was fixed." Measurements confirmed that both A2 and P2 were delayed nearly equally on inspiration.[6] The description of reversed splitting of the second sound in left bundle branch block was an easy step from our knowledge of physiological splitting. The discoveries that the delay of P2 gave an exact estimate of the severity of pulmonary stenosis and that the Eisenmenger ventricular septal defect and single ventricle gave a single second heart sound had to await Paul Wood's work at the National Heart Hospital.[7][8]

Classification of systolic murmurs

At the London Hospital, the influences of Mackenzie and then Parkinson meant that systolic murmurs were almost ignored ... and were certainly regarded as unimportant. This was an overreaction to the diagnostic abuse and unnecessary "cardiac invalidism" (one of William Evans's famous phrases) that the presence of a systolic murmur had prompted in earlier years. Parkinson's reaction to a systolic murmur is reflected in the case notes of a patient with this condition. The diagnosis was given as "mitral systolic murmur (mitral stenosis)." Indeed, William Evans said of mitral incompetence that it was a description of the physician who diagnosed it. One wonders what he would have said of mitral valve prolapse and the fiasco that minor degrees produced! Thirty years later the patient with the systolic murmur died of coronary disease and proved to have mild rheumatic mitral regurgitation.

It was soon clear from our high frequency phonocardiograms that the systolic murmur of aortic stenosis finished before the aortic component of the second heart sound – as indeed it had to, bearing in mind the cessation of forward flow before closure of the valve.[9] It seemed logical to label these and similar murmurs as "ejection" murmurs.[5] On the other hand, the systolic murmur of mitral regurgitation always reached A2 or beyond it, and so was termed "pansystolic." Sometimes, with minimal mitral regurgitation, it was maximal or even confined to late systole. In this way, apical systolic murmurs could be separated into left ventricular outflow ejection murmurs and mitral regurgitant murmurs, an important step forward in trying to produce order in a confused subject and to select patients for catheterisation and surgery.

With Wallace Brigden and the help of the Bernhard Baron Institute of Pathology, we studied the natural history of "pure" mitral regurgitation in 30 patients with loud apical pansystolic murmurs and enlargement or systolic expansion of the left atrium on *x* ray screening.[10] Apart from the risk of infective endocarditis, the course of the disorder was long and benign until the onset of left ventricular failure. In nine necropsy examinations, only one showed definite evidence of rheumatic valvulitis; in most of the others there was a parachuting mitral valve from an unknown cause, which we now appreciate was due to a floppy mitral valve. From this background, later confirmed by a 9 to 22 year follow up of patients with a late systolic murmur,[11] we could easily see that the threat of sudden death due to Barlow's syndrome and mitral valve prolapse would prove to be wildly exagerated in all but the most exceptional cases.[12]

Work at the National Heart Hospital

In 1951, I moved to the National Heart Hospital, where Paul Wood was director of the Institute of Cardiology. John Norman, the chief technician, found another 1918 vintage Cambridge table model string electrocardiograph on which we mounted a second string and two mirror galvanometers (with the aid of the Cambridge Instrument Company) (fig 1). Each of the four galvanometers had a separate light source, and these four sources had to be matched up to obtain an evenly illuminated recording. This was particularly difficult because the colour of the light sources varied. The falling plate camera used film that was far better than the usual recording paper because of its greater density range. The length of the recording was limited to 15 cm, but the speed of fall of the plate could be varied infinitely to suit the requirements of the particular recording. This system was ideal for composing a suitable length of recording to fit a page of the *British Heart Journal*. The quality of the sound recordings made with this apparatus has never been surpassed (see figure 3); it cannot even be equalled with modern apparatus.

Studies on components and intensity of the first heart sound

The final and most difficult problem was identification of the components of the first heart sound. From our first high frequency recordings at the London Hospital, it was clear that there were two components. Bearing in mind the precedence of left ventricular contraction over right, it seemed reasonable to guess that the first component, which was by far the larger, and was maximal at the apex, was due to mitral closure. The second component was maximal at the lower left sternal edge over the tricuspid valve and occurred too late in relation to the carotid upstroke to be mitral closure.

Working with Edgar Haber from the Massachusetts General Hospital, who spent a year at St George's, we produced support for a tricuspid origin by finding further delay in the second component with right bundle branch block and left ventricular ectopic complexes, and by pacing the left ventricle.[13] Opposition to a tricuspid origin came from Luisada in Chicago, who could not record tricuspid closure with intracardiac phonocardiograms. In addition, destruction of the right ventricle in dogs had failed to alter the first sound, which they attributed solely to the left side of the heart. When they found that the pressure crossovers of the ventricles and atria occurred before the sound, they deduced that valve closure was noiseless. They seemed to be unaware of the lag between a pressure crossover and the final halt of the valve. Even James Shaver's Pittsburgh group, with superb sound and pressure correlates, denied a tricuspid origin to the second component of the first sound. They attributed this sound to aortic ejection ("root sound"), although the ejection sound in aortic stenosis was later and related to aortic valve opening.

Splitting due to mitral followed by tricuspid closure

Until the development of echocardiography, we were unable to obtain the exact timing of valve movement. In the early days, it was difficult to obtain an echo reflection from the normal tricuspid valve, so we chose patients

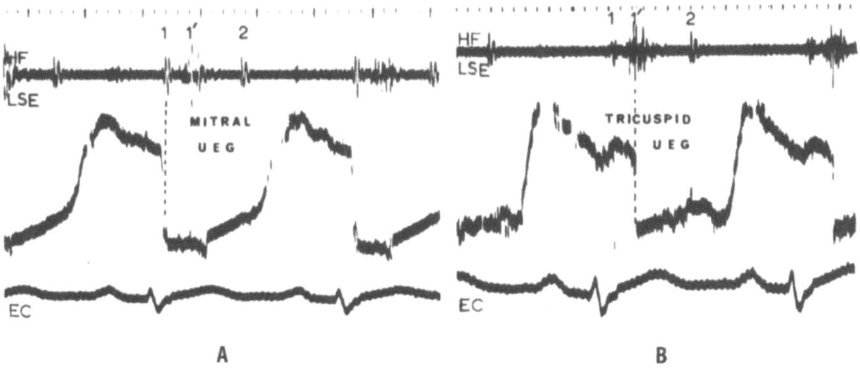

Figure 4 Ebstein's anomaly. Wide splitting of the first heart sound. **A**. The first component of the first sound coincides with mitral closure on the echo. **B**. The loud late high frequency component of the first sound (1′) coincides with tricuspid valve closure on the echo. (Reproduced with permission from reference [14]).

with Ebstein's anomaly, who had a large anterior tricuspid leaflet.[14] The loud, late component of the first sound, which we had assumed to be tricuspid closure delayed by the almost invariable right bundle branch block, was shown to coincide exactly with the final halt of the tricuspid valve on Ronald Pridie's primitive apparatus at Hammersmith (see figure 4). Subsequently, with apparatus improved by Graham Leech, and simultaneously with Ernest Craige of Chapel Hill, North Carolina (and St George's Hospital), it was shown that splitting of the first heart sound, as heard in most normal subjects, was indeed due to mitral closure followed by tricuspid closure. There was synchrony between the final halt of the closing movement of the mitral leaflets on the echocardiogram and the first component of the first heart sound, and the closing tricuspid valve coincided with the second component.

This led to work with Nicholas Brooks and Mark Dancy on bundle branch block.[15] Tricuspid closure was confirmed to be late in patients with isolated right bundle branch block; however, when right bundle branch block was associated with generalised conducting tissue disease, closure of the tricuspid valve was not delayed, indicating that the conduction block occurred at the peripheral arborisation level. This accorded with the site of histological change that was shown by Michael Davies.

The mechanism causing variation in the intensity of the first heart sound has been of interest for many years. The relation to the PR interval was emphasised by Samuel Levine of Boston, who did so much to stimulate clinical cardiology. I remember him discussing the mysteries of the first heart sound in front of the painting of the Mona Lisa in the Louvre during an early World Congress of Cardiology in Paris. Many years later, echocardiography showed conclusively that atrial contraction not only opened but also closed the atrioventricular valves, provided that the PR interval was long enough. With a long PR interval, the first sound was soft because the valve was already nearly closed. When the PR interval was short, the valve was still wide open at the onset of ventricular contraction, and the first sound was loud.[3]

But why should the distance of travel of this flimsy structure influence the intensity of sound that results from its final closure? From the early days of phonocardiography, researchers had appreciated that the first sound was late as well as loud in mitral stenosis. It seemed to Nicholas Brooks and me that if valve closure were delayed to a steeper part of the climb of the left ventricular pressure pulse, the velocity of closure would be increased. Using high speed echophonocardiography, we found that the same principle applied to normal subjects. With a short PR interval, the mitral valve, wide open at the moment of contraction, was late in reaching its final halting point and this coincided with a loud first sound. With a long PR interval, the valve was nearly closed at the slow rising start of ventricular contraction, and this was associated with a soft first sound.[16]

Studies on early systolic sounds

Finally, a few words about early systolic sounds, which Vogelpoel and I termed "ejection sounds" – despite the superb French expression "claquement protosystolique."[17] The early ejection sound occurring in pulmonary root dilatation (early with pulmonary valve stenosis and later when pulmonary hypertension causes a prolonged isovolumic time of the right ventricle) had been useful in diagnosis. However, there was great debate about aortic ejection sounds.

In the early days before echocardiography, we were puzzled by the lateness of the aortic ejection sound. This occurred during the upstroke of the aortic pressure pulse, rather than earlier when the valve opened. We had already used cineangiocardiography to examine the mitral valve, and had shown that its final halt coincided with the loud first sound of mitral stenosis. We were contemplating using a similar technique for the aortic valve when Richard Ross and O'Neil Humphries (an ex-fellow from St George's) gave us the answer from the Johns Hopkins Hospital. The sound coincided with the final halt of the upwardly moving valve visualised on the cineaortogram – a point easily confirmed by echocardiography.

Thus, an aortic ejection sound is produced by the sudden cessation of movement of an abnormal valve (for example, bicuspid), presumably one with abnormal prominence carried rapidly upward by systolic ejection. The sound disappears if the valve is immobilised, particularly by calcium deposition. Aortic root dilatation by itself does not seem to produce such a sound; the aortic "root sound" described by Shaver coincided with closure of the tricuspid valve on our high speed echocardiograms. Thus, there seems to be no aortic parallel to the pulmonary root sound that occurs with pulmonary artery dilatation (though we still do not know the mechanism of the ejection sound with the dilated aortic root of pulmonary atresia).

In aortic regurgitation, an ejection sound indicates an abnormal valve (most commonly bicuspid) rather than primary aortic root dilatation, the most common cause of isolated severe aortic regurgitation in the United Kingdom. Recognition of an aortic ejection sound has also been of great value in studying the course of the bicuspid aortic valve and calcific aortic stenosis. A long follow up study with Peter Mills of patients with isolated aortic ejection sounds has shown a bicuspid valve as the cause of the sound, and in many patients calcification and stenosis developed later.[18] We still do not know how often calcification develops and whether it can be prevented.

In conclusion

The evolution of ideas on the origins of heart sounds and murmurs is a striking example of the value of clinical research conducted over a long period. In this area at least, clinical research has yielded more information than isolated experiments in the laboratory. Unfortunately, there is a tendency nowadays to shorten the history taking and physical examination and go straight to echocardiography. This is not only a waste of expensive resources but provides results that are less informative because the echocardiographer does not know what to look for. Furthermore, the test only gives information about that particular moment in time and nothing about the course of any pathological process. Over enthusiastic interpretation by technician and physician looking solely at these tests leads to errors in management. It is sad and unfortunate that careful auscultation is seldom practised now and its main value seems to be to correct technician's reports on regurgitant valves in normal subjects.

References and notes

1. Mair A. *Sir James Mackenzie, MD. 1855–1925 general practitioner*. London: The Royal College of General Practitioners, 1986.
2. Mackenzie J. Observations on the process which results in auricular fibrillation. *BMJ* 1922;2:71–3.
3. Leatham A. Phonocardiography. *Br Med Bull* 1952;8:333–42.
4. Leatham A. Auscultation and phonocardiography: a personal view of the past 40 years. *Br Heart J* 1987;57:397–403.
5. Leatham A. Auscultation of the heart. *Lancet* 1958;ii:703–8; 757–65.
6. Leatham A, Gray I. Auscultatory and phonocardiographic signs of atrial septal defect. *Br Heart J* 1956;18:193–208.
7. Leatham A, Weitzman D. Auscultatory and phonocardiographic signs of pulmonary stenosis. *Br Heart J* 1957;19:303–17.
8. Sutton G, Harris A, Leatham A. Second heart sound in pulmonary hypertension. *Br Heart J* 1968;30:743–56.
9. Leatham A. The phonocardiogram of aortic stenosis. *Br Heart J* 1951;13:153–8.
10. Brigden W, Leatham A. Mitral incompetence. *Br Heart J* 1953;15:55–73.
11. Allen H, Harris A, Leatham A. Significance and prognosis of an isolated late systolic murmur: a 9 to 22 year follow up. *Br Heart J* 1974;36:525–32.
12. Leatham A, Brigden W. Mild mitral regurgitation and the mitral prolapse fiasco. *Am Heart J* 1980;99:659–64.

13. Haber E, Leatham A. Splitting of heart sounds from ventricular asynchrony in bundle branch block, ventricular ectopic beats and artificial pacing. *Br Heart J* 1965;27:691–6.
14. Crews TL, Pridie RB, Benham R, Leatham A. Auscultatory and phonocardiographic findings in Ebstein's anomaly. Correlation of first heart sound with ultrasonic records of tricuspid valve movement. *Br Heart J* 1972;34:681–7.
15. Brooks N, Leech G, Leatham A. Complete right bundle branch block. Echophonocardiographic study of first heart sound and right ventricular contraction times. *Br Heart J* 1979;41:637–46.
16. Leech G, Brooks N, Green-Wilkinson A, Leatham A. Mechanism of the influence of PR interval on loudness of first heart sound. *Br Heart J* 1980;42:138–42.
17. Leatham A, Vogelpoel L. The early systolic sound in dilatation of the pulmonary artery. *Br Heart J* 1954;16:21–33.
18. Leech G, Mills P, Leatham A. The diagnosis of a non-stenotic bicuspid aortic valve. *Br Heart J* 1978;40:941–50.

Chapter 9

The Chest X Ray in Cardiac Diagnosis, 1930–60

Derek Gibson

To anyone brought up in the last third of the 20th century, the essentials of a cardiac opinion consist of a carefully taken history and clinical examination, supplemented by a chest *x* ray and electrocardiogram. By 1960, the two latter investigations were readily available in all cardiac departments; the basic methods were standardised and stable, and have remained so ever since. Though obviously useful, a quality of immutability now invests both. Neither is seen as an area in which change is likely to occur.

Early use of the chest *x* ray

The physical basis of both the chest *x* ray and electrocardiogram developed late in the 19th century. For the chest *x* ray this can clearly be dated to the work of Roentgen in 1895. However, from then on their history diverges. In the early years of the 20th century, Einthoven decisively established the clinical value of the electrocardiogram, and the technique was taken up with particular interest in this country. Not only can this interest be documented in the experimental work of Thomas Lewis and his colleagues, it also appears in the discussions of the Cardiac Club, a group of physicians founded in 1922 to continue collaboration started in the first world war and to discuss the practice of cardiology.[1] The subjects of these discussions were recorded in detail; they involved the electrocardiogram on five occasions, but never radiology.

The reason for this omission is not obvious. The report of the Medical Research Committee on "Soldiers returned as cases of disordered action of the heart (DAH) or valvular disease of the heart (VDH)," written by Thomas Lewis and published in 1917, states that 50 of these patients were examined radiologically.[2] "Minute precautions were adopted to render these records accurate and uniform, and no (cardiac) outline was accepted unless it was repeated on more than one occasion and found to give an error no greater than ½ cm." Lewis found that the size of the heart, estimated in terms of the transverse diameter, was rather less than average (by approximately 6 mm) and the heart rate was consistently higher in patients than in normal controls. He concluded that these results supported the hypothesis that some, if not all, of these soldiers were suffering from a condition then described as "heart strain." Furthermore, by 1923 Lewis was using the chest *x* ray to show cardiac enlargement in a series of patients with coarctation of the aorta.

Improvement in radiological methods

Interest in cardiac radiology was not maintained. As late as 1929, Terence East reviewed the subject, pointing out that methods of screening had lagged far behind those on the continent, particularly in France, Germany, and Austria.[3] He was not enthusiastic about its merits: "The radiologist may require elaborate consideration of many small points to arrive at a diagnosis of a lesion obvious to the clinician. . . . We can only suppose that the rather antiquated apparatus usually available in this country has prevented much progress being made."[3]

In fact, East was able to cover what seems in retrospect to have been an impressive body of work that had been carried out in continental Europe. This was summarised in detail in Assmann's textbook of radiology – a superb production, particularly in its reproduction of chest radiographs.[4] These seem to have been reproduced by a direct photographic process, far ahead of the grey photogravure reproductions published elsewhere at the same time, and performers of classical music will be interested to note that it was printed by the firm of Breitkopf and Haertel of Leipzig.

Problems of precision

With standardisation of the distance between the tube and the patient to 2 metres, it was possible to detect cardiac enlargement and to develop criteria for defining enlargement of the left atrium, the left ventricle, and the great arteries. In fact, much of the work undertaken in continental Europe and the United States during the 1920s was concerned with detecting cardiac enlargement. Although the simple cardiothoracic ratio was described as early as 1921, the problem was felt to be very much more complex than this. A series of measurements of the heart shadow was described and was related to age, position, and body weight in a complex table. In retrospect, it seems that the main problem was not in obtaining diagnostic images; it was a lack of diagnostic precision in both anatomy and physiology, which would come only with cardiac catheterisation.

First techniques

The practice of cardiac radiology at the end of the 1920s differed appreciably from that later in the century. Four techniques were available: fluoroscopy, kymography, orthodiagraphy, and teleradiology.

Fluoroscopy

Fluoroscopy was the most popular technique. It depended on examining the image of the patient, in various projections, on a fluoroscopic (lead sulphide) screen.[5] Because energy levels were low, distances from the source to the patient and screen were correspondingly small (50 cm), and this distorted the radiographic field. The patient was examined first in the anterioposterior view and then in one or both oblique views. Finally, the patient would swallow a small amount of barium ("barium sulphate with a little cocoa or chocolate mixed with water until it is a thickish cream but not a stodgy paste"[5]) to outline the position of the oesophagus so that any enlargement of the left atrium could be detected. No objective record was made, but much useful information was obtained in respect of heart size and the relative prominence of different chambers. The relative motion of various cardiac structures as the patient was rotated gave a much clearer impression of the superposition of anatomical entities than does the standard chest *x* ray. Calcium in the heart valves or pericardium could be detected.[5]

Cardiac motion could also be appreciated. This might involve the activity of the ventricles, expansile pulsation of the left atrium in the presence of severe mitral regurgitation or of the hilar blood vessels in the presence of pulmonary congestion or plethora. The hilar dance was described in 1925 by Pezzi and Silingardias as "un phénomène que nous n'avons jamais constaté, c'est a dire une véritable danse ... d'un véritable pouls artèrial hilaire" (quoted by Campbell [6]). Its cause was not clear in the days before catheterisation, when most cardiac diagnosis was uncertain. Initially attributed to pulmonary regurgitation, the hilar dance was subsequently considered to occur in what would now be termed pulmonary venous hypertension as well as in plethora, with which it was finally associated.

Fluoroscopic apparatus was still used well into the 1950s. In 1954, Maurice Campbell described its value in assessing pulmonary blood flow in the presence of a left to right shunt, a disorder that is now confirmed by cardiac catheterisation.[6] He introduced the term pulmonary oligaemia, which was coined for him by EL York, classical tutor at New College Oxford. The contrasting term, pleonaemia, was never accepted. Routine screening took 5 minutes at most, and was felt, even in the late 1950s to supplement information available from the standard chest *x* ray. A "séance" followed each outpatient clinic when all new referrals were examined by fluoroscopy. At a time when there were *x* ray pedoscopes in all shoe shops, no thought was given to the radiation that the patient or the operator was exposed to.

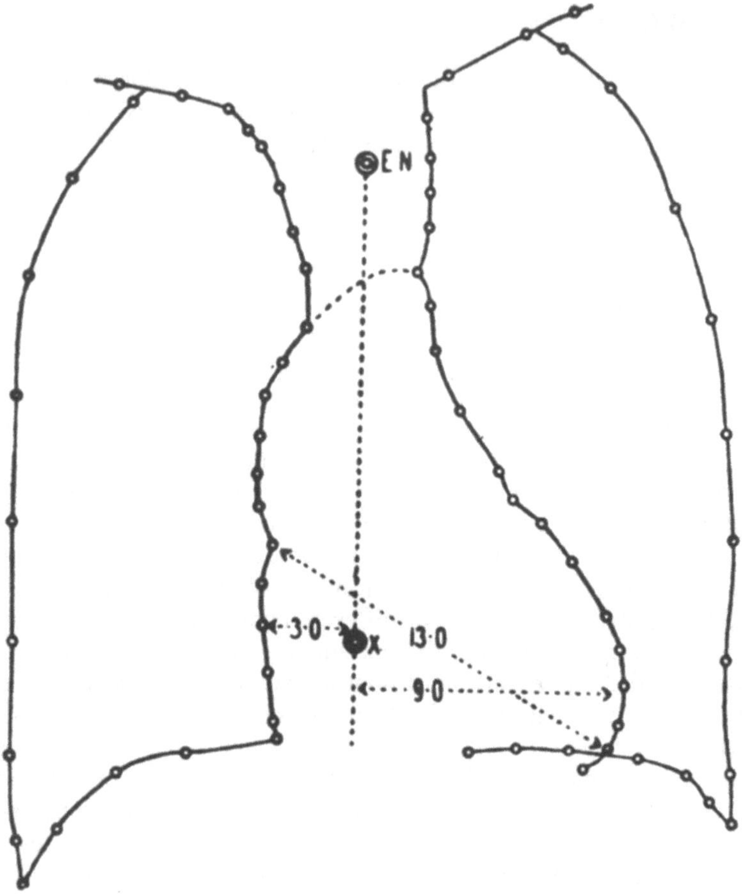

Figure 1 Anterioposterior orthodiagram (at one-fifth scale) of the chest of a patient with coarctation of the aorta by Thomas Lewis. The measurements used to assess cardiac size are shown. EN = episternal notch, X = base of xiphisternum. (Reproduced with permission from *Heart* 1933;16:205–61).

The main disadvantages of fluoroscopy were its limited energy output and the absence of any permanent record. The low level of illumination of the screen required adaptation to the dark. Parkinson recommended 15–30 minutes, so that before the introduction of image intensifiers in the early 1960s, red goggles were as characteristic of the radiologist then as head mirrors are of the ear nose and throat surgeon of the popular press today.

Kymography

Kymography was an attempt to capitalise on the ability of fluoroscopy to detect cardiac motion. Multiple slits were placed over the border of the heart, and recorded as a zigzag, representing local pulsation. Images were hard to interpret and the method was never widely accepted. In retrospect, this can be regarded as the first attempt to display the extent and timing of the motion of the heart, a problem that has still not been completely solved.

Orthodiagraphy

In orthodiagraphy, a permanent record was contrived by tracing the outline of the heart and great vessels against the fluoroscopic screen, assisted by the central rays of the *x* ray tube (thus avoiding distortion) and making use of a special lever and small diaphragm (figure 1). The points were marked with a grease pencil, and were subsequently traced. The whole procedure took "but a few minutes, sometimes as little as two or three."[5] From these outlines a series of measurements was made of oblique and transverse dimensions of the heart. This approach was used by Lewis in 1917, and he still recommended it as late as 1944 in the third edition of his *Diseases of the heart*.[7]

Teleradiography

The third technique, teleradiography, was the forerunner of the current standard, posterioanterior chest radiograph. It was originally described in 1905, but was not widely used until the early 1930s. Its introduction was delayed because the distance from the tube to the chest had to be at least 6 feet for distortion to be minimised, and power levels were low with the *x* ray generators then available. In addition, photographic technology was not advanced and glass plates had to be used initially. In retrospect, it is interesting that the main disadvantage of the technique at the time was felt to be the distortion it introduced into the assessment of heart size. By 1930 it was judged to be useful in difficult cases, although orthodiagraphy was considered preferable for routine work.

Cardiac enlargement and the pulmonary blood vessels

Progress in the United Kingdom became much more rapid during the 1930s. By 1933, Peter Kerley[8] was discussing the chest *x* ray in terms that might have been used half a century later: "It is not so much in the diagnosis of mitral stenosis as in the diagnosis of its complications that radiography is of great help."[9] Not only did he cover the causes of cardiac enlargement (mainly valvular or congenital disease, coarctation of the aorta, and nephritis), he also discussed in detail changes in the lung fields. In pulmonary oedema, the hila are enlarged, and translucency is lost through compression of the alveoli by distended capillaries. The interlobar fissures are thickened by transudation of fluid. After an attack of pulmonary oedema, "the shadows of the pulmonary lymphatics persist as fine, sharp lines, most marked at the bases and near the hila" – appearances now universally described as Kerley B lines.[9]

Three years later, Sir John Parkinson devoted the Lumleian Lectures to an account of enlargement of the heart, again mainly in valvular and congenital heart disease.[10][11] He considered the question of whether coronary thrombosis was a cause, but concluded that it was of little importance, except when cardiac aneurysm developed. Overall, though, the change in attitude towards radiology over 7 years was profound: "radiology can contribute to direct and exact knowledge in almost every variety of heart disease. By radiocardiology we reach a more vital anatomy and physiology – a dynamic pathology of the living heart."[10][11] This change in attitude was consolidated in the masterly chapter on cardiac radiology produced by Kerley in 1938, covering changes in the configuration of the heart shadow in nearly all common conditions.[12] How the standard of illustration had improved in a relatively few years so that it no longer seemed to be a limiting factor is also noteworthy.

Cardiac radiology made a greater contribution during the second world war than it had in the first. Medical examination of potential recruits was an important field of medical service, and many were rejected because of heart disease.[13] Of 2500 recruits referred to Sir John Parkinson on these grounds, 609 were found to have rheumatic heart disease, and approximately one third of these men had symptoms. In 80%–90% of these cases, convincing *x* ray support for the diagnosis was found. A large left atrium proved to be as sensitive in making the diagnosis as a presystolic murmur.

Heart failure

Viewed from 50 years on, consideration of heart failure seems a notable omission in the early publications. In his authoritative account of cardiac radiology, Kerley devotes less than a 10th of the space allotted to mitral stenosis to the subject of heart failure, giving only a cursory account of the changes of pulmonary congestion.[12] The exhaustive monograph on heart failure written by Fishberg in 1941, mentions only hilar enlargement associated with hilar dance, increased prominence of the lung markings, clouding of the lung fields, and oedema of the visceral pleura which may simulate pleural effusion.[14] In 1941, however, Evan Bedford and Lovibond showed that hydrothorax visualised radiologically was a major feature of heart failure.[15] It was present in up to 40% of cases and regressed after treatment with mercurial diuretics. In common with previous studies, Bedford and Lovibond noted that a left sided effusion was commoner in left heart failure and hypertension, while in mitral stenosis the effusion was bilateral.

Cardiac catheterisation helps interpretation

From the early 1940s, cardiac radiology entered a second phase of development, with increasing understanding of the importance and physiological basis of changes in the lung fields. This was an area to which the United Kingdom made a major contribution. The change in interest partly reflected the increasing use of the standard chest *x* ray rather than fluoroscopy, but, more importantly, it relied on the increased diagnostic accuracy and more complete physiological information supplied by cardiac catheterisation. Up to 1942, there were differences of opinion about the nature of the shadows in the lung fields in normal radiographs; some authors still considered them to be bronchi. However, in 1946, Lodge concluded from anatomical studies that "the linear shadows traversing the lung fields in normal radiographs are produced by the blood filled arteries and veins of the lung."[16] He also established that many of the lobar and segmental arteries and the main pulmonary veins could be identified on the plain chest radiograph. Lodge proposed criteria by which blood vessels could be identified. Thus, the emphasis of interpretation shifted from non-specific comments on the pulmonary markings to positive identification of pulmonary arteries and veins, and to detecting abnormalities in their calibre or distribution.

From the cardiological point of view, the most important of these changes to be clarified were those of pulmonary hypertension and congestion. Davies and his colleagues at the Hammersmith Hospital, London used cardiac catheterisation to measure the pulmonary artery pressure and to perform pulmonary angiography in patients with mitral stenosis, and compared the results with the chest radiograph.[17] A rise in the systolic or mean pulmonary artery pressure was associated with increasing dilatation of the proximal pulmonary arteries and narrowing and tortuosity of the distal branches. These abnormalities could also be recognised on the chest *x* ray, allowing semiquantitative estimates of pulmonary artery pressure to be made in individual patients. These radiographic criteria proved to be more reliable than those based on the history, clinical examination, or electrocardiogram. The authors pointed out that changes seen in pulmonary artery morphology were not those which would be expected with simple "congestion," but looked to be the result of active narrowing of the smaller branches. They further suggested that their presence correlated so closely with pulmonary hypertension that "cardiac catheterization may therefore be omitted in many patients, unless special problems are present" – an idea which still troubled the cardiological establishment a quarter of a century later.

Investigating pulmonary blood flow and oedema

Radiographic changes associated with pulmonary oedema were described in detail by Jackson in 1951.[18] He paid particular attention to hilar distension, lung shadows, and hydrothorax and their relation to treatment. Whether there were specific forms of pulmonary oedema associated with renal failure and mitral stenosis remained uncertain. By 1954, Carmichael et al. were able to assert that when "lines B were present, the pulmonary capillary pressure was almost invariably above 30 mm Hg."[19] In 1956,

Short extended these findings in patients with left heart failure to include lymphatic lines and distension of the upper lobe pulmonary veins.[20] Indeed his view of radiographic changes of left ventricular failure would be accepted by many today. Short pointed out that radiographic changes might precede the onset of symptoms in patients with severe hypertension, coronary artery disease, or aortic regurgitation. He even raised the possibility that "radiology following exercise might prove an even more sensitive test of ventricular competence that the standard radiogram at rest"; an early foreshadowing of stress imaging.[20] In the previous year, Short had also studied pulmonary changes in patients with mitral stenosis. The severity of the stenosis was, for the first time, documented against the mitral valve area determined either at surgery or at autopsy. This was a less comprehensive investigation than his study of heart failure.

In 1958, Morris Simon described in greater detail the changes in the pulmonary veins in patients with mitral stenosis, correlating these with pulmonary venous (wedge) pressure obtained at cardiac catheterisation.[21] He showed how veins could be distinguished from arteries (based on tomography) thus avoiding the necessity of having to refer to "vascular markings." While arteries and veins to the upper lobes are parallel to one another, with the veins lying lateral, the orientation of the veins to the middle and lower lobes is quite different to that of the arteries. On this anatomical basis, the concept of selective dilatation of the upper lobe veins in mitral stenosis was developed. Dilatation proved to be maximum when wedge pressure was in the range 24–26 mm Hg, and tended to be less when pressure was either lower or high. Thus hydrostatic pressure alone was an unlikely explanation, and the possibility of active vasoconstriction in the lower lobes was raised. As pulmonary venous hypertension becomes more severe, so other abnormalities can be recognised. Lymphatic lines appear, the main pulmonary artery and its proximal branches enlarge, while the peripheral vessels become narrow and tortuous.

Pulmonary hypertension

Similar changes in the pulmonary arteries with increased pressure and blood flow had been described in congenital heart disease by Campbell in 1951.[6] In two landmark papers, Evans et al.[22] and Heath et al.[23] used cardiac catheterisation and pulmonary angiography and autopsy findings to clarify the diagnosis of primary pulmonary hypertension and show the characteristic histological changes in the pulmonary vascular bed. The classic radiological features – proximal arterial dilatation, even to the extent of aneurysm formation, peripheral pruning, and clear lung fields – were present. By 1958, therefore, Steiner was able to produce a comprehensive review of all these changes in pulmonary vasculature, in a form which has altered little over the succeeding 40 years.[24]

In conclusion

During a period of just less than 30 years that included the second world war, cardiac radiography developed from a technique of little perceived practical value to one which formed an essential part of any cardiological assessment. Many factors have contributed to this progress. Initially, these included technical improvements in equipment and the ability to obtain standardised records rather than the subjective judgements of fluoroscopy. The rapid progress made during the early 1950s directly reflects the revolution introduced by cardiac catheterisation, both in terms of accurate diagnosis and associated disturbances of physiology. As the century has progressed, new imaging procedures of increasing complexity and expense have followed one another, more and more rapidly, each claiming to supplant its predecessor. In this context, it is difficult to overestimate the value of a method such as simple chest radiography, which provides so much information relevant to patient management, is based on intermediate technology, is standardised in its technique and interpretation throughout the world, and has been stable in relation to both these latter points for more than 40 years. It is only to be hoped that this happy state of affairs will be maintained, and that such uniformity as has been achieved over time and space will not be sacrificed to the apparently relentless pressure of misplaced digital technology.

References and notes

1. Cowan J. Some notes on the Cardiac Club. *Br Heart J* 1939;1:97–104.
2. Lewis T. *Report upon soldiers returned as cases of "disordered action of the heart" (D.A.H.) or "valvular disease of the heart" (V.D.H.).* London: HMSO, 1917:1–100. (MRC special report series no 8.)
3. East CFT, Bain CWC. *Recent advances in cardiology.* London: Churchill, 1929:299–311.
4. Assmann H. *Die Klinische Roentgendiagnostik der Inneren Erkrankungen.* Berlin: Vogel, 1929:1–213.
5. Parkinson J. The radiology of rheumatic heart disease. *Lancet* 1949;i:895–922.
6. Campbell M. Visible pulsation in relation to blood flow and pressure in the pulmonary artery. *Br Heart J* 1951;13:438–456.
7. Lewis T. *Diseases of the heart.* London: Macmillan, 1944:140–1.
8. Sir Peter James Kerley (1900–79) was a leader of British radiology. He was on the staff of the Westminster Hospital and the National Heart Hospital. Having qualified in Dublin, he studied radiology in Vienna in 1924. There he developed his special interest in the radiology of the heart and lungs, on which he became a world authority. He initiated the series *Recent advances in radiology* and his many original papers included the St Cyres lecture on "Radiology in the pulmonary circulation." Sir Peter had a long association with the Royal family after his diagnosis in 1952 of cancer of the lung in King George VI. For this service he was appointed a Knight Commander of the Royal Victorian Order.
9. Kerley P. Radiology in heart disease. *BMJ* 1933;2:594–7.
10. Parkinson J. Enlargement of the heart. *Lancet* 1936;i:1337–45.
11. Parkinson J. Enlargement of the heart. *Lancet* 1936;i:1391–400.
12. Kerley P. Cardiovascular system. In: Shanks CS, Kerley P, Twining EW, eds. *A text-book of x ray diagnosis by British authors.* London: HK Lewis, 1938:3–96.
13. Parkinson J, Hartley R. Early diagnosis of rheumatic valvular disease in recruits. *Br Heart J* 1947;8:212–32.
14. Fishberg AM. *Heart failure.* London: Henry Kimpton, 1940:218–21.
15. Bedford DE, Lovibond JL. Hydrothorax in heart failure. *Br Heart J* 1941;3:93–111.

16. Lodge T. The anatomy of the blood vessels of the human lung as applied to chest radiography. *Br J Radiol* 1946;29:1–13.
17. Davies LG, Goodwin JF, Steiner RE, van Leuven BD. The clinical and radiological assessment of the pulmonary arterial pressure in mitral stenosis. *Br Heart J* 1953;13:393–400.
18. Jackson F. The radiology of acute pulmonary oedema. *Br Heart J* 1951;13:503–17.
19. Carmichael JHE, Julian DG, Jones GP, Wren EM. Radiological signs of pulmonary hypertension. The significance of lines B of Kerley. *Br J Radiol* 1949;27:393–7.
20. Short DS. Radiology of the lung in left heart failure. *Br Heart J* 1956;18:233–40.
21. Simon M. The pulmonary veins in mitral stenosis. *J Faculty Radiol* 1958;9:25–32.
22. Evans W, Short DS, Bedford DE. Solitary pulmonary hypertension. *Br Heart J* 1957;19:93–116.
23. Heath D, Whitaker W, Brown JW. Idiopathic pulmonary hypertension. *Br Heart J* 1957;19:83–92.
24. Steiner RE. Radiological appearances in pulmonary hypertension. *Br J Radiol* 1958;31:188–200.

Chapter 10

Electrocardiography, Electrophysiology, and Arrhythmias

Dennis M Krikler

Until the middle of the 19th century the physician could feel the pulse and describe irregularities, but their significance was impossible to ascertain. Mechanical recordings of the pulse were developed in France and Germany in the mid-19th century and were further refined by Sir James Mackenzie while he was still in practice in Burnley, Lancashire just over 100 years ago (see chapter 1). Mackenzie obtained a considerable amount of information from his clinical polygraph, but diagnostic accuracy awaited the invention of the electrocardiograph.

Electrocardiography

Electrocardiography was a British invention. In 1887, Augustus Desiré Waller (head of the department of physiology at St Mary's Hospital, London) used a modified Lippmann capillary electrometer to demonstrate the electrical activity of the heart in intact animals. Waller also applied this technique to man. Using the capillary electrometer, a light beam was interrupted by the mercury column, enabling records to be made on photographic plates mounted on slowly moving toy train wagons.[1] Willem Einthoven from Leiden, who was present at Waller's first demonstration, was inspired to use and improve the method. Waller later became professor at the newly founded physiological laboratory of the University of London (in the Imperial Institute, South Kensington), and subsequently also became consulting physician to the National Heart Hospital.[2]

Einthoven's string galvanometer

In 1901, Waller's "laboratory tool" was supplanted by the string galvanometer, which had been developed in Holland by Einthoven. The first models were developed by the Edelmann company in Germany, but from 1904 Einthoven arranged for the Cambridge Scientific Instrument Company to

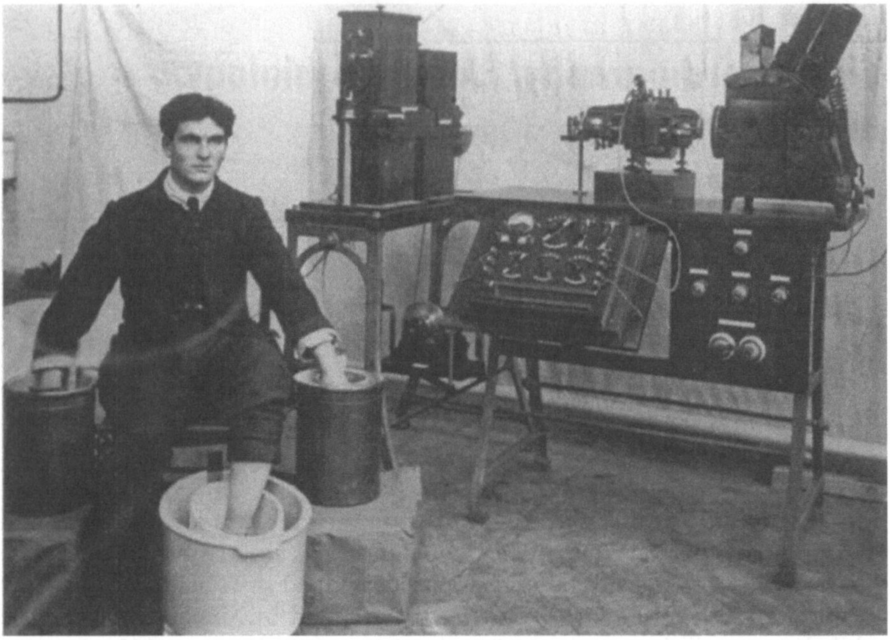

Figure 1 The first British clinical electrocardiograph apparatus made in 1911 by the Cambridge Instrument Company and used by Dr Thomas Lewis at University College Hospital, London. The apparatus comprised (from left to right) two cameras, one with a glass plate and other with continuous paper recording; Einthoven string galvanometer; and an arc lamp. The patient's limbs were in pots of saline.

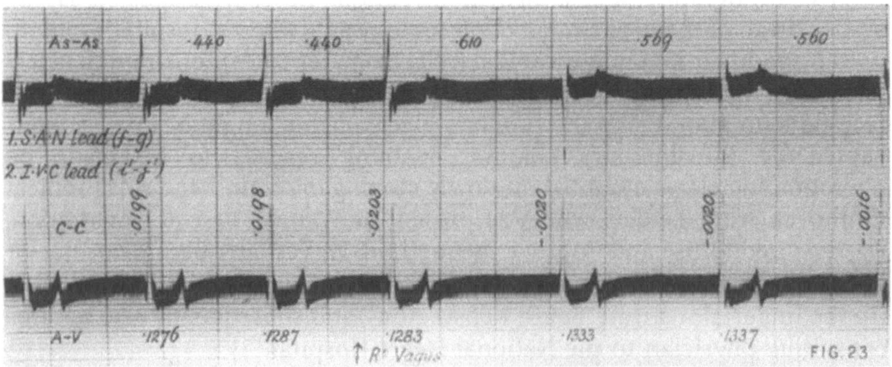

Figure 2 A superb recording of an electrocardiograph made with a twin string galvanometer by Dr Thomas Lewis in 1914.

produce a new version, and the first instrument was made in the following year. The early models of the galvanometer were used for physiological work. It was 1908 before Cambridge manufactured a complete electrocardiograph, and only in 1911 was the apparatus available for clinical use.[3] (figures 1 and 2)

Sir Thomas Lewis's work

In 1908, together with Arthur S Macnalty, Thomas Lewis published his first paper on arrhythmia.[4] The article included a single electrocardiogram. This had been recorded using Waller's apparatus and depicted a ventricular escape complex. During the following year, Lewis obtained an Edelmann electrocardiograph and embarked upon a series of studies in which he defined the major arrhythmias. He showed that the rapid irregular cardiac arrhythmia, which was thought by Mackenzie to be nodal rhythm and was described by Hering as *pulsus irregularis perpetuus*, was actually a result of atrial fibrillation.[5] An article by Rothberger and Winterberg of Vienna (of whose work Lewis was not at that time aware) pre-empted by 5 months the publication of Lewis' work. However, Lewis's book on electrocardiography was the first to be published in English.[6]

Over the next 15 years, Lewis and his colleagues published extensively and demonstrated electrocardiographic signs of sinoatrial and atrioventricular block, as well as atrial, junctional, and ventricular arrhythmias. The work showing that ventricular fibrillation could be induced by the combination of chloroform and adrenaline was of particular interest.[7] All Lewis's studies were discussed extensively in his series of articles and books, culminating in his classic work, the third edition of the *Mechanism and graphic registration of the heart beat*, which was published in 1925.[8] Interestingly, it did not contain any examples of atrioventricular tachycardia caused by pre-excitation, though the appearances had first been described by Cohn and Fraser.[9] This syndrome was subsequently recognised as a specific entity by Wolff et al.,[10] who did not themselves appreciate the fact that the appearances resulted from an accessory atrioventricular pathway. Other workers in the United States and Sweden defined pre-excitation during the next decade. Another omission was Lewis's failure to recognise the electrocardiographic signs of myocardial infarction or ischaemia, which had been noted in the United States some 7 years before his book was published.[8] There were isolated UK reports of myocardial infarction in the early 1920s, but the first definitive series of cases was reported by Parkinson and Bedford.[11]

Lewis was not the only physician to describe specific arrhythmias. In 1911, Jolly and Ritchie described the electrocardiographic appearances of atrial flutter in a patient with complete heart block,[12][13] and in 1915, GES Ward showed that this could occur with a 4:1 atrioventricular response.[14]. However, it was Lewis who, having recognised the arrhythmia (with the more usual 2:1 atrioventricular response) in 1912, was the first to describe circus movement as the mechanism of both atrial flutter and fibrillation in man.[15] In 1915, Lewis relied on his own experimental work when sectioning the left and right bundle branches in dogs. He did not appreciate the difference in the bundle branches in man and dogs, and mixed up right and left bundle branch block – an error carefully analysed by Hollman.[16] Although Lewis moved into other areas of work,[17] his postgraduate fellow Craib made the important contribution of defining the electrical activation of the myocardium by electrical doublets.[18][19] This work was expanded by Frank Wilson in the United States. He labelled the activation unit as a dipole, and this rapidly became the preferred term.

Electrocardiographic leads

The three standard electrocardiograph limb leads introduced by Einthoven remained in sole use for nearly 40 years, even though, in teaching, William Evans advocated the use of IIIR, lead III with held inspiration. This was very close to the subsequent augmented unipolar limb lead aVF. Evans' powerful advocacy meant that this lead remained popular in the United Kingdom. Although chest leads were used by a number of workers, and Frank Wilson in the United States had used them widely, their precise standardisation and positions were introduced only in 1937, with the publication of the joint recommendation of the American Heart Association and Cardiac Society of Great Britain and Ireland.[20] A bipolar chest lead in which the exploring electrode was placed in the designated position on the chest while the indifferent electrode was connected to the right arm, was preferred by Evans,[21] and was also favoured by Wood and Selzer.[22] In the United States, the configuration CL or CF (with the left arm or left leg being connected to the indifferent electrode) was often preferred. It was only after the second world war that the unipolar chest leads advocated by Frank Wilson came into more general use. From the 1950s, these became accepted practice, together with the augmented limb leads recommended by Emanuel Goldberger in the United States. Their adoption in the United Kingdom was rather more gradual. Even in 1950, William Evans referred only to bipolar leads.[23]

Recording methods

The method of recording the electrocardiogram was on the whole somewhat behind in the United Kingdom. Wet glass plates were used for the records and this practice persisted in some institutions until well after the first world war. Although Siemens and Halske in Berlin had introduced continuous rolls of film for recording as early as 1913, this only became more popular in the United Kingdom (albeit not in general use) in the late 1920s. Direct writing electrocardiographs, in which a heated stylus produced a tracing on coated paper, were a feature of the US Sanborn apparatus. However, it was only in the 1950s that these were introduced into the United Kingdom on any scale, and it was some time before they were used universally. This apparatus then proved more robust and more popular than the Swedish Elema-Schonanders ink jet method, whose greater frequency range lent itself best to phonocardiography.

Exercise testing

While the resting electrocardiogram provided interesting information on the fixed or evolving changes of cardiac ischaemia, exercise electrocardiography aimed to reproduce angina and then take a tracing. It was first carried out in Vienna by Scherf and Goldhammer in 1928.[24] Several years later exercise testing became more widely used in the United States through the influence of Master and Dack, who developed the two step test. In one early British report on exercise electrocardiography, 5 or 10 minutes of brisk walking preceded the recording, but only the three limb leads plus CR4 or CF4, or both, were recorded, and a comparison was made with anoxaemia.[25] The series was small (20 patients) and positive results were obtained in a few patients, although analysis was rendered difficult by the restricted number of leads used. It was only in the 1960s that exercise protocols using treadmills or bicycle ergometers, which were developed in the United States and Germany, in particular, came into use in the United Kingdom, and these have become the standard methods of assessing reversible ischaemia using the electrocardiogram. It took more than another decade before this had an impact on practice, and it is only in the past 20 years that these standardised exercise tests have become the norm. The use of atrial pacing to show ischaemia is discussed by Leatham and Rickards in chapter 17.

Analysis

Parkinson et al. described the different electrocardiographic appearances in Adams-Stokes attacks,[26] and Parkinson and Papp[27][28] described repetitive tachycardia, which had earlier been identified by Gallavardin in Lyons. Another major contribution was that of David Short, of Aberdeen, then working at the National Heart Hospital. He described what was later called the sick sinus syndrome, a disorder presenting with alternating bradycardia and tachycardia.[29] While others had reported elements of the disorder, including sinoatrial block, Short's comprehensive work provided a more complete account. Peter Macfarlane of Glasgow pioneered the development of computerised systems for electrocardiographic analysis which have become commercially available during the past 15 years. Unfortunately, there is now no UK manufacturer of electrocardiographs as the Cambridge Scientific Instrument Company and its successors left the field or sourced equipment from abroad.

Vectorcardiography was used by some. However, it never developed into an established technique of general application.

Intracardiac electrocardiography

Although intracardiac electrocardiograms had been recorded by Lenègre and Maurice in occupied France during the second world war, these authors' published work did not receive the attention it deserved in other countries. In the United Kingdom, Watson et al. made the first recordings of intracardiac electrograms.[30] The wider importance of this technique was first demonstrated to UK cardiologists by Dirk Durrer of Amsterdam in his Thomas Lewis lecture in 1967.[31] Durrer's work was soon enhanced by technical improvements in recording His bundle activity reported from the United States, and awareness of the value of this technique followed a number of presentations from French and Dutch workers (Puech, Coumel, and Wellens) at the World Congress of Cardiology held in London in 1970.

Charles Smithen, an American research fellow at the National Heart Hospital, was the first to apply these techniques systematically to four patients under my care who had the Wolff–Parkinson–White syndrome.[32] After Smithen returned to the United States, this work was continued in conjunction with Roworth Spurrell at Guy's Hospital, and then by Spurrell and John Camm at St Bartholomew's Hospital. Electrophysiological work in Camm's unit continued when he moved to the chair of cardiology at St George's Hospital. At the same time, extensive studies were carried out at the Hammersmith Hospital, initially in conjunction with Paul Curry and later with Edward Rowland. In these studies, several electrophysiological problems were defined[33] and the mechanisms of a number of treatments, particularly with calcium antagonists, were explored.[34][35] During the subsequent decades, electrophysiological units were created in many institutions throughout Great Britain, including Newcastle, Birmingham, and Edinburgh.

Developments in surface electrocardiography

The use of ambulatory electrocardiographic recordings has become widespread. British manufacturers of the apparatus include the Oxford Instrument Company and companies developed by Pat Reynolds. The technique of signal averaging has been used, particularly to detect after-depolarisations following the QRS complex, which might indicate a risk of ventricular arrhythmias, particularly in people experiencing myocardial infarction, but there has been no ground-breaking British contribution to this technique, which is still being refined. An important contribution from the late Ronald Campbell at Newcastle was the concept of QT dispersion, indicated by differences in the duration of the QT interval in different leads.[36] Whether this reliably predicts the likelihood of ventricular tachycardia remains uncertain.

Antiarrhythmic therapy

Medication

In the early years of the century, James Mackenzie rediscovered the ability of digitalis to reduce the pulse rate in those who were soon recognised as suffering from atrial fibrillation. The next major British contribution was the recognition of the antiarrhythmic properties of β adrenergic blockers in the 1960s.[37] Although these observations were generally unsystematic, and save for sotalol the role of these drugs has remained uncertain, they continue to be used widely.

An important contribution to the understanding of how to use antiarrhythmic agents was the classification propounded by Vaughan Williams of Oxford in 1970.[38] He initially described three classes of drugs:

- I. Quinidine and other drugs with a similar ("local anaesthetic") action;
- II. The β adrenergic blockers;
- III. Agents that prolong the refractory period.

In 1970, following observations in Germany that verapamil tended to prolong atrioventricular conduction, we investigated the antiarrhythmic activity of this agent when given intravenously to patients with paroxysmal supraventricular tachycardia and published the results 2 years later.[39] We postulated that the antiarrhythmic action of verapamil reflected the drug's ability to interrupt re-entry atrioventricular tachycardias at the atrioventricular node through its calcium antagonist properties (shown experimentally by Albrecht Fleckenstein in Germany). In subsequent electrophysiological studies, we showed that verapamil did indeed work by slowing conduction in the atrioventricular node, and that diltiazem, but not nifedipine, had similar properties.[34][35] In 1972, on the basis of animal studies, Singh and Vaughan Williams had expanded the latter's classification and had listed verapamil as the prototype of a fourth drug class.[40] The basic principles outlined by Vaughan Williams continue to be useful, but since many drugs have more than one class of action, there is considerable overlap.

Amiodarone, developed in Belgium and introduced there and in France for angina, was found by French workers to have useful antiarrhythmic properties, and to be especially valuable in patients with atrial fibrillation complicating the Wolff-Parkinson-White syndrome. In 1973, Douglas Chamberlain of Brighton was the first physician in the United Kingdom to prescribe amiodarone for patients with this disorder.[41] Several agents with class I properties, including flecainide and propafenone, were developed elsewhere in the 1970s and were then further evaluated and used in Britain.

Pacing

Leatham, Rickards and Gold discuss the use of pacemakers for bradycardias in chapter 17. In 1975, extrapolating from American studies in which pacemakers were activated externally to overdrive or underdrive (rapid or slow pacing respectively) in order to interrupt a re-entry atrioventricular circuit, we devised a dual demand pacemaker.[42] This was a totally implantable device in which the magnetic reed switch that activated the underdrive function responded to the tachycardia itself. Promising initial results were not sustained as the system depended on the electrophysiological variables pertaining when the unit was implanted, and these tended to change. This stricture may also explain the lack of long term response to burst pacing and similar modalities.

Implantable defibrillators, developed in the United States by Michal Mirowski, were welcomed cautiously at first in the United Kingdom. This was largely because these defibrillators were very expensive and, as they were not generally supplied by the NHS, individual funding had to be sought.

Ablation

Surgical ablation of accessory pathways, pioneered in the United States, was carried out in the United Kingdom from 1975 onwards. Although it was soon supplanted by catheter based ablative techniques, the value of surgical ablation was well demonstrated in the series of patients operated on at the Hammersmith Hospital by Hugh Bentall.[43] Catheter based ultrasound and, subsequently, radiofrequency techniques for ablation were developed outside the United Kingdom, but became widely used here during the 1980s.

Conclusion

In little more than a century, electrocardiography using Waller's initial apparatus has evolved into a technically refined tool that can be applied non-invasively to produce an immense amount of useful information. This has been supplemented by a variety of techniques through which arrhythmias, conduction disturbances, and chamber enlargement can be identified and the effects of ischaemia can be studied and modified, yielding many advances in the management of the disorders.

References and notes

1. Waller AD. A demonstration on man of electromotive changes accompanying the heart's beat. *J Physiol* 1887;8:229–34.
2. Marshall R. Early days in Westmoreland Street. *Br Heart J* 1964;26:140–5.
3. Barron SL. The development of the electrocardiograph in Great Britain. *BMJ* 1950;i:720–5
4. Lewis T, Macnalty AS. A note on the simultaneous occurrence of sinus and ventricular rhythm in man. *J Physiol* 1908;37:445–58.
5. Lewis T. Auricular fibrillation: a common clinical condition. *BMJ* 1909;ii:1528.
6. Lewis T. *The mechanism of the heart beat.* London: Shaw and Sons, 1911.
7. Levy AG, Lewis T. Heart irregularities, resulting from the inhalation of low percentages of chloroform vapour, and their relationship to ventricular fibrillation. *Heart* 1911;3:99–112.

8. Lewis T. *The mechanism and graphic registration of the heart beat.* 3rd ed. London: Shaw and Sons, 1925.
9. Cohn AE, Fraser FR. Paroxysmal tachycardia and the effect of stimulation of the vagus nerve by pressure. *Heart* 1913–14;5:93–105.
10. Wolff L, Parkinson J, White PD. Bundle-branch block with short P-R interval in healthy young people prone to paroxysmal tachycardia. *Am Heart J* 1930;5:93–105.
11. Parkinson J, Bedford DE. Successive changes in the electrocardiogram after cardiac infarction (coronary thrombosis). *Heart* 1927–8;14:195–212.
12. Jolly WA, Ritchie WT. Auricular flutter and fibrillation. *Heart* 1910–11;2:177–221.
13. William Adam Tasker Jolly (1877–1939) worked with Einthoven in 1908, and on his return to Edinburgh carried out the work on atrial flutter. In 1911 he took up the new chair of physiology at the South African College (precursor of the University of Cape Town). There he installed a Cambridge electrocardiograph which he used for several projects, including a study of the electrocardiogram of the tortoise (Belonje PC. William Jolly: father of medical science in South Africa. *SAMJ* 1997;80:156–8).
14. Somerville W. The auricular arrhythmias. *Arch Middlesex Hosp* 1952;2:204–14.
15. Lewis T. Observations upon a curious and not uncommon form of extreme acceleration of the auricle. 'Auricular flutter.' *Heart* 1912;4:171–220.
16. Hollman A. The history of bundle branch block. *Med Hist* 1985;suppl 5:53–76.
17. Hollman A. *Sir Thomas Lewis. Pioneer cardiologist and clinical scientist.* London: Springer, 1997.
18. Craib WH. *The electrocardiogram.* London, HMSO, 1930. (MRC special report series no 147.)
19. William Hofmeyr Craib (1895–1982) was born in South Africa where he graduated in mathematics and physics. After military service in France (1914–18), during which he was awarded the Military Cross and Bar, he took up medical studies, qualifying at Guy's Hospital. He developed an interest in electrocardiography while on a Rockfeller Scholarship at Johns Hopkins University, and joined Lewis in a Medical Research Council post in 1926. Because of discord with Lewis, Craib resigned and returned to South Africa in 1931, where he became professor of medicine at the University of the Witwatersrand. He did not continue with his electrocardiographic research. This episode is chronicled by Hollman [17].
20. Cardiac Society and American Heart Association. Praecordial leads in electrocardiography. Memorandum by the Cardiac Society and the American Heart Association. *Br Heart J* 1939;1:45–8.
21. Evans W. Chest lead $(CR)_1$ electrocardiograms in auricular fibrillation. *Br Heart J* 1941;3:247–58.
22. Wood P, Selzer A. Praecordial leads in electrocardiography. *Br Heart J* 1939;1:45–80.
23. Evans W. *Cardiology.* London; Butterworths Medical Publications, 1950:6–10.
24. Krikler DM. Historical aspects of electrocardiography. Cardiol Clin 1987;5:349–55.
25. Evans C, Bourne G. Electrocardiographic changes after anoxaemia and exercise in angina on effort. *Br Heart J* 1941;3:69–74.
26. Parkinson J, Papp C, Evans W. The electrocardiogram of the Stokes-Adams attack. *Br Heart J* 1941;3:171–99.
27. Parkinson J, Papp C. Repetitive paroxysmal tachycardia. *Br Heart J* 1947;9:241–62.
28. Cornelio Papp (1903–74) was a Hungarian emigré who, having qualified in Italy, settled in London before the outbreak of the second world war. He became clinical assistant to Parkinson at the London Hospital, and later to Kenneth Shirley Smith at the Charing Cross Hospital. During Shirley Smith's editorship of the *British Heart Journal*, he served on the editorial committee.
29. Short DS. The syndrome of alternating bradycardia and tachycardia. *Br Heart J* 1954;16:208–14.
30. Watson H, Emslie-Smith D, Lowe KG. The intracardiac electrogram of human atrio-ventricular conducting tissue. *Am Heart J* 1967;74:61–70.
31. Durrer D. Electrical aspects of human cardiac activity: a clinical electrophysiological approach to excitation and stimulation. *Cardiovascular Res* 1968;2:1–8.
32. Smithen CS, Krikler DM. Aspects of pre-excitation and their elucidation by His bundle electrography. *Br Heart J* 1972;34:735–41.
33. Curry PVL, Rowland E, Fox KM, Krikler DM. The relationship between posture, blood pressure and electrophysiological properties in patients with paroxysmal supraventricular tachycardia. *Arch Mal Coeur* 1978;71:293–9.
34. Rowland E, Evans T, Krikler D. Effects of nifedipine on atrioventricular conduction as compared with verapamil. Intracardiac electrophysiologic study. *Br Heart J* 1979;42:124–7.
35. Rowland E, McKenna WJ, Gülker H, Krikler DM. The comparative effects of diltiazem and verapamil on atrioventricular conduction and atrioventricular re-entry tachycardia. *Circ Res* 1983:52-I:163–8.
36. Day CP, McComb JM, Campbell RWF. QT dispersion: an indication of arrhythmia risk in patients with long QT intervals. *Br Heart J* 1990;63:342–4.
37. Stock JPP. Beta-adrenergic blocking drugs in the clinical management of cardiac arrhythmias. *Am J Cardiol* 1966;18:444–51.

38. Vaughan Williams EM. Classification of anti-arrhythmic drugs. In: Sandøe E, Flensted-Jensen E, Olesen KH, eds. *Symposium on cardiac arrhythmias.* Södertalje: AB Astra, 1970:449–72.
39. Schamroth L, Krikler DM, Garrett C. Immediate effects of intravenous verapamil in cardiac arrhythmias. *BMJ* 1972;1:660–2.
40. Singh BN, Vaughan Williams EM. A fourth class of antidysrhythmic action? Effects of verapamil on ouabain toxicity, on atrial and ventricular intracellular potentials, and on features of cardiac function. *Cardiovasc Res* 1972;6:109–19.
41. Chamberlain DA, Clark ANG. Atrial fibrillation complicating Wolff–Parkinson–White syndrome treated with amiodarone. *BMJ* 1977;2:1519–20.
42. Krikler D, Curry P, Buffet J. Dual-demand pacing for reciprocating atrioventricular tachycardia. *BMJ* 1976;1:1114–6.
43. Rowland E, Robinson K, Edmondson S, Krikler DM, Bentall HH. Cryoablation of the accessory pathway in Wolff–Parkinson–White syndrome: initial results and long-term follow-up. *Br Heart J* 1988;59:453–7.

Chapter 11

Cardiac Catheterisation

Malcolm Towers and Simon Davies

Major advances in surgery or invasive medicine are made by a few individuals with the courage to introduce a new technique despite the misgivings or open opposition of their colleagues. Thereafter, the technique is refined by developments in apparatus and instrumentation, and wider applications are found for it. Advances in surgery spurred the development of cardiac catheterisation. This review focuses on cardiac catheterisation in Britain; fuller accounts are given in the books of Mendel, Verel and Grainger, and Miller.[1–3] Many of the major developments in catheterisation took place in other countries, especially the United States and Sweden.

Early work

Although Carl Wiggers had studied the cardiovascular system extensively in animals,[4] cardiac catheterisation in humans began in 1929 with Werner Forssmann, who wanted a means of injecting adrenaline directly into the heart. With the unsuspecting assistance of his nurse – Gerda Ditzen – he exposed his own antecubital vein and passed a ureteric catheter to his axilla. Gerda Ditzen took fright, and Forssmann walked to the *x* ray department, where, with a radiographer holding a mirror in front of the screen, he advanced the catheter into his right atrium.[5] Forssman continued experiments on himself (including angiography) until he had used up all his superficial veins.[6] He contacted Professor Sauerbruch, the leading surgeon in Berlin, to see what use could be made of the technique, but Sauerbruch remarked that he "ran a clinic, not a circus!"

Others continued with catheterisation and angiography in a small way. The early investigators were beset with fears about clotting in the catheter, provoking arrhythmias, and harming patients in ways that could not be foreseen. André Cournand and colleagues in New York reported catheterisation of the right atrium in four patients in 1941,[7] and John McMichael and Peter Sharpey-Schafer performed their first cardiac catheterisation at Hammersmith Hospital in November 1942. Little more than a year later, they had catheterised 135 patients (mainly normal volunteers) to advance their studies of cardiac output using the Fick principle and to investigate the effects of postural change, digitalis, atropine, and adrenaline.[8] The catheter was manoeuvred without *x* ray control just into the right ventricle, and then withdrawn to the atrium. Saline manometry was used to record pressures, and the oxygen saturation of blood samples was measured with the Haldane blood gas apparatus. Other investigators in the United States had catheterised more patients, but John McMichael and Peter Sharpey-Schafer established it as a safe and rewarding investigation in the United Kingdom.

The Hammersmith team went on to study congenital heart disease.[9] Alfred Blalock, who had pioneered the "blue baby" operation with Helen Taussig, visited Guy's Hospital in London in 1947 and carried out 10 operations. This was a great stimulus to the Guy's group and Russell Brock. Congenital heart disease was studied by Baker et al. and by Holling et al., who catheterised 70 children and undertook angiograms in some of them.[10][11] (Chavez and colleagues had introduced selective angiocardiography in 1947.[12]) It took two doctors and one technician a whole day to investigate one patient. Pressure in the cardiac chambers was recorded with saline manometers, and because of the inertia of the saline column, only mean pressures could be measured. However, capacitance manometers and, later, strain gauge manometers were coming into use.

The Paul Wood era

The advent of mitral valvotomy in the 1940s called for better understanding and assessment of mitral valve disease. Dexter's team in Boston had shown that the "wedge" pressure mirrored the left atrial pressure,[13] but this was not universally accepted until 1953 when Epps recorded the left atrial pressure (using Philip Allison's technique of transbronchial puncture) and the wedge pressure sequentially.[14] When "closed" valvotomy was the only form of mitral surgery, it had to be determined whether stenosis or regurgitation was "dominant" in mixed mitral valve disease. In 1955, Owen et al. at the National Heart Hospital studied the rate of left atrial 'y' descent to help solve this problem.[15] Melville Arnott's group in Birmingham did physiological studies in patients who had undergone valvotomy.[16] Paul Wood defined the varieties of pulmonary hypertension, and in 1958 reported his classic investigations into the Eisenmenger syndrome.[17][18] The pulmonary vascular resistance is still calculated in "Wood units." Wood's integration of careful history taking, the precise assessment of physical signs at the bedside with the newer knowledge from phonocardiogaphy and cardiac catheterisation was one of the most exciting developments in the whole of medicine. Complex valve defects in rheumatic heart disease and the simpler forms of congenital heart disease could be now diagnosed and assessed at the bedside.[19] Coronary heart disease was of lesser interest at that time.

In the 1950s, there was great interest in indicator dilution curves, and catheters were placed at various sites within the heart to inject and sample the indicator. The technique was used to measure cardiac output, to detect shunts, and, it was hoped, to quantify valvular regurgitation.[20] Many hospitals offered a general catheter service but developed special investigative interests. John Goodwin at Hammersmith Hospital began a long term study of the cardiomyopathies.[21] Matthias Paneth at the Brompton Hospital, by operating on patients with massive pulmonary embolism, awakened interest in the pathophysiology of this condition.[22] Congenital heart disease was being investigated at Guy's, the Brompton, and the Hospital for Sick Children, Great Ormond Street.

Procedures and problems in the 1950s

By the middle 1950s, right heart catheterisation was established in most major cardiac units, though there were many technical problems. The two operators wore lead aprons and were gowned and gloved. One wore black goggles to adjust to darkness and the other would expose an antecubital vein and insert the catheter. The room would then be plunged into darkness except for a dim red light over the technician's instruments. The operator's goggles were removed and *x* ray screening began. The catheter would be manipulated into the superior vena cava. Often it could be not seen within the heart shadow. It would then be advanced into the lung fields and a wedge pressure recorded.

Catheters were reused; they were sterilised in cabinets using tablets that released formalin vapour when heated. However, eventually they became rigid and difficult to manoeuvre. Capacitance manometers and thermionic valve amplifiers were prone to drift, and technicians were continually having to balance and recalibrate them. If a shunt were suspected, six or more blood samples would be drawn from various sites, and it took a skilled technician at least 20 minutes to analyse each sample for oxygen content. A general anaesthetic was often given for angiography, and films frequently jammed in hand operated changers or the Elema machine. Sometimes films were ruined by static electricity. The main risks were ventricular fibrillation, paradoxical embolism, and rigors due to pyrogens in reused catheters that had not been cleaned completely. Left bundle branch block (because of the risk of catheter induction of right branch block causing complete heart block) and Ebstein's anomaly (because of the risk of malignant arrhythmias) were considered absolute contraindications to catheterisation. Alternate current defibrillators were unreliable and hazardous to operators. Contrast media had a high osmolality and were potentially dangerous in patients with high pulmonary vascular resistance or poor cardiac reserve.

John Norman, chief technician at the National Heart Hospital, writes of 1951–52:

> We had a senior registrar called Jimmy Lowe (who later went back to Green Lanes in New Zealand). He was very interested in angiocardiography. I remember spending

> two weeks making the hand operated film changer which carried several full sized X ray film cassettes. The dye would be injected and the operator would very quickly push the cassette carrier forwards so that it would stop at the patient, fire the X ray tube, and the exercise would be repeated until all the films were used. Jimmy Lowe and I and a couple of the technicians would attach this device to the X-ray table on Friday evenings, load it and have timed practice runs. Jimmy was a powerfully built Rugby player and was probably the only person on the staff with the stamina to achieve the speeds which he did!

Equipment manufacturers

In the early days, British companies supplied the electronic equipment – New Electronic Products made amplifiers for manometry, Cardiac Recorders made monitors and later direct current defibrillators, and Devices made multichannel recorders and later pacemakers. However, these companies did not prosper in the longer term, and most equipment is now manufactured abroad.

Left heart studies

Left heart studies began in the 1950s. Suprasternal puncture was used occasionally to obtain left atrial pressures.[23] In 1956, Russell Brock described direct left ventricular puncture with a needle to obtain gradients in the assessment of aortic stenosis.[24] Peter Nixon learned Ross's technique for transeptal puncture at the National Heart Institute, Bethesda in 1960.[25] Pericardial tamponade was a serious complication and the technique was not widely adopted. These procedures were gradually replaced by retrograde femoral arterial catheterisation, and it was usually possible to cross the aortic valve with a catheter, especially with the assistance of a guide wire. The Seldinger percutaneous technique developed in 1953 allowed easier access to the arterial circulation.[26]

Work in the 1960s and 1970s

Coronary angiography begins

Aubrey Leatham visited the United States in the late 1950s to study the surgery of coronary artery disease. After meeting Vineberg, Leatham was introduced to Mason Sones, and, later, Keith Jefferson visited Sones in Cleveland. In 1960, the St George's Hospital group began coronary angiography in dogs.[27] Sones in 1962,[28] reported his first coronary angiograms in man, and Leatham described coronary angiography in 26 patients in his St Cyres Lecture of 1963.[29] Coronary angiography was then started at the National Heart Hospital and spread rapidly, especially when the Judkins technique was introduced in 1967.[30] These and other developments led to a sea change in cardiology. Rheumatic valve disease was becoming uncommon. Coronary disease, which had been managed by

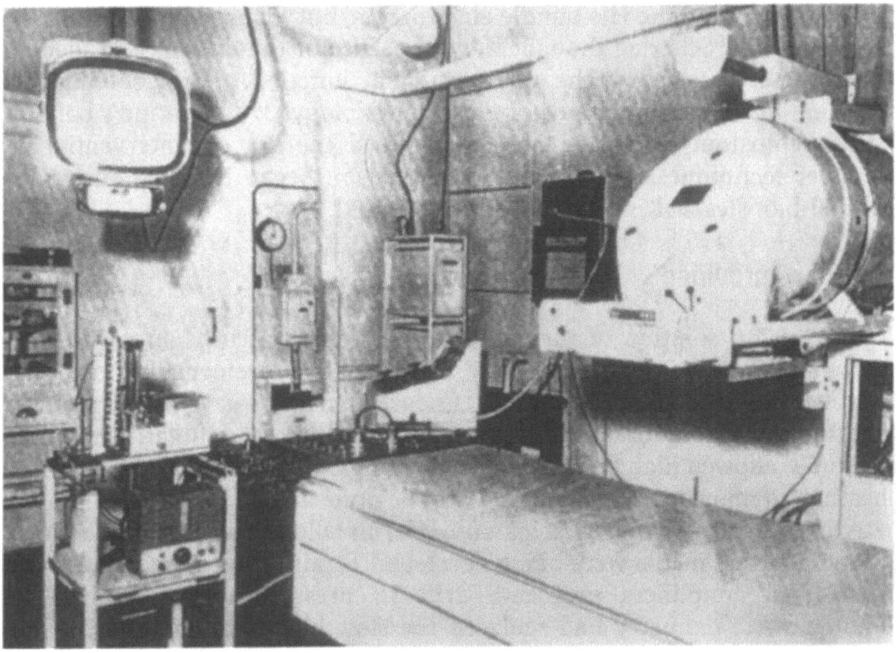

Figure 1 Catheter room at the National Heart Hospital in 1963. Right to left, amplifier for capacticance manometer (Sanborn, later Hewlett-Packard) and mercury manometer for calibration; *x* ray display monitor; at end of table, Sanborn four channel direct writing recorder; behind, *x* ray console; above, Honeywell chart recorder for dye dilution curves and image intensifier.

general physicians and, increasingly, by cardiologists, became the province of cardiologists.

Manometry

The Sharpey-Schafer influence persisted at St Thomas's Hospital. In 1964, Ronald Bradley used Statham strain gauge manometers, which required minimal fluid displacement, to measure the pulmonary artery pressure with a microcatheter at the bedside, and learned about fluid volume control in severely ill patients.[31] The Swan-Ganz catheter was a development of this technique.[32] David Mendel used catheter tip manometers for intracardiac phonocardiography and to measure the rate of rise of left ventricular pressure – a measure of ventricular function.[33]

Early catheter based techniques

Other catheter based techniques were being developed. Geoffrey Davies at St George's Hospital reported pacing by catheter in 1959.[34] Hamish Watson, working in Dundee in 1962, used to record the intracardiac electrocardiogram to help identify the site of the catheter tip in infants.[35] In

1967, he recorded the His bundle electrogram, but managed it only once in 700 cases.[36] Scherlag thought it was because of the difficulty in placing the catheter precisely at the atrioventricular junction, and by solving this problem laid the foundations of electrophysiology.[37] Rashkind's balloon atrial septostomy, reported in 1966, opened the era of "interventional" catheter techniques. In 1974, Peter Richardson began to carry out endocardial biopsies at King's College Hospital.[39]

Solutions provided

By the 1970s, solution of the technical problems was in sight worldwide. Catheters could be cleaned properly, and single-use, preformed, and special purpose catheters were used more. Image intensifiers gave better pictures and the catheter laboratory did not have to be darkened. Rotating anode *x* ray tubes allowed high pulsed currents for angiography and prevented overheating, so many procedures would now be done in a day. Cine-angiography was in general use and C arms and U arms allowed special projections. Better contrast media were being developed. Strain gauge manometers and solid state amplifiers overcame drift in pressure recording systems. Photoelectric oximetry had replaced the slow blood gas methods. Direct current defibrillators were available. These advances allowed paediatric cardiologists to investigate ever more complex congenital heart diseases at ever younger ages. Pacing and electrophysiology became an established subspecialty.

Classification of congenital heart disease

Most British doctors regard themselves as bedside cardiologists with an interest in catheterisation. Graham Miller, who trained at the Mayo Clinic and worked full time in the catheter laboratory at the Brompton Hospital from 1966 to 1989, mastered the whole range of catheter techniques and trained a generation of operators. He outlined a framework of physiological principles underlying the classification and coding of congenital heart disease, which became the basis of the present European coding system,[40] and in 1970 he set up a database to provide audit of cardiac catheterisation.

Coronary angiography becomes routine

The arrival and acceptance of percutaneous coronary revascularisation – especially stenting – has fuelled a further increase in demand for coronary angiography, and a broadening of the indications. In some ways, this is reminiscent of the way in which coronary angiography co-evolved with coronary artery surgery in the 1960s. In the United Kingdom, all cardiologists in training now undertake cardiac catheterisation and, specifically, coronary angiography. In 1994, the British Cardiac Society introduced a log book to document the experience of individual trainees in cardiac catheterisation.[41]

Catheter laboratories in general hospitals

As the indications for coronary arteriography became broader and the demand for this investigation increased throughout the 1980s, there was a move to establish cardiac catheterisation laboratories in general hospitals, not just in teaching centres and regional centres. Initially, there was some debate as to the safety of performing cardiac catheterisation in district general hospitals, but with careful patient selection and technique, the incidence of complications that would require urgent on-site surgery is very low indeed.[42] From about 1990 onwards, a new generation of cardiologists appointed to the district general hospitals have established cardiac catheterisation facilities, often shared with radiologists.[43] Despite this expansion of facilities, many areas of the United Kingdom still have long waiting lists for coronary angiography: no matter how clear the case for further expansion this seems an inevitable problem of a centrally funded healthcare system such as the NHS.

Basic technique

There have been few changes in the basic technique of cardiac catheterisation. In most British catheter laboratories, this is now performed via the femoral artery using the Judkins technique. The development of new plastics and manufacturing techniques has allowed us to use smaller calibre catheters while retaining an adequate lumen for injection and good mechanical properties. Virtually no British operators now use 8 French gauge femoral catheters, the routine catheter sets vary from 7 down to 5 French guage. In addition to the basic Judkins preshaped catheters, some new designs have found favour, including the hooked tip IMA catheter, and catheters with out-of-plane curves such as the Williams and Pryczinski catheters to help canulate difficult right coronary ostia.

The brachial approach is now used less often in the United Kingdom, perhaps because the introduction of smaller femoral catheters allows patients catheterised by this route to be treated as day cases. The significant proportion of patients undergoing angiography who have had previous coronary bypass surgery with internal mammary grafts also favours this approach. The Sones brachial technique requires more detailed training than the femoral approach, but remains useful in a number of clinical situations. A few centres continued to use predominantly the brachial approach throughout the 1980s and early 1990s – the chief proponents were Raphael Balcon at the London Chest Hospital and Graham Miller at the Royal Brompton Hospital.

Cardiac catheterisation via puncture of the radial artery at the wrist has been adopted in a number of centres since 1990. It was devised principally to reduce the local vascular complications of angioplasty at a time when oral anticoagulation with Warfarin was routine after stent implantation. However, very few transradial procedures are now performed in the United Kingdom for diagnostic purposes alone.

Current role of cardiac catheterisation

Although diagnostic coronary angiography has expanded, and there is a demand to increase it yet further, cardiac catheterisation of adult patients for other reasons has remained static. This is probably due to the widespread adoption of other methods of imaging, particularly transthoracic echocardiography. In adult patients with valvular or congenital heart disease, cardiac catheterisation might now be performed only when there is a clinical need to define any concomitant coronary artery disease. Occasionally, it might also be undertaken as a preliminary to transcatheter treatments such as mitral balloon valvoplasty or the implantation of an atrial septal defect closure device, neither of which procedures is performed in large numbers in the United Kingdom. Similarly, in paediatric cardiology and congenital heart disease, echocardiography has largely replaced invasive cardiac catheterisation, except where catheter based treatment is to be performed at the same time.

Although the last two decades have seen little in the way of innovation compared with the early days of cardiac catheterisation, there has been a steady improvement in technique, radiographic equipment, and safety. Left heart catheterisation is now performed routinely in many centres and district general hospitals, with very satisfactory results. Some of those involved in the early days of coronary angiography have remained active – Kurt Amplatz has recently designed a type of atrial septal defect occluder – but the basic approach to diagnostic catheterisation has changed little.

Angioplasty

The entire direction of adult invasive cardiology has been changed by the emergence of angioplasty and other percutaneous interventions. Coronary artery disease comprises most of the clinical workload for British cardiologists, and while the only option for revascularisation was coronary artery surgery, angiography was largely the handmaiden of cardiac surgery. This was equally true of the investigation and management of valvular disease. However, the emergence of percutaneous, catheter-based coronary and valve interventions has given cardiac physicians the ability to treat many patients without recourse to surgery.

The first coronary angioplasty was performed by Andreas Grüntzig of Zurich in 1979, and interest in this technique spread rapidly. The first coronary angioplasties in the United Kingdom were performed in 1980 by Raphael Balcon at the London Chest Hospital, by Tony Rickards at the National Heart Hospital, and by Edgar Sowton at Guy's Hospital. Initial experiences were mixed, as the balloon dilatation catheters then available were stiff, high in cross sectional profile, and difficult to steer. As guidewires and balloons improved rapidly, more operators adopted the technique, and a number of centres soon reported large case series at the British Cardiac Society annual meetings.

British Cardiovascular Intervention Society

In the early 1980s, the British Cardiovascular Intervention Society was formed and started to meet regularly as a forum for case presentations, discussion, and training. Initially, these meetings were small, informal, and separate from the Cardiac Society. The early contributors included Peter Hubner, Man Fai Shiu, Howard Swanton, and colleagues. Subsequently, the British Cardiovascular Intervention Society became affiliated to the Cardiac Society and one of its meetings forms an integral part of the annual British Cardiac Society Meeting.

Intracoronary stenting

The experience of acute coronary dissection and closure in 2% to 5% of cases tempered enthusiasm for balloon angioplasty, and careful case selection of straightforward lesions was the rule. Coronary angioplasty advanced appreciably with the introduction of intracoronary stents. The first coronary stent procedure was performed by Ulrich Sigwart (now of the Royal Brompton Hospital) in Lausanne in 1984. The stent forms a circular internal scaffolding which holds the lumen open, greatly reducing the risks of acute closure and roughly halving the rate of subsequent restenosis. The word "stent" can be traced to 14th century English, where it describes a framework of poles used to spread fishing nets across rivers and estuaries.

In the United Kingdom, the first coronary stent procedures were performed by Ulrich Sigwart at the National Heart Hospital and the London Chest Hospital. The original Wallstent was a self expanding stent with some technical limitations; shortly afterwards the balloon expanded Palmaz-Schatz stent was introduced, and was widely used in the early 1990s. Subsequently, over 80 different designs of balloon expandable stent have been introduced which are more flexible, of lower crossing profile, and easily used.

The British Cardiovascular Intervention Society publishes annual audit data. Stent implantation is performed in over 60% of percutaneous coronary intervention procedures in the United Kingdom. As well as undertaking audit of all coronary interventions each year, the British Cardiovascular Intervention Society is now responsible for recommendations on training and continuing competence in coronary intervention. The society also runs the annual "advanced angioplasty" series of meetings for dissemination of the latest information and for critical discussion of the place of new devices and stents in British clinical cardiology.

Other coronary interventional devices

Aside from stents, other coronary interventional devices such as lasers, rotating drills, and cutting devices have been used – generally in small numbers of patients for particular indications. Most of these devices have been designed and manufactured abroad, but one new device is the

"X-ciser" which is a safe drilling and aspiration device designed by Man Fai Shiu in Coventry. At the same time, stent design has advanced with new antithrombotic coatings, delivery of localised radiation to reduce restenosis, and improved mechanical properties. The successful short and long term results of stenting, combined with relative ease of use, has led to a widening of indications for angioplasty. Indeed, the role of surgery versus angioplasty in multivessel disease is being examined in the ARTS trial, which is based in Rotterdam, but involves a number of British centres, and in the stent or surgery (SOS) trial, based at the Royal Brompton Hospital. The ascendancy of stents has also led some interventional cardiologists to become involved in carotid and aortic stenting, and sometimes renal and peripheral arterial interventions also.

Angioplasty in myocardial infarction

In the United States and some large European centres, angioplasty as the initial treatment for patients presenting with acute myocardial infarction has been a vogue. Some trials have suggested advantages of primary angioplasty over intravenous thrombolysis with streptokinase or tPA. Current British practice is to use percutaneous coronary intervention when there are specific contraindications to thrombolysis, when thrombolysis has failed, when there is early recurrent ischaemia, and sometimes when the patient is in cardiogenic shock. The pioneers of percutaneous coronary intervention for myocardial infarction in Britain include David Ramsdale at Liverpool, LDR Smith in Exeter, and Mark de Belder in Middlesborough. However, at present, most patients with acute infarction are admitted to hospitals that have no invasive facilities, and only selected cases will be transferred urgently for early angioplasty.

Financial constraints

The principal limitation to the further expansion of angioplasty seems to be the financial and organisational constraints of the NHS. In the United Kingdom in 1998, British Cardiovascular Intervention Society figures indicate that about 25 000 coronary interventions were performed, compared with 450 000 in the United States (which has about four times the population). There are fewer coronary interventions performed per million of the population per year in the United Kingdom than in almost all other countries of western Europe.

The new generation of cardiologists is now being trained in coronary intervention as a routine part of cardiology. They are often appointed to posts based in district general hospitals with a number of sessions at the regional centre in which they can undertake elective angioplasty on their patients. We hope that the success of this approach will lead to a more appropriate level of angiography and angioplasty in the future, but no doubt there will still be a struggle for adequate funding and wider provision of invasive facilities.

Non-coronary interventions

Non-coronary interventions are performed in smaller numbers than coronary angioplasty. Aortic balloon valvuloplasty has doubtful results, mitral balloon valvuloplasty is beneficial in selected cases but the incidence of rheumatic mitral disease in Britian is low. Several devices have been tried to close septal defects non-operatively, and the results for atrial septal defects are encouraging.

Quality if not quantity

British expertise in congenital heart disease is mostly concentrated in a few large centres such as Guy's Hospital, the Hospital for Sick Children (Great Ormond Street), Southampton, and the Brompton Hospital. This has allowed a few operators in each of these centres to gain the necessary experience with the devices, which seems to be the best approach to complicated techniques in paediatric and adult cardiology. Thus, while the UK may not perform large total numbers of interventions, its centres have been relatively successful in attaining good clinical results and in publishing audit and research into interventions. The clinical use of new coronary and non-coronary devices is now regulated by the Medical Devices Agency, which is based in London but takes a lead in approval of devices across the European Union.

In conclusion

In future, it seems that the development of new interventional devices will continue apace, combined with new drugs to treat thrombosis and lipids. British cardiology will undoubtedly continue to contribute to clinical research and development, but the challenge of limited healthcare resources may slow the delivery of these technologies to the wider UK patient base.

References and notes

1. Mendel D. *A practice of cardiac catheterisation*. 2nd ed. Oxford: Blackwell Scientific Publications, 1968.
2. Verel D, Grainger RG. *Cardiac catheterisation and angiography*. 1st ed. London: Churchill Livingstone, 1969.
3. Miller GAH. *Invasive investigation of the heart*. Oxford. Blackwell Scientific Publications, 1989.
4. Wiggers CJ. *Physiology in health and disease*. 2nd ed. London: Henry Kimpton, 1937.
5. Forssmannn W. The catheterisation of the right side of the heart. *Klin Wochenschr* 1929;8:2085–87.
6. McMichael J. Foreward. In: Verel D, Grainger RG, eds. *Cardiac catheterisation and angiography*. 1st ed. London: Churchill Livingstone, 1969.
7. Cournand A, Ranges HA. Catheterisation of the right auricle in man. *Proc Soc Exp Biol* 1941;46:462–6.
8. McMichael J, Sharpey-Schafer EP. Cardiac output in man by a direct Fick method. *Br Heart J* 1944;6:33–40.
9. Howarth S, McMichael J, Sharpey-Schafer EP. Cardiac catheterisation in cases of patent inter-

auricular septum, primary pulmonary hypertension, Fallot's tetralogy and pulmonary stenosis. *Br Heart J* 1947;9:292–303.

10. Baker C, Brock RC, Campbell M, Suzman S. Morbus coeruleus. *Br Heart J* 1949;11:170–200.
11. Holling HE, Zak GA. Cardiac catheterisation in the diagnosis of congenital heart disease. *Br Heart J* 1950;12:153–82.
12. Chavez I, Dorbeckker N, Celis A. Direct intracardiac angiocardiography – its diagnostic value. *Am Heart J* 1947;33:560–93.
13. Hellems HK, Haynes FW, Gowdy JP, Dexter L. The pulmonary capillary pressure in man. *J Clin Invest* 1948;27:540.
14. Epps RG, Adler RH. Left atrial and pulmonary capillary venous pressure in mitral stenosis. *Br Heart J* 1953;15:298–304.
15. Owen SG, Wood PH. The degree of mitral obstruction. *Br Heart J* 1955;17:41–55.
16. Donald KW, Bishop JM, Wormald PN, Wade,OL. Haemodynamic and ventilatory studies in mitral stenosis before and two years after mitral valvotomy. *Br Heart J* 1956;18:566.
17. Wood PH. Pulmonary hypertension. *Br Med Bull* 1952;8:348–53.
18. Wood PH. The Eisenmenger syndrome. *BMJ* 1958;2:701–9, 755–62.
19. Wood PH. *Diseases of the heart and circulation.* 1st ed. London: Eyre and Spottiswoode, 1950.
20. Korner PI, Shillingford JP. The quantitiative estimation of valvar incompetence by dye dilution curves. *Clin Sci* 1955;14:553–7.
21. Goodwin JF. Cardiac function in primary myocardial disorders. *BMJ* 1964;1:1527–34, 1595–7.
22. Miller GAH, Sutton GC. Acute massive pulmonary embolism. Clinical and haemodynamic findings in 23 patients studied by cardiac catheterisation and pulmonary angiography. *Br Heart J* 1970;32:518–23.
23. Radner S. Suprasternal puncture of the left atrium for flow studies. *Acta Med Scand* 1954;148:57–60.
24. Brock RC, Milstein BB, Ross DN. Percutaneous left ventricular puncture in the assessment of aortic stenosis. *Thorax* 1956;11:163–71.
25. Nixon PG. The transeptal approach to the left atrium in mitral regurgitation. *Thorax* 1960;15:225–8.
26. Seldinger SI. Catheter replacement of the needle in percutaneous arteriography. *Acta Radiol* 1953;39:368–76.
27. Sloman G, Jefferson K. Cine-angiography of the coronary circulation in living dogs. *Br Heart J* 1960;22:54–60.
28. Sones FM, Shirey EK. Cine coronary arteriography. *Mod Concepts Cardiovasc Dis* 1962;31:735.
29. Hale D, Dexter D, Jefferson K, Leatham A. The value of coronary arteriography in the investigation of ischaemic heart disease. *Br Heart J* 1966;28:40–54.
30. Judkins MP. Selective coronary arteriography. 1. *Radiology* 1967;89:815–24.
31. Bradley RD. Diagnostic right heart catheterisation with microcatheter in severely ill patients. *Lancet* 1964;ii:941–2.
32. Swan HJC, Ganz W, Forrester J, Marcus H, Diamond G, Chonette D. Catheterisation of the heart in man with use of a flow directed balloon tipped catheter. *N Eng J Med* 1970;283:447–51.
33. Mendel D. Instantaneous measurement of the rate of change of pressure pulses. *Br Heart J* 1965;27:950.
34. Davies JG, Leatham A, Robinson BF. Ventricular stimulation by catheter electrode. *Lancet* 1959;i:583–4.
35. Watson H. Intracardiac electrocardiography in the investigation of congenital heart disease in infancy and the neonatal period. *Br Heart J* 1962;24:144–56.
36. Watson H, Emslie-Smith D, Lowe KG. The intracardiac electrocardiogram of human atrioventricular conducting tissue. *Am Heart J* 1967;74:66–70.
37. Scherlag BJ. The development of the His Bundle recording technique. *Pacing Clin Electrophysiol* 1979;2:230–3.
38. Rashkind WJ, Miller WW. Creation of an atrial septal defect without thoracotomy: a palliative approach to complete transposition of the great arteries. *JAMA* 1966;196:991–2.
39. Richardson PJ. King's endocardial bioptome. *Lancet* 1974;i:660–1.
40. Miller GAH, Anderson RH, Rigby ML. *The diagnosis of congenital heart disease.* Tunbridge Wells, Kent: Castle Publications, 1985.
41. Hall RJC, Boyle RM, Webb-Peploe M, Chamberlain D, Parker DJ. Guidelines for specialist training in cardiology. *Br Heart J* 1995;73(suppl 1):1–24.
42. Mills P. Should coronary angiography be performed in district hospitals? *Br Heart J* 1990;63:73.
43. BCS Council Statement. Strategic planning for cardiac services and the internal market: role of catheterisation laboratories in district general hospitals. *Br Heart J* 1994;71:110–12.

Chapter 12

Nuclear Medicine and Cardiology

Peter J Ell

The work of Norman Veall et al., as early as 1954, heralded the first British applications of the radioactive tracer in investigating a cardiac patient.[1] Veall described to a meeting of experts a method for determining cardiac output that was simple, ingenious, and ahead of its time. Similar methodology led later to the development of the so-called nuclear stethoscope which was to be used to measure cardiac function.[2] The nuclear stethoscope represented one of the very first attempts to obtain pathophysiological information on cardiac performance with a truly non-invasive approach based on radioactive tracers. Time-activity curve data were recorded from a detector placed over the chest. The cardiac probe was born. Although the *British Heart Journal* had published Nylin's work on determining blood volume with radioactive phosphorus in 1945[3] and Blumgart's use of radioactive gases in detecting cardiac shunts in 1962,[4] cardiology was to turn its attention to invasive methods of cardiac investigation. The golden era of cardiac catheterisation and heroic cardiac surgery was to make its mark in the ensuing years, and it would take some time before the interest of the invasive cardiologist was drawn to the newer non-invasive methods of imaging.

Early scanners

Imaging technology for radioactive tracer applications began in 1951. In that year, work with the Cassen scanner was described[5] and details of the Mayneord scanner, developed at the Royal Marsden Hospital, London, were published in *Nature*.[6] Yet it was the gamma camera developed by Anger in 1952, that was to have the most profound impact on nuclear medicine, including cardiology.[7] Furthermore, the arrival of the computer and modern data processing were to enable nuclear medicine to achieve its present status as a routine clinical tool.

The MRC medical cyclotron unit

In 1957, the Medical Research Council funded the world's first, hospital dedicated, medical cyclotron facility at the Hammersmith Hospital, London. This permitted fundamental work to take place that would lead to the application of short lived positron emitting radionuclides in man. In 1960, Dollery and West published an article in *Nature* on the metabolism of oxygen-15.[8] These authors produced an important body of work, using radioactive tracers to study the pathophysiology of the lung and circulatory system.[9][10] Clark et al. at the Hammersmith Hospital reported on an extensive programme for using cyclotron produced isotopes at the hospital.[11] In parallel, Dacie and Lewis were to make extensive use of the radioactive tracer method to change completely the practice of haematology. As early as 1963, a third edition of what was to become their classic text – *Practical haematology* – was published.[12] (It is interesting to note that the first edition had appeared in 1950!)

Seminal work emerged from the MRC cyclotron unit. In 1970, Jones and Clark developed the krypton-81m generator, equipment that is still shipped to many users.[13] In 1977, Lavender et al. described the use of krypton-81m in the continuous monitoring of regional myocardial perfusion,[14] while in 1979 Selwyn et al. used krypton-81m to investigate the patency of coronary artery bypass grafts.[15] Myocardial ischaemia in man was first investigated by Allan et al. in 1981, using rubidium-82 and carbon-11 acetate.[16] Three years later the relation between silent ischaemia and stress was studied with this positron emitter.[17] Still at the MRC cyclotron unit, Yamamoto et al. investigated the metabolic rate of oxygen-15,[18] and carbon-11 labelled ligands were used in the first studies of cardiac β receptor activity in patients with cardiomyopathy.[19]

Cardiac imaging

Imaging of the heart began somewhat hesitantly in the mid to late 1950s. Progress was hampered by the shortage of suitable radiopharmaceuticals and imaging detectors. Data processing of time-dependent parameters was yet to make its mark. Radioactive iodine labelled human serum albumin was used to delineate the cardiac chambers. The initial diagnostic dilemma associated with this technique was the differential diagnosis of pericardial effusions in patients with enlarged cardiac silhouettes.

Progress abroad

Clinical progress had to wait for suitable technology, and developmental work began to move abroad, where greater emphasis was being placed in the development of the gamma camera and computer dedicated systems. The only manufacturer of gamma cameras in the United Kingdom (Nuclear Enterprises) was unable to stay ahead of the field, inevitably real progress in nuclear cardiology could only be made when modern equipment was available in this country. Much of the development of radiopharmaceuticals also occurred abroad, and technetium-99m labelled phosphonates as well as the most important potassium analogue thallium-201 were first investigated outside the United Kingdom.

Scintigraphy

It is remarkable that scintigraphy of the cardiac chambers and cardiac muscle developed almost simultaneously. Techniques for investigating wall motion, ejection fraction, and ventricular volumes were investigated, and the now well established methods of first pass and equilibrium radionuclide ventriculography emerged. Scanning the cardiac muscle led to the emergence of tracers able to visualise the damaged or necrotic myocardium and, more relevantly, to study regional myocardial perfusion, where defects in tracer uptake reflected regional impairment of myocardial blood flow. Much good work in this area was accomplished in the United Kingdom. Tracers labelled with technetium-99m and, in particular, the phosphates were seen to concentrate in areas of acute myocardial necrosis. Ell and Joseph reported early work in this area from 1976 onwards.

Mobile gamma cameras

Mobile gamma cameras made their appearance in intensive and coronary care units from 1979[20][21][22][23], and were available on the wards in 1987.[24] These methods meant that in the coronary care unit, acute transmural and subendocardial infarction could be detected with sensitivities of 95% and 75% respectively.

Radionuclide ventriculography

The use of first pass radionuclide ventriculography to study the cardiac chambers at rest and during stress was described by Dymond et al. among others in 1979,[25] and by Walton et al. in the early 1980s.[26][27][28] The first data looking at myocardial perfusion and at ventricular wall motion in three dimensions were published by Dymond et al. in 1979[29] and by Underwood et al. in 1985.[30]

Applying the Fourier transformation to time-activity curve data from the heart enabled researchers to investigate the cardiac chambers in terms of the amplitude and timing of contraction. This allowed the imaging of myocardial aneurysms and abnormalities of wall motion in attractive colour coded maps. Parametric maps of amplitude, phase, and time of end systole could be displayed. Measuring the ventricular ejection fraction during stress and at rest became a routine procedure.

Risk stratification

The merit of using radionuclides with a very short half life to assess sequentially ventricular function was investigated.[31] Nuclear cardiology was now equipped to address practical clinical problems such as the assessment of ventricular reserve and the response to treatment of patients with left ventricular aneurysms,[32] and investigation of the hypertensive patient and the demonstration of early diastolic dysfunction.[33] It became possible to stratify patients with ischaemic heart disease into categories of low, moderate, and high risk, and the value of nuclear cardiology as a tool for prognosis was enhanced.[34][35]

Technological progress

Nuclear cardiology has, of course, depended greatly on technological progress, and this features prominently. In 1984, Lahiri et al. reported on ambulatory methods for the continuing monitoring of ventricular function with a new solid state detector,[36] and on the dual use of gold-195m and thallium-201 in studying simultaneously ventricular pump performance and myocardial perfusion.[37] Rodrigues et al. described the infusion of xenon-127 in the study of the right ventricle.[38] Jain et al. and Senior et al. discussed the efficacy of indium-111 labelled antimyosin in investigating acute myocardial infarction and detecting myocyte damage.[39][40]

New tracers

Since 1975, thallium-201, a potassium analogue, had been the principal radiopharmaceutical for investigating myocardial perfusion. The advantages of technetium-99m as the radionuclide of choice made it inevitable that new tracers for myocardial perfusion and for single photon emission tomography would become available. DuPont and Nycomed-Amersham played a decisive part here with the development of 2-Methoxy-isobutyl-isonitrile (MIBI) and tetrofosmin – both labelled with technetium-99m. In 1993, Sridhara et al. published a report comparing tetrofosmin and thallium.[41] A multicenter trial confirmed these findings,[42] and a very large trial comparing all three tracers (tetrofosmin, MIBI, and thallium) was recently reported by Kapur et al.[43] The added advantage of the technetium-99m labelled tracers was that they allowed myocardial perfusion to be investigated at the time of their intravenous administration, since they stayed in the cardiac cell without significant redistribution. Thus, acute coronary syndromes and their perfusion patterns could be investigated at the time of the acute event provided that a tracer was administered, while allowing for the imaging of perfusion at a later, safer stage. Triage of patients who presented with acute chest pain was to become a reality and possibly part of rapid access chest pain clinics.

Emission tomography

Emission tomography was born with the positron scanner in the early 1970s. Emission tomography with standard radionuclide tracers was to begin much later, and the first rotating Anger gamma camera in the United Kingdom was installed at the Institute of Nuclear Medicine, University College London in 1978. Tomographic maps of cardiac function or metabolism, or both, were to make their impact on the non-invasive investigation of patients. Various new tracers for myocardial perfusion scintigraphy and individually tailored stress protocols that allowed stress testing in nearly all patients (whether limited by symptoms or with other conditions that precluded conventional stress testing) helped to transform nuclear cardiology into an indispensable modern tool for investigating patients with myocardial ischaemia.

Gamma cameras with an *x* ray source

The initial gamma camera tomograms were based on a single, rotating, radiation detector. Modern instruments now use several detectors, which facilitates and speeds up data acquisition. Purpose built cardiac gamma cameras have emerged. The addition of a transmission source has permitted further improvements in the accuracy of data acquisition and processing.[44] Very recently, gamma cameras incorporating an *x* ray source have been developed so that a computed tomography type scan can be obtained together with a standard single photon emission computed tomogram. This will permit anatomical and functional tomograms of the human heart to be "fused" easily.

British Nuclear Cardiology Society

A British Nuclear Cardiology Group was established and renamed the British Nuclear Cardiology Society in 1997. An early survey in 1988 estimated that between 0.58/1000 and 0.66/1000 nuclear cardiology procedures per year were being undertaken. In 1994 this figure had risen to 0.82/1000 per year.[45] By 1994, the British Cardiac Society recommended that a target should be aimed at with an activity ceiling for procedures of 2.2/1000 per year, close to the European average level of activity of 2.6/1000 per year. The Calman training programme for specialist registrars in cardiology now acknowledges the need for specialised training in nuclear cardiology.

Cost-benefit analysis of scintigraphy

The United Kingdom took a European lead in analysing the cost and benefit of myocardial perfusion tomography. Original data were published in the *European Heart Journal* in 1999.[46] For the first time, a study on 400 patients showed that myocardial perfusion scintigraphy achieved a cheaper and more reliable diagnosis than other diagnostic techniques. Users of scintigraphy achieved greater prognostic power at the point of diagnosis and also had a lower normalcy rate for coronary angiography. Revised guidelines for the investigation and management of stable angina drawn up by the British Cardiac Society and the Royal College of Physicians of London also stress the useful role of myocardial perfusion scintigraphy.[47]

In conclusion

Nuclear cardiology now has an established place in the investigation of the cardiac patient. The use of radionuclides for therapeutic purposes is also in progress, and the topic of restenosis and coronary revascularisation is an important one. A number of devices are being manufactured with the aim of reducing proliferation of the intima via energy deposition. Balloon catheters with rhenium-188 have been reported, but other sealed, source based, radionuclide technology is also under investigation. Nuclear cardiology continues to make a substantial contribution to the management of patients.

References and notes

1. Veall N, Pearson JD, Hanley T, Lowes AE. A method for the determination of cardiac output (preliminary report). In: *Proceedings of the second radioisotope conference Oxford* 1954, vol 1. London: Butterworth Scientific Publications, 1954:183.
2. Wagner HN, Wake R, Nickoloff E, Natarajan TK. The nuclear stethoscope: a simple device for the recording of left ventricular volume curves. *Am J Cardiol* 1976;8:747–50.
3. Nylin G. Blood volume determinations with radioactive phosphorus. *Br Heart J* 1945;7:81.
4. Blumgart HL, Yens DC. Studies on velocity of blood flow: method utilized. *J Clin Invest* 1927;4:1.
5. Cassen B, Curtis L, Reed C, Libby R. Instrumentation for I-131 use in medical studies. *Nucleonics* 1951;9:46–50.
6. Mayneord WV, Turner RC, Newbery SP, Hodt HJ. A method of making visible the distribution of activity in a source of ionising radiation. *Nature* 1951;168:762.
7. Anger HO. Scintillation cameras. *Rev Sci Instrum* 1958;29:27–33.
8. Dollery CT, West JB. Metabolism of oxygen-15. *Nature* 1960;187:1121.
9. Dollery CT, West JB, Wilcken DEL, Goodwin JF, Hugh-Jones P. Regional pulmonary blood flow in patients with circulatory shunts. *Br Heart J* 1961;23:225–35.
10. Dollery CT, West JB. Regional uptake of radioactive oxygen, carbon monoxide and carbon dioxide in the lungs of patients with mitral stenosis. *Circulation Res* 1960;8:765–71.
11. Clark JC, Matthews CME, Sylvester DJ, Vonberg DD. Using cyclotron produced isotopes at Hammersmith Hospital. *Nucleonics* 1967;25b:54.
12. Dacie JV, Lewis SM. *Practical haematology*. 3rd ed. London: J & A Churchill Ltd, 1963:435.
13. Jones T, Clark JC. Kr-81m generator and its uses in cardiopulmonary studies with the scintillation camera. *J Nucl Med* 1970;11:118–24.
14. Lavender JP, Selwyn AP, Turner JH, Jones T. Continuous imaging of regional myocardial perfusion by krypton-81m. *Herz* 1977;2:23–6.
15. Selwyn AP, Sapsford R, Forge S, Fox K, Myers M. Assessment of coronary venous bypass graft function using krypton-81m. *Am J Cardiology* 1979;43:554–9.
16. Allan RM, Horlock PL, Pike VW, Jones T, Selwyn AP. Myocardial ischaemia: detection and investigation. In: Rafflenbeul W, Lichtlen PR, Balcon R eds. *Unstable angina pectoris*. Stuttgart: Georg Thieme Verlag, 1981:45–50.
17. Deanfield JE, Shea M, Kensett M, Horlock P, Wilson RA, De Landshere CM, Selwyn AP. Silent myocardial ischaemia due to mental stress. *Lancet* 1984;ii:1001–4.

18. Yamamoto Y, de Silva R, Rhodes CG, Iida H, Lammerstma AA, Jones T, Maseri A. Non invasive quantification of regional myocardial metabolic rate of oxygen by $15O_2$ inhalation and positron emission tomography. *Circulation* 1996;94:808–16.
19. Lefroy DC, deSilva R, Choudhury L, et al. Diffuse reduction of myocardial beta adrenoceptors in hypertrophic cardiomyopathy: a study with positron emission tomography. *J Am Coll Cardiol* 1993;22:1653–60.
20. Ell PJ . Scan analysis in myocardial infarction. *Nuklearmedizin* 1976;XV:157–9.
21. Joseph S, Ell PJ, Ross P, Donaldson R, et al. Tc-99m imidodiphosphonate. A superior radiopharmaceutical for in vivo positive myocardial infarct imaging. II. Clinical data. *Br Heart J* 1978;40:234–41.
22. Ell PJ, Donaldson RM. Cardiovascular nuclear medicine. *Intens Care Med* 1978;4:119–22.
23. Joseph SP, Pereira-Prestes AV, Ell PJ, Donaldson R, Somerville W, Emanuel RW. The value of positive myocardial infarct imaging in the coronary care unit. *BMJ* 1979;1:372–4.
24. Dymond DS, Jarritt PH, Britton KE, Langley D, Spurrell RAJ. Positive myocardial scintigraphy at the bedside-evaluation using a portable gamma camera. *Postgrad Med J* 1978;54:641–8.
25. Dymond DS, Jarritt PH, Britton KE, Spurrell RAJ. Detection of post infarction left ventricular aneurysms by first pass radionuclide ventriculography using a multicrystal gamma camera. *Br Heart J* 1979;41:68–78.
26. Walton S, Jarritt PH, Brown NJG, Ell PJ, Swanton, RH. Phase analysis of regional ventricular emptying in coronary artery disease. *Br Heart J* 1981;45:348–50.
27. Walton S, Yiannikis S, Jarritt PH, Brown NJG, Swanton RH, Ell PJ. Phasic abnormalities of left ventricular emptying in coronary artery disease. *Br Heart J* 1981;46:245–53.
28. Walton S, Ell PJ, Jarritt PH, Swanton RH. Phase analysis of the first pass radionuclide angiogram. *Br Heart J* 1982;48:441–8.
29. Dymond DS, Stone DL, Elliott AT, Britton KE, Spurrell RAJ. Cardiac emission tomography in patients using 201-thallium: a new technique for perfusion scintigraphy. *Clin Cardiol* 1979;2: 192–6.
30. Underwood SR, Walton S, Laming PJ, Jarritt PH, Ell PJ, Emanuel RW, Swanton,RH. Left ventricular volume and ejection fraction determined by gated blood pool emission tomography. *Br Heart J* 1985;53:216–2.
31. Dymond DS, Elliott AT, Flatman W, Stone D, et al. Clinical validation of gold-195m: a new short half-life radiopharmaceutical for rapid, sequential first pass radionuclide angiocardiography in man. *J Am Coll Cardiol* 1983;2:85–92.
32. Dymond DS, Foster C, Grenier RP, Carpenter J, Schmidt DH. Peak exercise and immediate post exercise imaging for the detection of left ventricular functional abnormalities in coronary artery disease. *Am J Cardiol* 1984;53:1532–37.
33. Caruna M, al-Khawaja I, Lahiri A, Lewis J, Raferty EB. Radionuclide measurements of diastolic function for assessing early left ventricular abnormalities in the hypertensive patient. *Br Heart J* 1988;59:218–26.
34. Rose EL, Liu XJ, Henley M, Lewis JD, Raferty EB, Lahiri A, Raval U. Prognostic value of non-invasive cardiac tests in the assessment of patients with peripheral vascular disease. *Am J Cardiol* 1993;71:40–4.
35. Senior R, Raval U, Lahiri A. Prognostic value of stress dobutamine technetium-99m sestamibi single-photon emission computed tomography (SPECT) in patients with suspected coronary artery disease. *Am J Cardiol* 1996;78:1092–6.
36. Lahiri A, Crawley JCW, Jones RI, Bowles MJ, Raferty EB. A non-invasive technique for continuous monitoring of the left ventricular function using a new solid state mercuric iodide radiation detector. *Clin Sci* 1984;66:551–6.
37. Lahiri A, Zanelli GD, O'Hara MJ, Bowles MJ, Jones RI, Cave APD, Raferty EB. Simultaneous measurement of left ventricular function and myocardial perfusion during a single exercise test: dual isotope imaging with gold-195m and thallium-201. *Eur Heart J* 1986;7:493–500.
38. Rodrigues EA, Lahiri A, Hinge DA, Smith T, Crawley JCW, Raferty EB. A new method of imaging the right ventricle using peripheral vein infusion of xenon-127. *Eur J Nucl Med* 1987;12:617–9.
39. Jain D, Lahiri A, Crawley JCW, Raferty EB. Post-mortem correlation between histopathologic and autoradiographic extent of myocardial necrosis detected by In-111 antimyosin imaging of a patient with acute myocardial infarction. *Am J Cardiac Imaging* 1988;2:158–61.
40. Senior R, Weston J, Bhattacharya S, Crawley JCW, Liu XJ, Lahiri A. Specific binding of Tc-99m antimyosin to necrotic human myocardium: clinical pathological correlates. *Am Heart J* 1991;122:857–9.
41. Sridhara BS, Braat S, Rigo P, Itti R, Cload AP, Lahiri A. Comparison of myocardial perfusion imaging with 99m-Tc-tetrofosmin versus 201-Tl in coronary artery disease. *Am J Cardiol* 1993;72:1015–9.
42. Zaret BL, Rigo P, Wackers FJT, et al. and the Tetrofosmin International Trial Study Group. Myocardial perfusion with technetium-99m tetrofosmin comparison to thallium-201 imaging and coronary angiography in a phase III multicenter trial. *Circulation* 1995;91:313–9.

43. Kapur A, Latus KA, Davies G, Jarritt PH, Young MC, Roussakis G, et al. The ROBUST study: a randomised comparison of three tracers for myocardial perfusion scintigraphy. *J Nucl Med* 1999;40: 85P.
44. Prvulovich E, Lonn AHR, Bomanji JB, Jarritt PH, Ell PJ. Transmission imaging for attenuation correction of myocardial ^{201}thallium images in obese patients. *Nucl Med Commun* 1997;18:207–18.
45. Pennell DJ, Prvulovich E, Tweddel A, Caplin J. British nuclear cardiology survey 1994. *Nucl Med Commun* 1998;19:305–13.
46. Underwood SR, Godman B, Salyani S, Ogle J, Ell PJ. Economics of myocardial perfusion imaging in Europe. The EMPIRE study. *Eur Heart J* 1999;20:157–66.
47. De Bono D. Investigation and management of stable angina: revised guidelines 1998. *Heart* 1999;81:546–55.

Chapter 13

Cardiovascular Magnetic Resonance

Donald B Longmore and S Richard Underwood

The phenomenon of magnetic resonance was described independently by Bloch and Purcell working in the United States just after the second world war.[1][2] It was first used in magnetic resonance spectroscopy, which became a routine analytical technique in chemistry, and later biochemistry, laboratories. However, it was not until the 1970s that magnetic resonance was used to produce images, and there is still debate over who was first to describe imaging.

Early days of imaging

In 1971, Damadian, working in the United States, suggested that it might be possible to distinguish tumour from normal tissue in an image because of its different magnetic relaxation properties, but he gave no details of an imaging technique.[3] In 1973, Lauterbur, also working in the United States, described a method of producing an image by applying a magnetic field gradient to encode positional information in the magnetic resonance signal.[4] He demonstrated the technique by creating a cross sectional image of two test tubes. In the same year, Mansfield and Grannell, working in Nottingham University, used a single frequency encoding gradient to resolve the signal from a number of parallel sample plates in their studies on nuclear magnetic resonance diffraction.[5] The concept of magnetic resonance imaging was treated with more scepticism than Hounsfield experienced when he described *x* ray transmission computed tomography,[6] and so it was left to a few far sighted groups, in particular those in Nottingham and Aberdeen Universities, to take an early lead.

The first magnetic resonance image of a live human was of a finger – it was produced by Mansfield and Maudesley at Nottingham University in 1976.[7] Edelstein and colleagues in Aberdeen also contributed to the development of imaging techniques.[8] Bydder and Young at the Hammersmith Hospital also showed the clinical value of the technique in whole body scans.[9][10] They collaborated with Longmore and colleagues from the

National Heart Hospital to implement electrocardiographic triggering and hence to acquire some of the first images of the heart.[11] In the United States, Higgins also showed the value of the technique for cardiac imaging at an early stage.[12] Other British workers with a major interest were Ian Isherwood's group in Manchester, who developed an early method of cine imaging,[13] and Smith and colleagues in Edinburgh, who exploited the ability of a very low field (0.05 tesla) scanner produced in Aberdeen to image myocardial T1 and its changes after acute infarction.[14]

Echo-planar imaging

An important aspect of cardiovascular magnetic resonance imaging is speed. Conventional imaging acquired data over, typically, 256 cardiac cycles. This meant that the patient would have to be as still as possible for 4 minutes. Problems also arose with arrhythmia and with the averaging of physiological changes. However, from an early stage, Mansfield was successful in developing echo-planar imaging, where a relatively low spatial resolution image was acquired in a fraction of a second. He first applied this in a small bore magnet to image the hearts of children,[15] and later implemented it on a full-sized magnet.[16] As with flow imaging, the technique was relatively slow to be implemented commercially because of the engineering problems of producing high magnetic field gradients with rapid rates of change.

CORDA

CORDA, the Heart Charity, was formed in 1975 by Donald Longmore and John Stevenson to obtain funding (which was then not readily available) for research into the secondary prevention of cardiovascular disease. The chairmen of CORDA have been Lord Carr of Hadley, Sir Cecil Clothier, Lord Rayner, Sir Richard Greenbury, and Professor Anthony Newman-Taylor.

The charity has principally funded research into atherogenesis and methods of detecting occlusive vascular disease at an early stage. In 1977, it funded a study of the biological effects of strong and fluctuating magnetic and radiofrequency fields using the ex vivo fetal mouse heart because of its extreme sensitivity to harmful agents.[17][18] No deleterious effect was found. In 1984, CORDA funded the purchase and installation at the Brompton Hospital of the first magnetic resonance scanner in the world dedicated to cardiovascular research, and the charity continues to provide funding alongside that provided by the NHS Trust, the Wellcome Foundation, and the British Heart Foundation.

Brompton Magnetic Resonance Unit

In 1984, what is now known as the Royal Brompton and Harefield NHS Trust, was the Brompton Hospital – with close links to its sister hospitals, the National Heart Hospital and the London Chest Hospital. The Brompton's Magnetic Resonance Unit was established by Donald Longmore, with joint funding from CORDA and from the hospital. A 0.26 tesla scanner was purchased from Picker International Ltd. Over the next decade, the scanner was modified extensively to optimise it for cardiovascular imaging, and it remained in full-time clinical and research use until 1999.

Initial research concentrated on the dimensional accuracy of the technique for measuring cardiac volumes and function.[19–21] The group also focussed on the ability of magnetic resonance imaging to illustrate anatomy and function in patients with grown up congenital heart disease, thus avoiding the need for invasive investigation in some.[22][23]

Functional aspects of cardiac imaging

An important distinction between the Brompton group and others was its concentration on functional aspects of cardiac imaging. The group developed a method of imaging blood flow by encoding velocity in the phase of the magnetic resonance signal – initially in collaboration with Ian Young at the Hammersmith, and then independently.[24] The same technique was implemented independently by Peter van Dijk in Holland, who used it to image myocardial velocity.[25] It was improved by the addition of even-echo re-phasing and by shortening the echo time[26] to make it more robust in rapidly flowing and turbulent blood.[27][28] The technique proved to be more reliable for quantitative flow imaging than other methods such as the one developed by the Aberdeen group.[29] Unfortunately, commercial manufacturers, who were relatively slow to appreciate the value of magnetic resonance imaging for the heart, did not implement it for many years, but it is now a routine part of the cardiovascular magnetic resonance examination. Nevertheless, the group showed its value in several clinical settings, including the assessment of flow in the great vessels,[30] valve function,[31] and even myocardial velocities.[32] The group was also the first to use pharmacological stress during imaging for the detection of coronary artery disease.[33]

In keeping with its aim of developing magnetic resonance as a tool for the early detection of atheroma, the Brompton group concentrated on developing methods of measuring aortic compliance as an indirect assessment of the effects of atheroma on the aorta,[34][35] and direct imaging of atheroma with chemical shift imaging to assess the amount of lipid within the plaque.[36] However, limitations in hardware meant that it was not possible to use these techniques clinically until much more recently. Groups in the United States and in France have extended these methods, and even promise glimpses of coronary atheroma.

Dedicated mobile scanner

Cardiovascular magnetic resonance imaging has particular requirements related to the need for high resolution imaging of a moving organ. Apart from the need for high magnetic field gradients with rapid and controllable rates of change, the cardiovascular machine requires real time acquisition and display and flexible image processing. This is still not available commercially in a robust format, but the Brompton group worked on a dedicated machine from an early stage. An actively shielded 0.6 tesla magnet was installed in a motorway coach converted by WH Bence and Co in 1988, and the radiofrequency and magnetic gradient components were designed specifically for rapid cardiovascular imaging. The machine was designed with flexibility in mind. The computer driving the image acquisition and display was based on a PC motherboard, with additional dedicated hardware designed by Surrey Medical Imaging Systems, a company developed by academics working in Guildford University. With this scanner, the group worked on modifications of Mansfield's echo-planar technique, such as zonal and spiral echo-planar imaging, and it was possible to acquire and reconstruct 64×64 pixel images in 100 ms, providing the first almost real time cardiac imaging.[37] The mobile machine is still in use today.

Magnetic resonance spectroscopy

The technical problems of introducing magnetic resonance imaging into clinical practice were large, but they were even larger for magnetic resonance spectroscopy. The relatively low sensitivity of the magnetic resonance technique was less of a problem for imaging, which, even now, limits itself to the hydrogen nucleus in fat and water (approximately 80 M in physiological systems). Until methods of suppressing the hydrogen signal were developed, spectroscopy concentrated on the phosphorus nucleus, which is five or six orders of magnitude less abundant.

In vivo cardiac spectroscopy also encountered problems in localising the signal to relatively small volumes and in distinguishing myocardial signal from that of blood and skeletal muscle. Much of this early work was carried out by George Radda's group in Oxford, mainly using animal models.[38] However, the first clinical application of magnetic resonance spectroscopy was in the detection of MacArdle's syndrome, an inherited defect of muscle metabolism.[39] Paul Bottomley and colleagues, working in the United States, also contributed significantly by developing techniques for whole body human cardiac spectroscopy.[40]

Coronary and myocardial perfusion imaging

British scientists and clinicians have played an important part in the development of cardiovascular magnetic resonance, and, as a result, magnetic resonance has a small but important role in routine cardiology. Further expansion is limited by the current inability of the technique to acquire reliable images of the coronary arteries and to assess the functional importance of disease either by direct imaging of coronary atheroma or by measuring coronary flow and myocardial perfusion. The United Kingdom has made some progress in these areas, but the lead has mainly come from abroad and from groups supported by the few commercial manufacturers who appreciated the importance of coronary imaging at an early stage.

Edelman and Manning in Boston (with a Siemens machine) were the first to use rapid breathhold gradient echo sequences to image the coronary lumen.[41] Wilke in Erlangen was the first to use similar techniques to image myocardial perfusion by following the myocardial passage of gadolinium tracers.[42] Both of these techniques are developing rapidly, with contributions from the Brompton group[43] and from Sheffield. Although it is now possible to acquire three dimensional images of the coronary arteries with a resolution of 0.1 mm, only history will tell if these techniques will ever replace *x* ray angiography, with its advantages of resolution and speed to set against its disadvantages of inflexibility and invasiveness.

Specialist societies

Cardiologists have traditionally performed their own imaging investigations, even though these may have been developed by other specialists. This applies to *x* ray angiography and to ultrasound imaging, but the "home" of nuclear cardiology and of cardiovascular magnetic resonance varies more. The development of cardiovascular magnetic resonance has been hindered by these political issues, since cardiologists – who manage the patients – have been slow to learn the value of magnetic resonance, and radiologists – who use magnetic resonance routinely for imaging of other organs – do not often assist in the care of cardiac patients.

In contrast, the specialist cardiac societies such as the British Cardiac Society, the European Society of Cardiology and the two American societies, were relatively quick to embrace magnetic resonance and support the technique in both teaching and research. The European Society of Cardiology, in particular, incorporated magnetic resonance into its working group on nuclear cardiology in 1990, and a task force produced the first summary of the clinical role of cardiovascular magnetic resonance.[44] The joint working group acted as a focus for activities in magnetic resonance until 1998, when the number of cardiologists working in the area was sufficient to justify the setting up of its own working group.

The one-stop shop

On the other side of the Atlantic, the Society for Cardiovascular Magnetic Resonance was founded in 1996, with Gerald Pohost as its first president. Pohost had worked in cardiac imaging since the early 1970s and is still a leading figure. Although his installation of the first clinical 4 tesla magnet in Birmingham, Alabama, was a notable achievement,[45] he will perhaps best be remembered for having popularised the term "the one-stop shop" to describe cardiovascular magnetic resonance as an imaging technique with the potential to provide all of the information necessary for clinical decision making. We hope that we do not have to wait another 50 years to discover whether magnetic resonance is the supermarket or the designer boutique of the future.

References and notes

1. Bloch F, Hansen WW, Packard ME. Nuclear Induction. *Phys Rev* 1946;69:127–9.
2. Purcell EM, Torrey HC, Pound RV. Resonance absorption by nuclear magnetic moments in a solid. *Phys Rev* 1946;69:37–8.
3. Damadian R. Tumour detection by nuclear magnetic resonance. *Science* 1971;171:1151.
4. Lauterbur PC. Image formation by induced local interactions. Examples employing nuclear magnetic resonance. *Nature* 1973;242:190–1.
5. Mansfield P, Grannell PK. NMR diffraction in solids? *J Phys Chem: Solid State Phys* 1973;6: L422–6.
6. Hounsfield GN. Computerised transverse axial scanning (tomography). Part 1: description of system. *Br J Radiol* 1973;46:1016–22.
7. Mansfield P, Maudsley AA. Planar and line scan spin imaging by NMR. *Proceedings of the XIXth congress.* Ampar Hiedelberg: 1976:247–52.
8. Edelstein WA, Hutchison JM, Johnson G, Redpath T. Spin warp NMR imaging and applications to human whole-body imaging. *Phys Med Biol* 1980;25:751–6.
9. Young IR, Bailes DR, Burle M, Smith DT, MacDonald MJ, Orr JS, et al. Initial clinical evaluation of a whole body magnetic resonance (NMR) tomograph. *J Comput Assist Tomogr* 1982;6:1–18.
10. Bydder GM, Steiner RE, Young IR, Hall AS, Thomas DJ, Marshall J, et al. Clinical NMR imaging of the brain. *Am J Roentgenol* 1982;139:215–36.
11. Steiner RE, Bydder GM, Selwyn A, Deanfield J, Longmore DB, Klipsten RH, Firmin DN. Nuclear magnetic resonance imaging of the heart. Current status and future prospects. *Br Heart J* 1983;50:202–8.
12. Higgins CB, Botvinick EH, Lanzer P, Herfkens R, Lipton MJ, Crooks LE, Kaufman L. Cardiovascular imaging with nuclear magnetic resonance. *Clin Cardiol* 1983;1: 527–39.
13. Waterton JC, Jenkins JP, Zhu XP, Love HG, Isherwood I, Rowlands DJ. Magnetic resonance (MR) cine imaging of the human heart. *Br J Radiol* 1985; 58: 711–716.
14. Smith MA, Ridgway JP, Brydon JW, Been M, Douglas RH, Kean DM, et al. ECG-gated T1 images of the heart. *Phys Med Biol* 1986;31:771–8.
15. Chrispin A, Small P, Rutter N, Coupland RE, Doyle M, Chapman B, et al. Echo planar imaging of normal and abnormal connections of the heart and great arteries. *Pediatr Radiol* 1986;16:289–92.
16. Chapman B, Turner R, Ordidge RJ, Doyle M, Cawley M, Coxon R, et al. Real-time movie imaging from a single cardiac cycle by NMR. *Magn Reson Med* 1987;5:246–54.
17. Armstrong SR, Longmore DB. The effects of cardio-active drugs on the performance of cultured foetal hearts. *Nature* 1973;243:350–2.
18. Hughes DM, Longmore DB. Relationship between the stage of development of foetal hearts and their survival in organ culture. *Nature* 1972;235:334–6.
19. Longmore DB, Klipstein RH, Underwood SR, Firmin DN, Hounsfield GN, Watanabe M, et al. Dimensional accuracy of magnetic resonance in studies of the heart. *Lancet* 1985;i:1360–2.
20. Underwood SR, Klipstein RH, Firmin DN, Fox KM, Poole-Wilson PA, Longmore DB, Rees RSO. Magnetic resonance assessment of aortic and mitral regurgitation. *Br Heart J* 1986;56:455–62.
21. Underwood SR, Gill CR, Firmin DN, Klipstein RH, Mohiaddin RH, Rees RSO, Longmore DB. Left ventricular volume measured rapidly by oblique magnetic resonance imaging. *Br Heart J* 1988;60:188–95.
22. Rees RSO, Somerville J, Underwood SR, Wright J, Firmin DN, Klipstein RH, Longmore DB. Magnetic resonance imaging of pulmonary arteries and their systemic connections in pulmonary atresia: comparison with angiographic and surgical findings. *Br Heart J* 1987;58:621–6.
23. Rees RSO, Somerville J, Warnes C, Underwood SR, Firmin DN, Klipstein RH, Longmore DB. Comparison of magnetic resonance imaging with echocardiography and radionuclide angiography in assessing cardiac function and anatomy following Mustard's operation for transposition of the great arteries. *Am J Cardiol* 1988;61:1316–22.

24. Bryant DJ, Payne JA, Firmin DN, Longmore DB. Measurement of flow with NMR imaging using a gradient pulse and phase difference technique. *J Comput Assist Tomogr* 1984;8:588–93.
25. Van Dijk P. Direct cardiac NMR imaging of heart wall and blood flow velocity. *J Comput Assist Tomogr* 1984;8:429–36.
26. Nayler GL, Firmin DN, Longmore DB. Blood flow imaging by cine magnetic resonance. *J Comput Assist Tomogr* 1986;10:715–22.
27. Firmin DN, Nayler GL, Klipstein RH, Underwood SR, Rees RS, Longmore DB. In vivo validation of MR velocity imaging. *J Comput Assist Tomogr* 1987;11:751–6.
28. Underwood SR, Firmin DN, Klipstein RH, Rees RS, Longmore DB. Magnetic resonance velocity mapping: clinical application of a new technique. *Br Heart J* 1987;57:404–12.
29. Redpath TW, Norris DG, Jones RA, Hutchison JM. A new method of NMR flow imaging. *Phys Med Biol* 1984;29:891–5.
30. Underwood SR, Firmin DN, Klipstein RH, Rees RSO, Longmore DB. Magnetic resonance velocity mapping: clinical application of a new technique. *Br Heart J* 1987;57:404–12.
31. Kilner PJ, Firmin DN, Rees RSO, Martinez J, Pennell DJ, Mohiaddin RH, et al. Valve and great vessel stenosis: assessment with magnetic resonance jet velocity mapping. *Radiology* 1991;178:229–35.
32. Karwatowski SP, Mohiaddin RH, Yang GZ, Firmin DN, St John Sutton M, Underwood SR, Longmore DB. Assessment of regional left ventricular long-axis motion with MR velocity mapping in normal subjects. *J Magn Res Imag* 1994;4:151–5.
33. Pennell DJ, Underwood SR, Ell PJ, Swanton RH, Walker MJ, Longmore DB. Dipyridamole magnetic resonance imaging: a comparison with thallium-201 emission tomography. *Br Heart J* 1990; 64:362–9.
34. Mohiaddin RH, Underwood SR, Bogren HG, Firmin DN, Klipstein RH, Rees RSO, Longmore DB. Regional aortic compliance studies by magnetic resonance imaging: the effects of age, training, and coronary artery disease. *Br Heart J* 1989;62:90–6.
35. Forbat SM, Naoumova RP, Sidhu PS, Neuwith C, MacMahon M, Thompson GR, Underwood SR. The effect of cholesterol reduction with fluvastatin on aortic compliance, coronary calcification and carotid intimal-medial thickness: a pilot study. *J Cardiovascular Risk* 1998;5:1–10.
36. Mohiaddin RH, Firmin DN, Underwood SR, Abdulla AK, Klipstein RH, Rees RSO, Longmore DB. Chemical shift magnetic resonance imaging of human atheroma. *Br Heart J* 1989;62:81.
37. Gatehouse PD, Firmin DN, Collins S, Longmore DB. Real time blood flow imaging by spiral scan phase velocity mapping. *Magn Reson Med* 1994;31:504–12.
38. Seymour AM, Bailey IA, Radda GK. A protective effect of insulin on reperfusing the ischaemic rat heart shown using 31P-NMR. *Biochim Biophys Acta* 1983;762:525–30.
39. Ross BD, Radda GK, Gadian DG, Rocker G, Esiri M, Falconer-Smith J. Examination of a case of suspected McArdle's syndrome by 31P. *N Engl J Med* 1981;304:1338–42.
40. Bottomley PA, Herfkens RJ, Smith LS, Brazzamano S, Blinder R, Hedlund LW, et al. Noninvasive detection and monitoring of regional myocardial ischemia in situ using depth-resolved 31P NMR spectroscopy. *Proc Natl Acad Sci USA* 1985;82:8747–51.
41. Edelman RR, Manning W, Burstein D, Paulin S. Coronary arteries: breath-hold MR angiography. *Radiology* 1991;181:641–3.
42. Wilke N, Simm C, Zhang J, Ellermann J, Ya X, Merkle H, et al. Contrast-enhanced first pass myocardial perfusion imaging: correlation between myocardial blood flow in dogs at rest and during hyperemia. *Magn Reson Med* 1993;29:485–97.
43. Pennell DJ, Keegan J, Firmin DN, Gatehouse PD, Underwood SR, Longmore DB. Magnetic resonance imaging of coronary arteries: technique and preliminary results. *Br Heart J* 1993;70:315–26.
44. Neubauer S, Revel D, Deroos A, Vanrossum AC, Vonschulthess GK, Sechtem U, et al. Task force report: the clinical role of magnetic resonance in cardiovascular disease. *Eur Heart J* 1998; 19: 19–39.
45. Hetherington HP, Luney DJE, Vaughan JT, Pan JW, Ponder SL, et al. 3D P-31 spectroscopic imaging of the human heart at 4.1T. *Magn Reson Med* 1995;33:427–31.

Chapter 14

The Development of Cardiac Ultrasound

Stewart Hunter

I am not sure who coined the term "echocardiography." Echo was a Greek nymph who fell in love with a beautiful youth called Narcissus. Her love was unrequited. Narcissus, gazing into a pool in the forest, fell in love with his own reflection and had no eyes for the adoring Echo. She pined and eventually disappeared, leaving only her voice, repeating words spoken by others. This classical myth always seems to me to be appropriate for a technique that sometimes is as much art as science. Used carefully, it is a technique that appeals to clinicians because it can be repeated as frequently as necessary during the clinical course of a cardiac illness and does not necessitate moving the patient to the machine. Although modern technology has greatly enhanced the diagnostic capability of ultrasound, the physics still imposes limits, and even with today's sophisticated techniques, echocardiography still depends more than most diagnostic methods on the operator's skill and experience.

Beginnings

As Peter Wells (one of the earlier echocardiographers in the United Kingdom) stated in a potted history of ultrasound, the importance of sound waves was known long before echocardiography – "everyone already knew that it was the sound of trumpets that destroyed the walls of Jericho and that bats, although blind, navigate by inaudible sound."[1] Indeed, the properties of sound within the cavities of the body had already been used by clinicians for many years when they percussed the chest, introducing sound waves whose pitch depended on the tissues through which they passed.

Edler and Herz

In scientific development, new techniques and advances are often spurred on by the needs of the military. There is a story (possibly apocryphal) of a French scientist who bombarded a ship moored off the coast of France with underwater sound waves. The ship appeared impervious to the bombardment but the surface of the water nearby was covered with stunned and dead fish. Whatever the truth of this tale, the development of ultrasound in cardiological practice was truly a European affair. Most texts refer to Edler and Herz whose descriptions of reflections from the heart were achieved by the earliest M mode echocardiography in 1954.[2] Using an ultrasound "reflectoscope" designed to discover metal weakness, they studied first the isolated heart and then live patients. Edler's first echoes from the anterior mitral valve were misinterpreted initially as coming from the wall of the heart. It was 10 years before the Swedish results were reproduced elsewhere in the world, despite the fact that several well known clinicians (among them Paul Wood) visited Sweden and had demonstrations of the new technique.

M mode echocardiography

A technological advance was responsible for the establishment of M mode echocardiography as a clinically useful tool. Echocardiograms were initially recorded on photographic paper. The introduction of fibreoptic strip chart recorders led to a sudden popularity of M mode for diagnosing valvar pathology and for the assessment of ventricular function. In the early 1970s, M mode machines of increasing sophistication began to be found in teaching hospitals through the United Kingdom.

Early British workers

Operators of M mode machines came from a number of backgrounds. Peter Wells already active in Doppler ultrasound was a physicist; Ron Pridie at the Hammersmith and later at Harefield was a cardiac radiologist; Graham Leech was an engineer working in the cardiology department of St George's Hospital; Derek Gibson was a cardiologist working in adult practice at the Brompton Hospital; and I was a paediatric cardiologist working in the Freeman Hospital. The different origins of the early workers were both a strength and a weakness in the development of cardiac ultrasound. It was useful to have a multi-disciplinary input, but for many years the development of regional and district services through the United Kingdom remained a patchy and incomplete process.

Looking back, the impact of echocardiography on clinical practice was remarkable considering how primitive the machines and the techniques were. The great strength of the M mode technique was – and is – the huge amount of information provided in unit time from a small circumscribed part of the heart. I remember very elegant demonstrations using M mode and strip chart recorders of the normal and abnormal function of a mechanical valve made by Graham Leech at St George's Hospital. About the same time, Derek Gibson at the Brompton Hospital was using M mode to perform detailed examination of left ventricular function in health and disease with a sophistication which is hardly matched even in these days of high resolution cross sectional echocardiography and tissue harmonics.[3]

Developments in the 1970s and 1980s

Serendipity always plays a part in the development of a technique. Contrast echocardiography, using various media including the patient's own blood, had been used in the early 1970s in the United States, but it failed to make a great clinical impact. Quite by chance, a young research worker in our own department, Carlos Mortera (now of Barcelona), was undertaking an M mode echocardiogram on a baby while the registrar flushed a peripheral venous line with dextrose saline. The contrast effect produced on the M mode echocardiogram was so dramatic that we started to use peripheral venous injection of dextrose to demonstrate intracardiac and extracardiac shunting and abnormalities of cardiac connection such as transposition of the great arteries with great success.[4] Contrast has now a much wider use in the assessment of myocardial perfusion and segmental function.

From 1975 onwards, Ron Pridie and I ran a bi-annual training course because there was great interest in the technique and a need for formal training. The first few meetings were small and quite contentious gatherings of lecturers and tutors who argued about the findings on the scans. Since the technique was still developing, we tried to include everything that was new and different. Doppler ultrasound had been around for some time but there was not much communication between the M mode echocardiographers and the Doppler ultrasonographers. Dan Tunstall Pedoe arrived and taught in a "Doppler session" during our echo courses, but in truth we were blind to the great value of this technique.

Doppler

Doppler ultrasound only started to take its rightful place in cardiac diagnosis following the work of Dr Liv Hatle and her colleagues in Norway. The ability to characterise stenotic lesions of the mitral and aortic valve using Doppler significantly reduced the need for invasive investigation in the adult population.[5][6]

Linear array and sector scanners

We greeted Klaas Bom's linear array, which he developed in Rotterdam in 1972 and demonstrated in our echo course, similarly – with interest but some scepticism.[7] Linear arrays are after all not ideal for peering between ribs. Nonetheless, this technique afforded the opportunity for looking at the whole heart and its function in a way that M mode could not. Within a very short time technology had overtaken us with the development in North America of the sector scanner, the phased array and duplex scanning heads which brought the two ultrasound techniques together finally. Thus, just as

M mode echocardiography had achieved acceptability as a clinical tool, it was pushed back into a subsidiary (although still useful) facility as the combined advances of sector scanning and Doppler ultrasound became available. The new echo machines did not immediately appear in every cardiological unit in the United Kingdom. They were very much more expensive than M mode machines and were therefore initially much more often found in radiology departments.

Cross sectional echocardiography and the increasing sophistication of the equipment allowed very different sorts of clinical practice to benefit from ultrasound. Len Shapiro in Cambridge studied the pathophysiology of ventricular hypertrophy and cardiomyopathy highlighting the potential similarities between idiopathic and secondary disease of the myocardium and the athlete's heart.[8]

Importance in paediatric cardiology

The combination of cross sectional scans with Doppler (particularly colour flow mapping) was avidly seized upon by paediatric cardiologists. More than any other branch of cardiology, the new techniques radically altered clinical practice. Paediatric cardiologists were able to spend more time in their beds at night, as it was not necessary to catheterise every new sick neonate admitted as an emergency. Even balloon septostomy for transposition of the great arteries could be carried out in special care baby units under ultrasonic control. Paediatric cardiologists in the United Kingdom produced a series of elegant comparative studies proving that in many ways ultrasound was not just an alternative technique but the best technique for investigating congenital malformations. This group including Michael Godman from Edinburgh, Geoff Smallhorn and Michael Rigby from London, George Sutherland and myself in Newcastle were greatly helped by the radical new approach to morphology and nomenclature of congenital heart anomalies promulgated by Bob Anderson from the Royal Brompton Hospital.[9]

If we could diagnose congenital heart disease in babies, why not in fetuses? The first fetal cardiological service was established and developed by Lindsay Allan working at Kings and Guy's Hospitals.[10] The implications of this development may be very significant in the long run as more and more complex congenital heart disease is recognised at an early gestational period, allowing the parents the possibility of termination of pregnancy.

Transoesophageal echo

Although ultrasound has always been sold as a non-invasive technique, it was not really surprising that it should be delivered from the end of an endoscope to study the heart via the oesophagus. Most of the early development of this transoesophageal echo was in Japan. Many of us learned the technique from Peter Hanrath in Germany or Jos Roelandt in Rotterdam. European development of transoesophageal echo was ahead of the United Kingdom. In the 1980s, I visited the Thorax Center in Rotterdam to study transoesophageal echo and was amazed to see that each of their cardiac theatres had dedicated echocardiography during every cardiac operation.

Ultrasound's role in cardiology

I think it is reasonable to claim that ultrasound has altered the practice of cardiology as much as any other technique. Today's cardiologists in training must be practised in, and conversant with, all aspects of echocardiography. Many cardiac technicians in the United Kingdom now specialise in echocardiography. In this again we differ from our European colleagues, In Europe, echocardiographers are much more likely to be clinicians rather than technicians or technologists probably for monetary reasons! In Britain, adult cardiologists have been slow to superspecialise in cardiac ultrasound. The practice of echocardiography is so time consuming and complex that in all large cardiological units there should be a consultant dedicated to providing a fully comprehensive ultrasound service, without a commitment to invasive work.

The next millennium

Arguably, the most common requirement for echocardiographers is to assess left ventricular function – the cardiological "staff of life". While cardiologists may still argue about the best index of ventricular function, the physician wants to know whether clinical appearances of cardiac decompensation are confirmed ultrasonically. Open echocardiography clinics are now quite widespread in the United Kingdom, with echo technicians once again providing an important service commitment.

For a period in the 1980s, Organon Technical made a small hand-held real time scanner. It was never successful, probably because it did not produce a particularly sophisticated image. The future must include portable bedside scanners capable of performing a triage function. We are already seeing the development of three dimensional reconstructions of the heart which seem likely to give valuable information to the clinician, particularly in valvar and congenital heart disease. Our images are now being enhanced using tissue harmonics, and there are other new techniques for handling Doppler information. We will, I think, continue look to North America and Japan for technological improvement.

Where we excel in the United Kingdom is in the clinical evaluation of the newer techniques and the teaching and training which we are now providing on an organised national basis. An important development was the foundation of the British Society of Echocardiography. It mirrors echocardiography in the United Kingdom, as it is a multidisciplinary organisation quite unlike the older colleges and societies. Members come from the ranks of cardiologists, radiologists, technologists, and representatives of the ultrasound manufacturers and allied professions. Training for technicians at least is now regulated on a national basis. When the organisation was set up in 1990, we were aware of the unfortunate similarity of our initials to a potential health problem for the nation's cattle. We stuck with BSE confident that the British Society of Echocardiography would be around long after bovine spongiform encephalopathy had become an item in the history books. We are still hopeful.

References and notes

1. Wells PT. History and development. In: Roelandt JRTC, Sutherland GR, Iliceto S, Linker DT, eds. *Cardiac ultrasound.* Edinburgh: Churchill Livingstone, 1993.
2. Edler I, Hertz CH. *The use of the ultrasonic reflectoscope for the continuous recording of the movements of the heart wall.* Fovhaulingav: Kungl Fysiografiska, Sallskapets I Lund, 1954:24, 40.
3. Gibson DF, Brown DJ. Assessment of left ventricular systolic function in man from simultaneous echocardiographic and pressure measurements. *Br Heart J* 1976;38:8–17.
4. Mortera C, Hunter S, Tynan M. Contrast echocardiography and the suprasternal approach in infants and children. *Eur J Cardiol* 1979;9:437–54.
5. Hatle L, Brubakk A, Tromsdal A, Angelsen B. Non invasive assessment of pressure drop in mitral stenosis by Doppler ultrasound. *Br Heart J* 1978;40:131–40.
6. Hatle L, Angelsen B, Tromsdal A. Non-invasive assessment of aortic stenosis by Doppler ultrasound. *Br Heart J* 1980;43:284–92.
7. Bom N. *New concepts in echocardiography.* Leiden: Stenfevr Kvoese 1972.
8. Shapiro LM, McKenna WJ. Distribution of left ventricular hypertrophy in hypertrophic cardiomyopathy: a two dimensional echocardiographic study. *J Am Coll Cardiology* 1983;2:437–44.
9. Silverman NH, Hunter S, Anderson RH, Ho SY, Sutherland GR, Davis MJ. Anatomical basis of cross sectional echocardiography. *Br Heart J* 1983;50:421.
10. Allan LD, Tynan MJ, Campbell S, Wilkinson J, Anderson RH. Echocardiographic and anatomical correlates in the fetus. *Br Heart J* 1980;44:444.

Chapter 15

Prevention of Heart Disease

Ross Lorimer

The prevention of heart disease in Britain received little attention in the first part of the century because of the scourge of infectious diseases. Treatment was essentially symptomatic since accurate diagnosis and the classification of disease entities were in their infancy. In the United States, by contrast, the leading American cardiologist Paul Dudley White wrote a paper in 1922 entitled "The diagnosis of heart disease, with especial reference to its importance in prevention".[1] In the 1951 edition of his textbook, *Heart disease*, White wrote, "By the early 1920s, the present day fundamental classification of cardiac diagnosis based primarily on aetiology had been well established. The major importance of this step was indicated not only by better diagnosis and treatment but especially by the directing of attention to the causes of heart disease, the elucidation of which will undoubtedly lead to effective preventive medicine, so much more important in the final analysis than research, interesting though it is, in abnormal physiology, and in therapy, both medical and surgical."[2] A review of White's work, published in 1973, included the statement "preventive medicine is the aim of every clear thinking physician who has the welfare of the race in his mind."[3]

The prevalence of the different forms of heart disease has changed remarkably over the years. In 1956, Davidson noted that coronary atheroma and hypertension had become the principal causes of heart disease in middle and old age.[4] Rheumatic fever was by far the commonest cause of heart disease in childhood, adolescence, and early adult life, but its incidence was falling. The approximate incidence of each form of heart disease seen in hospital practice in the Britain at that time is given in table 1.

Rheumatic heart disease

Those practising cardiology at this time were all too familiar with acute rheumatic fever and its consequences (see also chapter 23). Today, rheumatic fever has gone, and mitral stenosis is a rarity except in the immi-

Table 1 Approximate incidence of each form of heart disease seen in hospital practice in the early 1950s

Form	Proportion (%)
Ischaemic heart disease (coronary atheroma) and hypertensive heart disease	55
Rheumatic heart disease	25
Pulmonary heart disease (higher in industrial areas)	5
Thyrotoxic heart disease	3
Syphilitic heart disease	3
Others	6

grant population. Physicians cannot claim all the credit for curtailing this epidemic – medicine may have played a small part compared with environmental change. Social and economic factors are of primary importance in the aetiology of rheumatic fever. Improved housing, sanitation, and nutrition have reduced the spread of infection. The prompt treatment of upper respiratory infections, especially with penicillin, was important in reducing the consequences of haemolytic streptococcal infections.

Bywaters and Thomas reviewed the treatment of acute rheumatic fever and the prevention of recurrences in 1958.[5] Prophylaxis had first been introduced using sulphonamide drugs. These remained effective, but were gradually superseded by penicillin.[6] However, prophylaxis to reduce recurrences of rheumatic fever was not widely used until 1950, when the Royal College of Physicians of London recommended a 10-day course of penicillin (1.2 million units daily).[7]

Bywaters and Thomas had studied two comparable groups of rheumatic fever patients over five years.[8] Those seen in 1949–50 were not given prophylaxis while those presenting in 1950–1 were treated with sulphonamide. The incidences of recurrence per patient per year were 5.6% in the unprotected group and 1.2% in the treated group.

Why was prophylaxis not used sooner and with more enthusiasm in the United Kingdom? There was apathy and failure to appreciate its value and importance, and objections on the grounds of cost and the possible development of antibiotic resistance were raised. The work of Bywaters and Thomas showed that resistance was not a problem and that the drugs were cheap compared with the consequences of the disease.

Coronary heart disease

For many years "cardiologists" failed to recognise the possibility that coronary heart disease could be prevented – treatment aimed at symptom relief, but had little or no influence on prognosis. Efforts were concentrated on invasive investigation and treatment, although a few clinicians, epidemiologists, and biochemists were considering the potential of prevention. Things have now changed. Clinical and scientific evidence in primary and secondary prevention now supports the previously theoretical benefits of preventive measures. Moreover, it was once thought that a myocardial infarction ruled out measures to reduce recurrence or death since the major deterrent of prognosis was the extent of irreversible cardiac damage. Managing risk factors aggressively has now been shown to reduce mortality and morbidity.[9][10] The newer prevention programmes are multidisciplinary. Social circumstances and lifestyle and government policies have profound effects which are not always beneficial. Physicians participate but do not necessarily lead or control the programme. Nurses, physician's assistants, and paramedical groups all have a major role.

Inevitably fatal

Coronary thrombosis was well known in the 19th century, but until the report by McNee in 1925 it was largely regarded in Britain as inevitably fatal.[11] McNee (later Sir John McNee, but known as John Willy McNee to his colleagues in Glasgow, where he was professor of medicine) had seen three survivors of myocardial infarction during 1924–25, when he was working in Johns Hopkins University Hospital in Baltimore. He commented "embolism and thrombosis of large branches of the coronary arteries are everywhere recognised as causes of sudden death from myocardial infarction, but what requires emphasis is that, in the case of thrombosis at least, an immediate fatal issue does not always occur. On the contrary, patients who are presented with the symptoms and signs of thrombosis of a large branch may survive for years."[11]

The recognition that coronary thrombosis did not have to mean immediate death led to a worldwide interest in its diagnosis and management. Given the vital part played by interpretation of the electrocardiogram, it is somewhat ironic to read what McNee had to say about this. He wrote, "It is evident that there is no special electrocardiogram characteristic of coronary thrombosis, but many deviations from the normal may be found, and when grouped, they may with advancing experience have some localising significance and importance."

McCormick, in his 1975 review of Sir James Mackenzie's work, commented on the increased incidence and prevalence of coronary heart disease in the years after 1945.[12] McCormick believed that much had been written in terms that were highly emotional. He quoted Mackenzie as saying, "on going over my notes I find records of the deaths of 380 patients who had consulted me for attacks of angina pectoris. I have no doubt a great many have died whom I have not been able to trace."[13]

It was the role of risk factors for coronary heart disease that drew most attention in Britain. Cardiologists, with the notable exceptions of Michael Oliver in Edinburgh and Veitch Lawrie in Glasgow, were not in the forefront. Epidemiologists led the way.

Epidemiological studies

In 1954, Richard Doll and Austin Bradford Hill drew attention to the malign consequences of cigarette smoking.[14] At the end of 1951, some 40 000 men and women on the British medical register had replied to a simple questionnaire on smoking habits. Doll and Bradford Hill commented in their initial report that "although the number of deaths at present available is small, the resulting rates reveal a significant and steadily rising mortality from deaths due to cancer of the lung. There is also a rise in the mortality from death attributed to coronary thrombosis as the amount smoked increases."

Cholesterol and inactivity

Jeremy (Jerry) Morris, reviewing the aetiology of coronary heart disease in 1962, commented that coronary atherosclerosis involved two semi-independent processes – atheroma of the walls of the vessel and occlusion of the lumen.[15] He believed that it was occlusion of the lumen that was the main problem, since coronary atheroma was almost universal. What caused coronary thrombosis was a crucial question, since there was a persistent hope that changes in lifestyle might be able to control coronary occlusion and thus coronary heart disease. There was undoubtedly a role for cholesterol and a need to assess the value of a vegetable oil diet in men with a high cholesterol concentration.

Morris was also extremely concerned about the potential role of physical inactivity. His studies on London busmen showed that drivers in early middle age were three times as likely as conductors to die suddenly from coronary heart disease. Although the drivers were fatter overall, thin drivers still had a higher death rate than thin conductors.[16][17] Morris suggested that physical activity might be protective.

Stress

At this time, it was generally agreed that the increased incidence of coronary heart disease resulted partly from improved diagnosis in an ageing population and partly from changing patterns in death certification. However, much of the increase seemed to be real, and as the extent of atheroma did not seem greater, additional reasons had to be sought. Possibilities included an increased incidence of thrombosis, a disturbance of cholesterol metabolism, and the effects of stress. In addition, coronary heart disease was considered especially prevalent among executives and professionals rather than working class people and was related to disturbed endocrine function or autonomic control. This has now been disproved (figure 1).

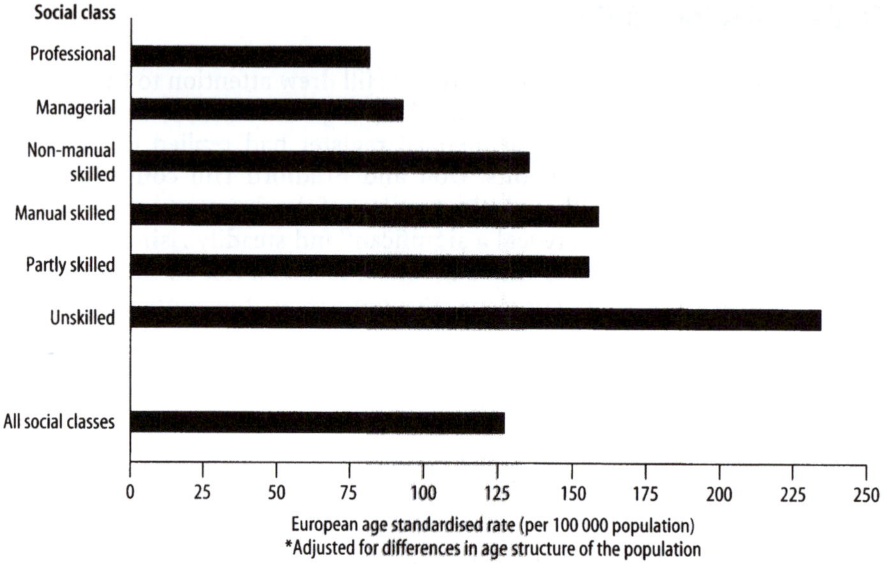

Figure 1 Mortality from coronary heart disease by social class in men aged 20–64 (England and Wales, 1991–3).

Genetic and environmental factors

In 1958, Bronte-Stewart concluded that although the serum cholesterol concentration and the nature of the dietary fat intake were closely related, the hypothesis that coronary heart disease resulted from a disturbance of fat metabolism was founded more on assumption than fact.[18] He felt that there was also an interplay of genetic and other environmental factors. The role of fat in the diet had considerable implications for animal husbandry, methods of food production, and food processing. The directing of food preferences and health education could well prevent or reduce coronary heart disease in the community.

Manipulating lipid concentrations

The possibility of lipid control as a preventive strategy now began to move on stage. In 1962, Oliver reviewed the importance of raised plasma lipid concentrations in prevention of coronary disease.[19] He asked two questions: will reducing raised plasma lipid concentrations to levels present in healthy individuals benefit patients or postpone or prevent coronary heart disease? and, what is the best way of correcting plasma lipid concentrations?

Changes in lipid patterns were related to age and sex. Plasma cholesterol, triglycerides, and phospholipid concentrations were often high in people developing coronary heart disease before the age of 40. The disease was rare in women before the menopause, but increased lipid concentrations and heart disease accompanied the menopause or premature oophorectomy. Epidemiological studies supported a relation between plasma lipids and coronary disease.[20] In terms of reducing plasma lipids, there was an implicit argument that the high intake of saturated fat could contribute to an increase in certain plasma lipids with detrimental effects both in terms of deposition in the arterial wall and increased thrombosis. Oliver pointed out that the suggestion that reducing lipid concentrations would prevent or reduce coronary heart disease was untested. Possible dietary measures were an increase in the intake of unsaturated fat and a low fat diet. An interesting conclusion was drawn from the study of oestrogen administration in men who had had a heart attack; there were no benefits in relation to mortality or morbidity. The comment was made that the continued reduction of plasma lipids would not improve prognosis once myocardial infarction had occurred.[20] Although this seems entirely logical, it has subsequently been proved wrong as secondary prevention has been shown to be effective. Oliver felt that pharmacological reduction of raised lipids would be valuable, but an effective agent was lacking until Imperial Chemical Industries developed Atromid S (ethyl-alpha-para-chlorophenoxyisobutyrate), which could lower triglyceride and cholesterol values and reduce platelet adhesiveness and plasma fibrinogen (see below).[21][22]

Work of Geoffrey Rose

No review of risk factors and possible prevention would be complete without emphasising the enormous contribution made by Geoffrey Rose and his colleagues at the London School of Tropical Medicine and Hygiene. Rose [23] was a brilliant advocate for clinical epidemiology and preventive medicine. In 1977, he and his colleagues reported on myocardial ischaemia, risk factors, and death from coronary heart disease.[24] The Whitehall study involved a five year follow up of 18 403 male civil servants aged 40–64, who were examined between 1967 and 1969. Altogether 277 died from coronary heart disease, and in half of these men, initial screening had suggested early myocardial ischaemia. At each level of the primary risk factors, the risk of death from coronary heart disease was much greater if ischaemia was suspected. The main risk factors still operated at the stage of early ischaemia. Quite rightly, the authors regarded that their findings had implications for studies of both primary and secondary prevention.

Importance of treating small risk

In 1986, Rose and Shipley published a further important paper on plasma cholesterol concentrations and death rates from coronary heart disease.[25] This paper pointed out that the treatment of a small risk affecting many was more important in terms of benefit than treating a large risk in a few. These authors reported that the 10 year mortality in 17 718 middle aged men was related to their initial plasma cholesterol concentration. The risk gradient was continuous over the whole range of cholesterol concentration; the lowest mortality being in men with concentrations below the lowest decile. It seemed, as with blood pressure, that the average cholesterol concentration on the population was too high. The lower the concentration, the better the prognosis would be. Although 25% of all deaths from coronary heart disease occurred in men whose concentrations were in the top decile, 55% occurred in men with concentrations in the middle three fifths of the distribution and these deaths could be reduced only by a policy aimed at lowering concentrations in the whole population.

Hard water

In the early 1960s, there was interest in an association between the hardness of drinking water and cardiovascular disease. Morris, Crawford, and Heady, in 1961, found striking negative correlations between water hardness and cardiovascular mortality in 83 county boroughs in England and Wales.[26] The British regional heart study was set up in 1975 to assess the role of water quality in determining regional variations in cardiovascular mortality, and also to determine the extent to which other risk factors could account for the regional variations. The first phase of the study related cardiovascular mortality to a variety of potential risk factors including drinking water quality, climate, air pollution, and socioeconomic factors in 253 British towns.[27] The highest mortality was in the west of Scotland, and the lowest in the south east of England. Cardiovascular mortality in areas with very soft water was estimated to be 10%–15% per cent higher than in the areas with medium hard water while any further increase in hardness had no effect on mortality. There was no increase in cardiovascular mortality in 13 towns which had deliberately softened their water supply. The report concluded that there was no immediate need for action regarding water supplies that were naturally soft. The potential risks from smoking, hypertension, and hypercholesterolaemia were regarded as far greater than the risk from drinking soft water.

British regional heart study

In 1981, Shaper et al. reported on the second phase of their British regional heart study.[28] They had measured cardiovascular risk factors in 7735 middle aged men in 24 towns throughout Britain and found that cardiovascular mortality was associated with systolic blood pressure, years of cigarette smoking, and heavy alcohol consumption. No relation was seen for serum cholesterol, possibly because of the small range of mean total cholesterol values. Cigarette smoking and alcohol consumption were related to the social class. Shaper et al. commented on the previous view that working class men had lower rates of coronary heart disease than men in non-manual occupations. In 1941, Price had written in his popular textbook that "Angina pectoris is much more common in those classes of society who are subject to exercise mental or emotional stress or strain, being relatively uncommon in those whose occupation is of a manual character."[29]

Social class differences

In 1981, Rose and Marmot commented that over the past 40 years in England and Wales, the rise in mortality from coronary heart disease had continued unabated among working class men, while it had changed little for 20 years in professional men.[30] Consequence, mortality from coronary heart disease was 26% higher in social class V than I. The difference between social classes was even higher in women – 152%. The social gradient for men was confirmed in Rose and Marmot's survey of 18 403 London civil servants aged between 40 and 64. When men in the lower employment grades were compared with those in the top, the age adjusted prevalence rate was 53% higher for angina. After seven and half years of follow up, coronary mortality was 3.6 times higher in the lower than in the top grades. The difference was partly explained by known coronary risk factors such as smoking, blood pressure, and exercise but much of it remained unexplained.

Prevalence

The prevalence of coronary heart disease was determined as part of the British regional heart study of men aged 40–59.[31] Overall, a quarter had some evidence of coronary heart disease. On questionnaire, 14% had possible myocardial infarction or angina but there was considerable overlap of the syndromes. Electrocardiographic evidence of coronary heart disease was present in approximately 15%, many of whom had had no symptoms. This national population study indicated that the prevalence of coronary disease in middle aged men was greater than previously thought. The apparently high prevalence should be considered along with the report of Rose et al.[32] Using their standard questionnaire, they had interviewed 1136 men in 1961 and re-interviewed 995 of them in 1962. The prevalence rates for angina were 3.3% in 1961 and 3.4% in 1962. Approximately half of those with angina in 1961 did not have angina in 1962 and half of those with angina in 1962 had not complained of this in 1961. However, men with consistently positive answers or those who had one positive answer were more likely to have electrocardiographic changes. In the study of Shaper et al., subjects were asked whether a doctor had ever told them they had any form of cardiovascular disease.[33] Only 50% of those with electrocardiographic evidence of myocardial infarction had recall. Indeed, only one in five of those regarded as having ischaemic heart disease were able to recall such a diagnosis, suggesting that ischaemic heart disease is common but that most of those affected seem to be unaware of it.

Isles and colleagues studied the relation between coronary risk and coronary mortality in Renfrew and Paisley (urban areas in the west of Scotland).[34] Their longitudinal survey included 15 399 subjects (8362 women), who were aged between 45–64 years when first examined between 1972 and 1976. The 15-year coronary heart disease mortality was related to plasma cholesterol, cigarette smoking, diastolic blood pressure, and low social class. In women, the absolute risk was less in that, for a given risk factor, women with a high individual risk generally had a lower coronary mortality than men with low risk. Thus, women with a cholesterol concentration above 7.2 mmol/l were at a lower risk of coronary heart disease than men with cholesterol values below 5.0 mmol/l. Trends were similar for blood pressure, smoking, and social class. Their conclusions included the important one that the threshold for introducing cholesterol lowering treatment might be higher in women than in men.

The changing situation with regard to coronary heart disease in Scotland and Northern Ireland was further examined by Tunstall-Pedoe et al. as part of the World Health Organization (WHO) MONICA project.[35] This study, which began in the mid-1980s, registered coronary events in 25–64 year old residents of north Glasgow and Belfast, and confirmed the fall in coronary events and mortality.

Prevention

The studies on prevalence and the importance of risk factors led to work on the effect of reducing risk factors – work that focused particularly on primary prevention at first. Studies were undertaken nationally and in Europe. Kornitzer and Rose, in 1985, reported results from a trial of multifactorial prevention of coronary heart disease in occupational groups.[36] This involved randomising 49 781 men employed in 66 factories in Britian, Italy, Belgium, and Poland to control and intervention groups. The average reduction in the intervention factors were 1.2% for plasma cholesterol, 8.9% in daily cigarette consumption, 2% in systolic blood pressure, and 11% for a combined risk estimate. There was an overall reduction of 7.4% in fatal coronary heart disease and a 2.7% reduction in total deaths. The benefits were greater in centres achieving larger reductions in risk factors, and in one country (Belgium) the net decrease in heart disease incidence and total deaths was significant at the 5% level. The conclusion was an important one – that risk in middle aged men is reducible by simple and cost effective means.

By this time, the possibility of preventing or postponing the onset of the disease was being recognised. An important conference took place at Canterbury in 1983.[37] This was to consider practical ways in which the WHO recommendations on the prevention of coronary heart disease could be implemented in the United Kingdom.[36] The conference was sponsored by many governmental, professional, industrial, and charitable organisations. Those taking part had wide ranging expertise in such areas as national policy, food and agriculture, health care, and health education. Geoffrey Rose was the conference chairman. The recommendations included:

- Establishment of a national strategy for the prevention of coronary heart disease. This should be promoted and coordinated by national organisations including the Royal Colleges, the Cardiac Society and Health Education Councils. The body created as a result of this recommendation is now called the National Heart Forum.
- Improved training in prevention.
- Production of healthy foods to be encouraged.
- Better control of smoking.

In 1987, a working party of the British Cardiac Society produced its first report on the prevention of coronary heart disease.[38]

Lipid lowering

In the late 1970s and early 1980s, the goal of primary prevention of coronary heart disease by lipid lowering therapy was being pursued with enthusiasm in Europe and in the United States.[39][40] The studies showed that lowering cholesterol concentrations in middle aged men could reduce the incidence of myocardial infarction but were unable to show an effect of treatment on total mortality. Indeed there were concerns that the risk of death from non-cardiovascular causes might be increased by treatment.[40] The use of fibrates declined but the introduction of a new class of more effective lipid lowering drugs, 3-hydroxy-3-methylglutaryl - coenzyme reductase inhibitors - provided an enormous impetus to the direction, investigation, and management of coronary heart disease. In terms of secondary prevention, these compounds were shown dramatically to reduce the incidence of coronary death in men who had sustained a previous myocardial infarction or who had angina pectoris.[10]

The role of lipid lowering in primary prevention was clarified by the west of Scotland study of coronary prevention (WOSCOPS) published in 1995.[9] (See also chapter 26.) This study was designed to establish whether the administration of pravastatin to men with raised cholesterol concentrations and no history of myocardial infarction reduced the incidence of deaths from coronary heart disease plus non-fatal myocardial infarction. Altogether 6595 men aged 45–64 with a mean plasma cholesterol concnetration of 7.0 mmol/l were randomly assigned to receive placebo or pravastatin (40 mg daily). The average follow up time was 4.9 years. Pravastatin was found to lower plasma cholesterol by 20% and low density lipoprotein cholesterol by 26%. There were 248 definite coronary events in the placebo group and 174 in the pravastatin treated group. The relative reduction in risk was 31% ($P < 0.001$). There was a 22% reduction overall in the risk of death from any cause. Treatment was associated with a comparable reduced frequency of coronary angiography and revascularisation procedures.

The British Cardiac Society undertook a survey of the potential for the secondary prevention of coronary disease in 1996.[41] It found that risk factors were recorded incompletely in hospital records. The review found 10–27% of patients were still smoking and 75% remained overweight. Up

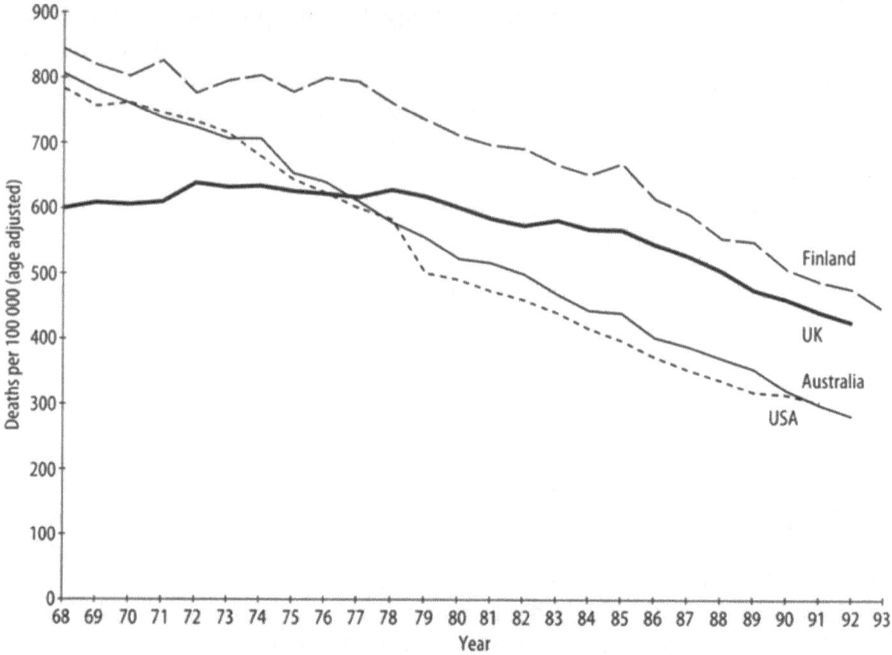

Figure 2 Death rates from coronary heart disease in men aged 35–74 in selected countries (1968–93).

to 25% remained hypertensive and more than 75% had a cholesterol concentration of more than 5.2 mmol/l. The potential for improvement was thus considerable.

Decreasing mortality from coronary heart disease

Deaths from coronary heart disease in the United Kingdom peaked in the mid-1970s and have been decreasing steadily ever since (figures 2 and 3). In men aged between 35 and 74, the age standardised death rate per 100 000 fell by 50%, from 554 in 1974 to 276 in 1997.[42] Comparable figures for women were 184 and 100. Although, at one time, coronary disease was considered an affliction of professionals and business men, it is now much more common in unskilled and manual workers.

Capewell and colleagues assessed the contribution of modern cardiovascular treatment and changes in risk factors to the decline in coronary deaths in Scotland between 1975 and 1994.[43] There were 15 234 deaths from coronary heart disease in 1994. In 1994, the total number of deaths prevented or postponed was estimated at 6747. Forty per cent of this benefit was attributed to treatment and 51% to measurable risk factor reduction.

Both primary and secondary prevention have thus been shown to have a definite role. There has been a sea change in our view of prevention of coronary heart disease. Since the successful Canterbury conference in 1983,

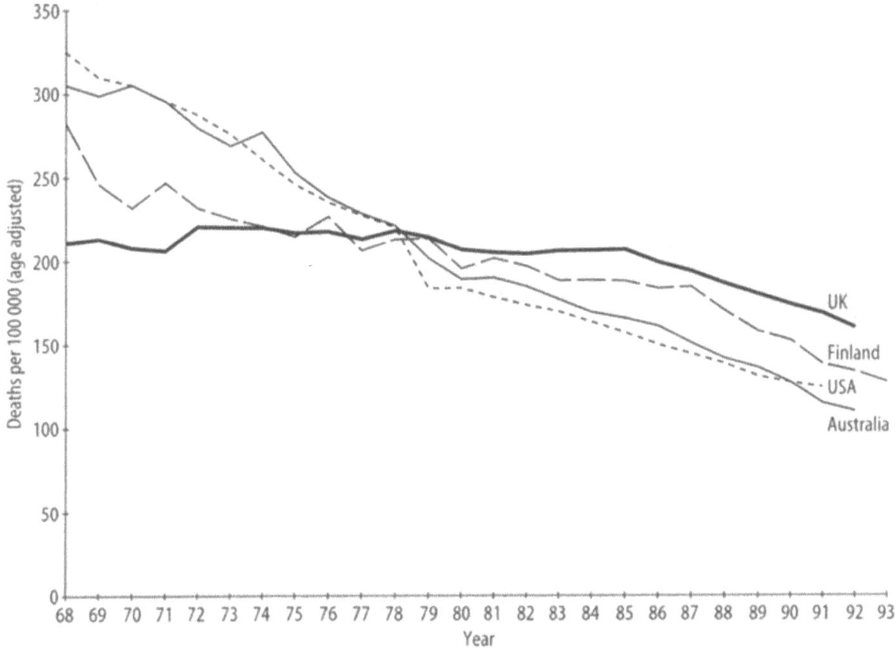

Figure 3 Death rates from coronary heart disease in women aged 35–74 in selected countries (1968–93).

new studies have been done and much more new information has accrued. Effective intervention both for the population as a whole and for high risk groups has become established on the basis of scientific evidence. The agenda is national and multifactorial.

Continuing further decline in mortality and morbidity requires changes in the lifestyle of the community at large and implementation of the primary and secondary prevention measures that are the responsibility of health-care professionals. These efforts need to be coordinated which is why the National Heart Forum, an alliance of over 40 national organisations concerned with the prevention of coronary heart disease has been set up. Its members are drawn from the health services, professional bodies, consumer groups, and voluntary organisations. Its report *Looking to the future* contributes substantially in pointing the way to making coronary heart disease an epidemic of the past.[44]

Hypertension

The importance of hypertension (see also chapter 25) has not always been recognised. Thus, Osler, in concluding an address to the Southern Medical Society of Glasgow in 1911, said "Don't let anyone take your blood pressure."[45] I suspect and hope that this was said more in jest than in seriousness. In 1956, Davidson stated that coronary atheroma and hypertension were the principal causes of heart disease in middle age men.[4] Their incidences were increasing, and were contributory factors in about 55% of patients admitted to hospital with heart disease.

High blood pressure was generally considered as benign, "essential," and associated with the ageing process. However, its importance was appreciated by Pickering.[46] He pointed out that, although cancer and cardiovascular disease were predominantly affections of an ageing population, they often struck people down at their most productive period. High blood pressure posed a twofold challenge to medicine – what could be done to prevent it and to mitigate its effects if it existed already? Pickering believed that successful treatment demanded a clear appreciation of what it should and could achieve. Treatment aimed to prolong life and encourage a sense of wellbeing, objectives that were often in conflict. Pickering pointed out that past treatment of hypertension had been based on the negation of the scientific method called clinical pharmacology – treatment regimens in humans had been developed from studies that often used anaesthetised animals and therefore inappropriate drug dosages. Pickering questioned whether treatment of hypertension had so far increased life expectancy, but believed that it had certainly made it more difficult for patients to experience any "joie de vivre." He suggested that the rice diet prescribed in the MRC study (which contained less than 250 mg of salt per day) would certainly lower the blood pressure but also "disrupted social relations and was insipid and unappetising." Fortunately, help was at hand from the pharmaceutical industry. Methyldopa, thiazide diuretics, β adrenoceptor blockers meant that controlling blood pressure no longer required an intolerable lifestyle.

Salt restriction

Salt restriction as a treatment for hypertension has been considered for some time but remains controversial. The diet advocated by Kempner in 1948 was very low in sodium. It was a drastic and unpalatable regimen, which lowered the blood pressure, but not for long since long term compliance was by and large impossible. In 1983, Watt et al. reported that salt restriction had little effect on blood pressure, and was unlikely to be relevant in managing hypertension in general practice.[47] However, it is now agreed that salt intake in Britain has been far too high.

Tudor Hart, working in a rural Welsh practice, early realised that the detection and management of hypertension was best undertaken in the community.[48] He showed that by additional effort directed towards ensuring that all adults had their blood pressure recorded, the considerable number of people whose hypertension had previously been undiagnosed could be identified. In 1984, Tudor Hart wrote that a major attack on the main risk factors of coronary heart disease was essential in order to control it; in general practice, there was a real opportunity to control high blood pressure and smoking.[48]

Once again, Rose and his colleagues made an important contribution.[49] They compared systolic and diastolic blood pressures as predictors of death from coronary heart disease, using data on the 10 year mortality in the Whitehall study. Contrary to previous beliefs, systolic blood pressure at entry was a greater risk for coronary disease than was diastolic pressure.

Effects of treatment

The Medical Research Council set out to assess the effect of treatment in patients with mild idiopathic hypertension.[50] The study aimed to find out whether bendrofluazide or propranolol would improve life expectancy and reduce morbidity in patients aged 35 with mild to moderate hypertension (90–109 mmHg diastolic). Most of the 17 534 patients were recruited through group general practices. They were randomly allocated to bendrofluazide, propranolol, or placebo. Bendrofluazide seemed to be more effective than propranolol in reducing stroke, and propranolol but not bendrofluazide was associated with a reduction in myocardial infarction. The trial showed that 850 mildly hypertensive patients had to be treated for one year to prevent one stroke. The Medical Research Council concluded that such a policy of active intervention on a national scale would not justify the costs incurred. However, the position has changed. Large numbers of patients have been followed for longer times. We now know that just a few years of blood pressure lowering is effective in reducing the proportion of strokes and, although to a lesser extent, coronary heart disease events. In 17 trials of drug treatments, involving almost 50 000 individuals, and with mean follow up of 4.9 years, the average treatment reduced diastolic blood pressure by 5–6 mmHg was associated both with highly significant reductions in fatal and non-fatal stroke (38%) and fatal and non-fatal heart attacks (16%).[51]

In conclusion

Prevention has come a long way – no longer derided, its potential has been realised and accepted. Collaboration between specialties rather than isolationism has developed. The practice of evidence based medicine has brought together the British Cardiac Society, the British Hyperlipidaemia Association, and the British Hypertension Society, who, together with the British Diabetic Association, have published recommendations on prevention of coronary heart disease in clinical practice which provide a firm basis for use in primary and secondary care.[52]

We now have evidence of benefit in primary prevention and we now have effective treatment that can change risk factor levels. For patients with no clinical atherosclerotic disease, the possibility of reducing the absolute risk of developing coronary heart disease should strongly influence their lifestyle and possibly therapeutic intervention.

References and notes

1. White PD. The diagnosis of heart disease, with especial reference to its importance in preventive medicine. *Boston Med Surg J*, 1922;186:34–8.
2. White PD. *Heart disease*. 4th ed. New York: McMillan Co, 1951.
3. White PD. The early infancy of preventive cardiology. *Am Clin Climatol Soc* 1973;84:17–21.
4. Davidson LSP. Diseases of the cardiovascular system. In: *Principles and practice of medicine*. 3rd ed. Edinburgh, Livingston, 1956:57.
5. Bywaters EGL, Thomas GT. Prevention of rheumatic fever recurrences. *BMJ* 1958;2:350.
6. Perry CB, Gillespie WA. Intramuscular benzathine penicillin in the prophylaxis of streptococcal infection in rheumatic children. *BMJ* 1954;1:729–30.
7. Rheumatic Fever Committee of the Royal College of Physicians. *Further report*. London: Royal College of Physicians, 1957.
8. Bywaters EGL, Thomas GT. Treatment and prevention of rheumatic fever. In: Jones AM, ed. *Modern trends in cardiology*. London: Butterworths, 1961:100–114.
9. Shepherd J, Cobbe SM, Ford I, Isles CG, Lorimer AR, MacFarlane PW, et al. Prevention of coronary heart disease with pravastatin in men with hypercholesterolaemia. *N Engl J Med* 1995;333:1301–7.
10. Scandinavian Simvastatin Survival Study Group. Randomised trial of cholesterol lowering in 4444 patients with coronary heart disease: the Scandinavian simvastatin survival study. *Lancet* 1994;344:1383–89.
11. McNee JW. The clinical syndrome of thrombosis of the coronary arteries. *Q J Med*;44:1925.
12. McCormick J. James Mackenzie lecture. Fifty years of progress. *Practitioner* 1975;214:87–97.
13. MacKenzie J. *Angina pectoris*. Oxford: Medical Publications, 1923.
14. Doll R, Hill AB. The mortality of doctors in relation to their smoking habits. *BMJ* 1954;1451–7.
15. Morris JN. Aetiology of ischaemic heart disease. *Proc R Soc Med* 1962;33:693–5.
16. Morris JN, Heady JA, Raffle PAB, Roberts CG, Parks JW. Coronary heart disease and physical activity at work. *Lancet* 1953;264:1053–7.
17. Morris JN, Heady JA, Raffle PAB, Roberts CG, Parks JW. Coronary heart disease and physical activity at work. *Lancet* 1953;264:1111–20.
18. Bronte-Stewart B. The effects of dietary fats on the blood lipids. *Br Med Bull* 1958;14:243–51.
19. Oliver MF. Ischaemic heart disease. An assessment of the value of reducing raised plasma lipids. *Lancet* 1962;i:653–6.
20. Oliver MF. The significance of elevated plasma lipids in relation to the prevention of ischaemic heart disease. *Bull WHO* 1962;27:409–19.
21. Oliver MF. Current therapeutics CXCV. Atromid S and Atromid. *Practitioner* 1964;192:424.
22. A co-operative trial in the primary prevention of ischaemic heart disease using clofibrate. Report from the Committee of Principal Investigators. *Br Heart J* 1978;40:1069–1118.
23. Geoffrey Rose (1926–93) was an unconventional and uncompromising clinical scientist, whose role was seminal. Geoffrey Arthur Rose was a member of the very successful "family" of Sir George Pickering at St Mary's Hospital which made major contributions to our knowledge of hypertension. After training as a clinician he turned his attention to clinical epidemiology and was appointed in 1977 to the chair of epidemiology at the London School of Hygiene. Geoffrey Rose was a superb teacher and his skills were highly regarded in the United States.
24. Rose G, Hamilton PS, Keen H, Reid DD, McCartney P, Jarrett RJ. Myocardial ischaemia, risk factors and death from coronary heart disease. *Lancet* 1977;i:105–9.
25. Rose GA, Shipley M. Plasma cholesterol concentrations and death from coronary heart disease. *BMJ* 1986;293:306–7.
26. Morris JN, Crawford M, Heady JA. Hardness of local water supplies and mortality. From Cardiovascular Disease. *Lancet* 1961;i:860.
27. Pocock SJ, Shaper AG, Cook PG, Lacey RF, Powell P, Russell PF. British regional heart study: graphic variations in cardiovascular mortality and the role of water quality. *BMJ* 1980;280:1243–9.
28. Shaper AG, Pocock SJ, Walker M, Cohen NM, Wale CJ, Thomson AG. British regional heart study: cardiovascular risk factors in middle aged men in 24 towns. *BMJ* 1981;283:179–86.
29. Price FW, ed. *A text book of the practice of medicine*. 6th ed. London: Oxford University Press, 1941:981.
30. Rose G, Marmot M. Social class and coronary heart disease. *BMJ* 1981;45:13–19.
31. Shaper AG, Cook DG, Walker M, MacFarlane PW. Prevalence of heart disease in middle aged British men. *Br Heart J* 1984;51:595–605.
32. Rose GA. Variability of angina, some implications for epidemiology. *Br J Prevent Soc Med* 1968;22:12–15.
33. Shaper AG, Cook DG, Walker M, MacFarlane PW. Recall of diagnosis by men with ischaemic heart disease. *Br Heart J* 1984;51:606–11.

34. Isles CG, Hole DG, Hawthorne VM, Lever AF. Relation between coronary risk and coronary mortality in women of the Paisley and Renfrew survey: comparison with men. *Lancet* 1992;339:702–6.
35. Tunstall-Pedoe H, Kuulasmaa K, Mahonen M, Tolonene H, Ruokokoski E, Asmouyel P. Contribution of trends in survival and coronary-event rates to changes in coronary heart disease mortality: 10-year results from 37 WHO MONICA project populations. *Lancet* 1999;353:1547–57.
36. Kornitzer M, Rose GA. Who European collaborative trial of multifactorial prevention of coronary heart disease. *Prevent Med* 1985;14:272–8.
37. Rose G, Ball K, Catford J, James P, Lambert D, Maryon-Davis S, et al. Coronary Heart Disease Prevention: Plans for Action. Pitman, London 1984.
38. British Cardiac Society. Working group on coronary prevention. *Br Heart J* 1987;57:187–9.
39. Reduction in incidence of coronary heart disease. Lipid research clinics coronary prevention trial, Results 1. *JAMA* 1984;251:351–64.
40. Oliver MF. Might treatment of hypercholesterolaemia increase noncardiac mortality? *Lancet* 1991;337:1529–31.
41. British Cardiac Society. Survey of the potential for the secondary prevention of coronary disease. Aspire Steering Group. *Heart* 1996;75:334–42.
42. British Heart Foundation Health Promotion Research Group. *Coronary heart disease statistics.* London: British Heart Foundation, 1999.
43. Capewell S, Morrison CE, McMurray JJ. Contribution of modern cardiovascular treatment and risk factor changes to the decline in coronary heart disease mortality in Scotland between 1975 and 1994. *Heart* 1999;81:380–6.
44. National Heart Forum. *Looking to the future.* London: Stationery Office, 1999.
45. Osler W. Meeting of Southern Medical Society, Glasgow 5th October 1911. (Item by W Watson Buchanan). *Bull R Coll Physicians Surgeons Glasgow* 1999;28:18–21.
46. Pickering GW. *High blood pressure.* London: J and A Churchill, 1955.
47. Watt GC, Foy CJ, Hart JT. Dietary sodium and blood pressure in young people with and without familial predisposition to high blood pressure. *J Clin Hypertens* 1986;2:141–7.
48. Hart JT. Hypertension and the prevention of coronary heart disease in general practice. *Postgrad Med J* 1984;60:34–8.
49. Lichtenstein MJ, Shipley MJ, Rose G. Systolic and diastolic blood pressures as predictors of coronary heart disease mortality in the Whitehall study. *BMJ* 1985;291:243–5.
50. Medical Research Council. Trial of mild hypertension. *Lancet* 1985;325:92–5.
51. Collins R, McMahon S. Blood pressure, antihypertensive drug treatment and the risks of stroke and of coronary heart disease. *BMJ* 1994;50:272–8.
52. British Cardiac Society. Joint British recommendations on prevention of coronary heart disease in clinical practice. *Heart* 1998;80(suppl 2):51–29.

Chapter 16

Cardiac Surgery

Tom Treasure

Visitors to the operating theatres of Guy's Hospital in September 1948 had the opportunity to be present at two pioneering operations. In one theatre, they would have been able to watch Mr Russell Brock performing one of the six or so operations in that year for the relief of mitral stenosis.[1] In the other, Mr Hedley Atkins was performing thoracolumbar sympathectomy (Smithwick's operation).[2–4] These young surgeons went on to be eminent in surgery and in the medical establishment. Both became president of the Royal College of Surgeons of England. What happened to their operations? Whose method might visitors have chosen to follow in their own practice? If they had elected to view Mr Atkins's thoracolumbar sympathectomy, they would have been present at a dramatic and effective operation (hypertension was relieved – too effectively in many cases), but a procedure that has vanished without trace.[4][5] However, if they had chosen Mr Brock's valvotomy, they would be able to recall that day with increasing vividness as heart surgery developed from those brave but tentative beginnings to modern practice in which virtually no structural or mechanical problem of the heart is regarded as inoperable. And yet, a reading of contemporary textbooks indicates that valvotomy to relieve mitral stenosis was regarded as reckless and, of the two procedures, was the one considered to have no basis in science or logic.[6][7]

Within the 20th century, cardiac surgery has come from nothing to a high volume, high technology endeavour. Tens of thousands of patients in Britain have heart operations each year,[8] with benefits ranging from good palliation of disabling and distressing symptoms to near perfect total correction. Surgery is applicable to most congenital, valvular, and ischaemic heart disease. The overall survival rate is 95%, a figure that has now remained relatively stable over 20 years,[9][10] a plateau which probably represents the balance of hope and acceptable risk. As technical success is more often achieved, mortality tends to fall, and patients with higher risk conditions are offered an operation, therefore the mortality remains much the same.

Such has been the success of heart surgery that we have moved from a situation in which Sir Lauder Brunton was castigated in the *Lancet* in 1902 for suggesting that a surgeon might even touch the human heart [11] to one in which the public seems to expect faultless surgical correction with return to normal expectation of life for every child with congenital heart disease. The responsibility for death or brain damage has moved from fate, God, and nature to the hands of the surgeon.[12][13]

There is abundant evidence that at least 90% of patients who undergo cardiac surgery have an improved and extended life (many dramatically so), but in the closing years of the century heart surgeons are being vilified in the media. Surgical units are the subject of public enquiries. The "Bristol babies" and the "Wisheart affair" have filled many pages of local and national newspapers, the *British Medical Journal* has provided a web page especially for the purpose. This is not because the public or the press doubt that heart surgery is highly successful. On the contrary, the expectations of the public are extraordinarily high.

A history of the 20th century presents a problem of perspective. The last third of the century is easily within the memory of the authors of this book. The history of the middle third is a combination of some vivid and some old memories, and some that have been embellished in the telling. For the remote third, we can only rely on written material. These three epochs will inevitably be viewed unevenly, partly because the protagonists of the last third of the history are still with us.

Back to the beginning

In 1902, the *Lancet* published an article by Sir Lauder Brunton, a scientifically minded physician, in which he suggested that a surgeon might be able to open a narrowed and obstructed heart valve.[14] Brunton introduced his subject thus:

> Mitral stenosis is not only one of the most distressing forms of cardiac disease, but in its most severe forms it resists all treatment by medicines. On looking at the contracted mitral orifice in a severe case of this disease one is impressed by the hopelessness of ever finding a remedy which will enable the auricle to drive the blood in a sufficient stream through the small mitral orifice, and the wish unconsciously arises that one could divide the constriction as easily during life as one can after death.

One can sense Brunton's desire to simply fix the problem mechanically. Brunton had observed in the autopsy room that the two leaflets of the valve were easily freed with a finger and he proposed that this might be done within the living and beating heart to restore normal flow. Correspondents to the *Lancet* regarded the relief of mitral stenosis as unnecessary or impossible, or both.[15–17] The *Lancet* turned against Brunton, and in a stern editorial recommended that he develop his proposed operation on animals before publicising the idea further.[11]

In 1908, Sir James Mackenzie wrote in his *Diseases of the heart* of the "utmost confusion prevailing as to the significance of the signs detected in the heart," and expressed his concern about the dangers of mechanistic, technology-driven diagnosis. The Victorians, great engineers that they were, applied what they knew of pumps to the heart, to its valves, and to the noises these made. In the early years of the century, however, this gave way to an emphasis on the ability of the heart, and the patient, to compensate for disordered function.[18] We might now call this "holistic." The mechanistic approach returned with a vengeance after the second world war, gathering momentum through the 1960s and 1970s, before again facing a decline in support towards the end of the century.

Souttar's operation for mitral stenosis

Rheumatic heart disease and mitral stenosis, in particular, remained commonplace. Brunton's suggestion was set aside but not forgotten. In 1925, Henry Souttar reported his first and only operation for mitral stenosis, undertaken at the London Hospital.[19][20] The operation was performed in the way that Brunton had suggested, through the left atrium. This was the route that was to become established in the 1950s. With his right index finger introduced through the left atrial appendage into the beating heart, Souttar was able to appreciate the movements of the blood and the valve and to free the adherent edges, just as Brunton had predicted it could be done.[14] His patient lived several years, became a celebrity around the hospital, and was visited by royalty. However, this event did not advance the surgical treatment of mitral stenosis. Souttar never operated on another case.[21][22]

To place this in international context, a Boston surgeon, Elliot Cutler, had also reported a single case, in 1923, in which he had used a knife through the apex of the heart to cut the valve. The patient survived and improved.[23] Cutler operated on six more patients, but all died within days of surgery and he abandoned his attempts.[24] Of 10 patients operated on for mitral stenosis in the 1920s, only two survived to gain any benefit, one of them, the most successful operation of this era, was the one performed in London by Souttar.

Why did Souttar stop?

Why did Souttar not continue?[25] There were many more patients who might have benefited and his operation was seen as successful by the celebrity attention that his patient attracted later.[22] It is said that there were three obstacles to progress – heart surgery had to await blood transfusion, antibiotics, and improvements in anaesthesia. In fact, the evidence is to the contrary. Souttar had been successful without these, and none of Cutler's failures were a result of haemorrhage, infection, or anaesthetic failure. Furthermore, in 1925 antibiotics and blood transfusion simply did not exist.

Historical anecdote has it that Souttar was ostracised and physician colleagues would not send him patients. However, there is no evidence of

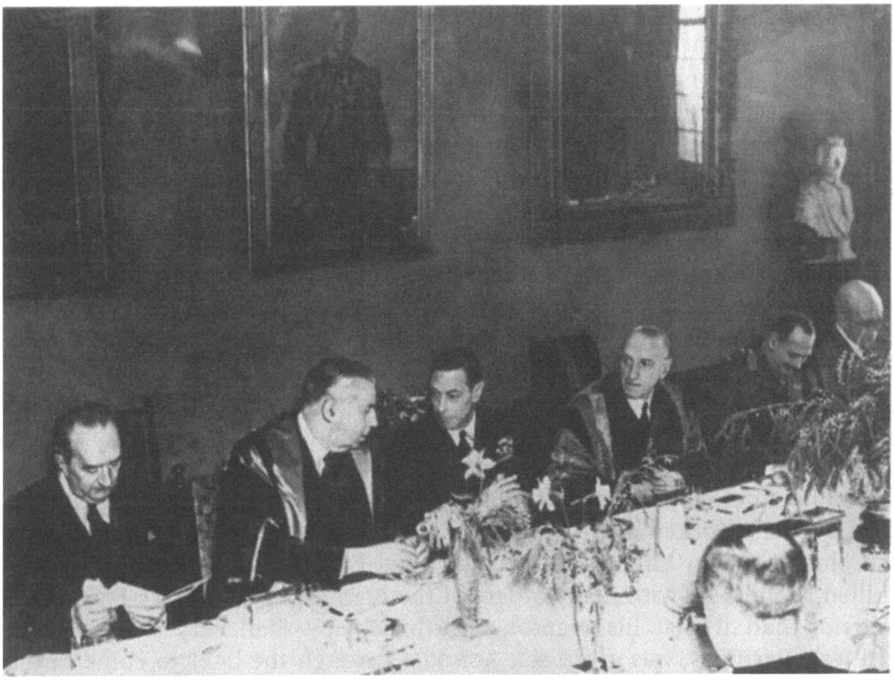

Figure 1 The King comes to luncheon – 8 March 1944. *Left to right*: unidentified; Sir Henry Souttar; King George VI; Sir Alfred (later Lord) Webb Johnson, PRCS; HRH Duke of Gloucester; Sir Girling Ball.

public criticism. Souttar had a long and successful career (figure 1). He was elected to the council of the Royal College of Surgeons and was its vice president in 1943–4. It is more likely that he was referred no cases, was warned off, and could see that this was not the route to success for a London surgeon in the 1920s. Souttars own version was that the "time was not yet ripe."[26] In April 1924, Mackenzie had written "I see the old notion of operating on mitral stenosis is being revised," pouring scorn on the idea.[18]

No further operations were performed on the mitral valve for about 20 years. Souttar's approach to the valve, his technique, and his observations were remarkably prescient, but the low success rate for all operations in the chest, the general ghastliness that probably surrounded them, and the failure rate of eight out of 10 for operations on mitral stenosis outweighed Souttar's single success.

The antimechanistic era

John Josias Conybeare was physician at Guy's Hospital and produced the first edition of his *Textbook of Medicine* in 1929.[27] On the subject of valvular heart disease he wrote:

> Before passing to a consideration of the effects produced by lesions of the various valves, it is necessary to lay stress upon the fact that valvular lesions in themselves

> do not produce any symptoms; the development of symptoms in valvular disease indicates that the myocardium in unable to carry on its work efficiently.[27]

Here we see a clear backlash in medical thinking, prompted by the knowledge that surgeons had become interested in the heart. It is almost as though it was considered that the best way to dissuade Souttar and his fellow surgeons from believing that they might have a role in mending broken hearts was to preclude the possibility that the illness could be understood in mechanical terms. From then until the second world war very little British surgery on the heart is recorded. An Irishman, Laurence O'Shaugnessy was making his name as a thoracic surgeon. In 1936, he proposed that mobilisation of the greater omentum from within the abdomen might bring a source of blood to the heart to relieve angina. He reported a series of cases in 1938.[28][29] In terms of surgical progress, however, it was a blind alley; the omentum does not readily form vascular adhesions.

O'Shaugnessy struck up a friendship with the German surgeon Ferdinand Sauerbruch, worked with him for a period, and translated Sauerbruch's surgical text into English. The war divided Europe and O'Shaugnessy was killed at Dunkirk with many others of the British Expeditionary Force. One version had it that his mentor, Sauerbruch, by then very influential in Hitler's Germany, was given safe conduct through the lines to come to the aid of his dying colleague. The French surgeon, Michel Ribet, who at the age of 12 fled his burning home in Dunkirk, corrected this account. O'Shaugnessy's name is on the war memorial at Dunkirk, but his body was never found.[30] That story has taught me to be wary of placing credence on oral history. Myth and folklore have their place – they are interesting – but they are not to be relied upon if we want to know the truth.

Opportunities of war

War provides opportunities for surgical innovation as young and adventurous surgeons cope with the acute injuries of fit young men. Souttar was an army surgeon in the first world war, which provided the material for his first book.[31] O'Shaugnessy was lost to British surgery in battle, but an American surgeon, Dwight Harken, was of particular interest in the second war. Harken worked at the 160th General Hospital of the US army, situated in Cirencester, Gloucestershire in the West of England. He used his opportunity to gain confidence in handling the heart and great vessels. He reported on 134 cases in which he had removed bullets, pieces of shrapnel, and other foreign bodies from in and around the heart and great vessels.[32] All patients in the series survived. Thirteen of the missiles were retrieved from within the chambers of the heart. Harken presented his work to a meeting of the Association of Surgeons of Great Britain and Ireland on 2 May 1945.[32]

Closing in on the heart

Although the medical texts denied the importance of the mechanics of the heart (the valves) congenital malformations around the heart were also of great interest to surgeons, who saw an opportunity to repair and restore structures. They were more accessible and amenable to operative correction. Throughout the world, surgeons were working closer and closer to the heart. In 1939, the American surgeon Robert Gross had successfully operated on ductus arteriosus. The London surgeon, Oswald Tubbs, successfully operated on an infected duct in 1939.[34] A coarctation was repaired by Clarence Crafoord in 1944.[33]

Some of the surgeons who started working in the chest, around the heart and great vessels, were still very much general surgeons. Some had already narrowed their field to thoracic surgery, working with empyema and tuberculosis. It is an interesting fact that while London had a specialised cardiological centre in the National Heart Hospital it had no surgeons to call upon. Since there was no heart surgery, how could a heart hospital employ a surgeon? On the other hand, the thoracic centres such as the Brompton and Harefield, and the general hospitals such as Guy's, the Middlesex, and Edinburgh, had specialist chest surgeons who were the first to operate on the heart. The National Heart Hospital was left behind for a time.

Specialisation develops

The identification of "specialist" is an important feature of the development of medicine. The general surgeons and the general physicians were the dominant force of the hospital in history. They controlled the "take" of urgent and emergency patients, and were therefore in charge of most of the beds, the teaching, and the examination of students. The orthopaedic surgeons had wrested the treatment of fractures from the general surgeons in the interwar years.[35][36] Thoracic surgery also became established.

In October 1947, Guy's Hospital medical committee agreed "to recommend that a Thoracic Surgical unit should be formed . . . under the charge of Mr. Brock," and in November the house committee (chaired by the same Sir John Conybeare) gave its approval.[37] In December 1947, it was minuted that "Dr. Maurice Campbell gave up being a Full Physician in order to devote himself entirely to be . . . Cardiologist" to deal with the large number of congenital heart disease patients coming to the hospital. Brock and Campbell were prepared to nail their colours to the mast as cardiac specialists.

By the end of 1947, Guy's had a medical and surgical infrastructure, formally established with the explicit approval of their consultant colleagues, ready to dedicate itself to heart disease, and, in particular, to heart surgery. It should be remembered that much of the work of a cardiologist is the identification and diagnosis of conditions amenable to surgical correction. This is particularly true of the structural abnormalities of congenital and valvular heart disease.

Anglo-American relationships

Alfred Blalock had been working with Dr Helen Taussig, at Johns Hopkins Hospital on the problem of cyanotic congenital heart disease.[38] Taussig had noted that patients with cyanotic heart disease in association with a persistent ductus arteriosus fared better than those in whom the ductus had closed – the flow of blood to the lungs providing better systemic oxygenation. With Alfred Blalock she devised an operation where a systemic artery, usually the left subclavian artery, was dissected from its position in the upper mediastinum and anastomosed to the left pulmonary artery.[39] This directed enough blood to the lungs to improve oxygenation.

Blalock taught Brock the operation during a visit under an exchange scheme between Guy's and Johns Hopkins. Between June 1948 and June 1949, Brock performed Blalock's operation in 21 cases of a total of 37 procedures to improve pulmonary blood flow.[37]

During Brock's visit to Baltimore in 1949, he also operated on mitral stenosis. This pattern of exchange was developed in many specialties and between many institutions. It became usual for British trainee cardiac surgeons to spend a year in America to gain the unofficial diploma of "BTA" (been to America). Britain continued to look to the Americans, and not until the forming of the European Association for Cardiothoracic Surgery in the late 1980s was there much exchange of ideas between Britain and the continent of Europe.

Cardiac surgical clubs

Brock was aware of the need to ensure support within his hospital. The American surgeon Charles Bailey had been officially barred from operating on mitral stenosis at several Philadelphia hospitals as one patient after another died. On Wednesday 21 April 1948, Brock convened a meeting at Guy's of those "concerned in the management of congenital disease of the heart." Those present included the physicians Dr Charles Baker and Dr Maurice Campbell, his anaesthetist Dr Rink, Medical Research Council clinical physiologists, pathologist, radiologists, and the dentist, Mr Kelsey Fry – in fact all who might be encouraged to take a special interest in these cases, and might want a "share of the action," or to whom he might turn for help. In current terms, they were stakeholders, and Brock was networking. Visitors to these meetings over the subsequent years included many prominent names in cardiac work in London, and from all over the world. Cases were discussed before surgery and were reviewed afterwards.

Peacock club

The group considered the name "The True Blues," alluding to the "blue" babies who were their initial interest, but at a meeting in July 1948 "Dr.

Campbell quoted from the work of Peacock," which seemed to carry the day, and so the club was named, the Peacock Club. Thomas P Peacock was the author of the first standard textbook on *Malformations of the Human Heart* 1855. Perhaps the hint of blueness was still important.[40]

The Peacock Club was confined to Guy's, but in subsequent years a whole succession of clubs grew up. These included Browns Club (after the hotel where they met), Charlies Club where members could only present errors or "Charlies," not triumphs. Others took the name of a founder or mentor – Pete's Club, Dave's Club, the Christopher Robin Club, McCormick's Club. They comprised a (more or less) closed circle of colleagues, often representing a cohort, who presented to each other their difficulties, problems, complications, and disasters for mutual support, sympathy, and edification.

The Peacock Club was built around Brock, deliberately to rally support and to bond his clinical team together. In all his writings Brock stressed the teamwork, the cases assessed by the cardiological physician, the surgeon supported by his anaesthetist, and here we see the evidence of a deliberate strategy. In his publications, Baker, Brock, Campbell, and later Wood, are in deliberate alphabetical order.

Blue babies had been there since the beginning of time. Peacock had studied the causes a century earlier. In 1934, the Canadian pathologist Maude Abbot had presented an exhibition of hearts with congenital abnormalities to the centennial meeting of the British Medical Association in London.[41] but until the time when a surgeon could relieve the pulmonary obstruction and physically divert the blood flow these hearts were of interest mainly as post mortem specimens.

Next wave of valvular surgery

Pulmonary valve stenosis

The first pulmonary valvotomy was performed by Thomas Holmes Sellors at Harefield Hospital.[42] His patient was a 20 year old man, deeply cyanosed as a result of tetralogy of Fallot. Holmes Sellors had intended to perform a Blalock–Taussig operation. After opening the left chest anteriorly through the third interspace, an incision which brings one directly onto the main pulmonary artery, he was impressed by finding "that a firm structure was thrust from the ventricle into the pulmonary artery with each heart beat." Holmes Sellors correctly interpreted this as being a barely perforate but mobile pulmonary valve and decided to do a direct operation on the heart. After placing several holding sutures, he incised the right ventricular infundibulum and "A long tenotomy knife was then thrust between the stitches till it engaged the resistant valve . . . which was . . . cut in two directions." The pulmonary blood flow was much improved and cyanosis largely relieved. The knife, a tenotome, had been borrowed from the nearby orthopaedic theatre.[43]

Holmes Sellors was a very fine surgeon who worked with deceptive rapidity and economy of effort. He rehearsed his operations step by step at home, practising the sequence of sutures for the Blalock anastomosis for example,[44] but he was a reluctant author and allowed 6 months to lapse before writing up this case.[45] By the time it was published, his friend and rival Russell Brock had published his results on three patients operated on subsequently.[46] The race to publish cases was part of the culture of the time but Holmes Sellors acknowledged Brock's paper with characteristic generosity in a footnote to his own article, saying that it was admirable and dealt with the subject more thoroughly.

The Guy's Hospital operating theatre books show that between June 1948 and June 1949 Brock performed operations for coarctation and persistent ductus arteriosus, and 14 operations for the relief of right ventricular outflow obstruction either at the valve itself or the infundibulum.[37]

Mitral stenosis

The cardiology textbooks remained steadfast in playing down the importance of the cardiac valves. There had been no evidence since the 1920s but the arguments had become ever more firmly entrenched. Conybeare's textbook (8th edition, 1946) states under "Mitral disease" that "No specific symptoms are associated with mitral stenosis unless the heart muscle is failing."[47]

Frederick Price at the National Hospital for Diseases of the Heart and the Royal Northern Hospital edited his book eight times between 1922 and 1950. His teaching on mitral valve disease became progressively more certain. In the seventh edition, published in 1946, he wrote: "Surgical treatment in the form of valvulotomy, both by the auricular and ventricular routes, has been performed in a number of cases of mitral stenosis, with the object of enlarging the orifice. This procedure is contra-indicated. The mortality is high." The auricular approach had been used only once, in fact, without mortality.[48]

The argument against surgery was put with characteristic vigour by Thomas Lewis in the 1946 (4th) edition of *Diseases of the Heart*:

> Surgical attempts to relieve cases of mitral stenosis . . . by cutting the valve have so far failed to give benefit. I think they will continue to fail, not only because the treatment is too drastic, but because the attempt is based upon what, usually at all events, is an erroneous idea, namely, that the valve is the chief source of the trouble.[7]

Then an editorial appeared in the *British Medical Journal* in the first half of 1948.

> What will be the next step in the development of surgery of the heart? It may, perhaps extend to acquired heart disease and it is worth recalling that Souttar, as long ago as 1925, attempted direct digital dilatation of the mitral valve in a patient with mitral stenosis. While it is the disease of the heart muscle that causes cardiac

> failure and death in the patient with chronic rheumatic carditis, it is possible that if the strain of the stenosed valve were removed from that muscle it might function for many years longer.[50]

This was coat trailing at the received wisdom about the futility of surgery on mitral stenosis in the textbooks of the day. Interest in mitral stenosis is also evident in the hand-written minutes of Brock's Peacock Club. At the fourth meeting in September 1948, details of the case of Doris Diggins were presented, including cardiac catheterisation and measurement of her circulation time. Until then the management would not have been any different whether or not there was a significant degree of regurgitation, but Brock knew that regurgitation had surprised Souttar in 1925. Doris Diggins was operated on three days later, on 16 September 1948 – this was Brock's first operation for mitral stenosis. His next three cases followed on 23 and 27 September. Note that he had three patients ready for surgery, and operated on them within a period of 8 days, unlike Bailey and Harken who took one case at a time, failed and tried again before their eventual first survivors.

In 1948, three surgeons independently performed valvotomy. The first was Charles Bailey in June 1948, followed within days by Dwight Harken who wrote to me as follows: "I rushed to Joe Garland, editor of the *New England Journal of Medicine*, and told him to get it published as soon as possible."[26] The third surgeon was Russell Brock who operated on nine patients, of whom seven survived, before he published his results.[51] Closed mitral valvotomy was, and still is, a brilliantly successful procedure in cases of pure stenosis with a mobile valve. These are now best dealt with by balloon valvotomy.

In December 1948, Guy's medical committee "agreed to recommend that Mr. Brock should visit the Johns Hopkins Hospital in 1949.[37] We know that during that visit he repaid them by performing the two first mitral valvotomies at Johns Hopkins, and series of six operations for pulmonary stenosis, an operation which, notwithstanding Holmes Sellors's precedence, he had pioneered and probably had the greatest worldwide experience.

Disseminating information

The surgical section of the Royal Society of Medicine devoted its meeting on 4 April 1951 to "Surgery of the heart and great vessels."[52] Crafoord reported on coarctation in 85 cases and persistent ductus in 282 cases. Brock spoke on pulmonary valvotomy in 57 cases, 28 for pure pulmonary valve stenosis and 29 as palliation in Fallot's tetralogy, with 10 deaths in the series (17.5%). He had operated on 48 cases for mitral stenosis; there had been 8 deaths (17%), but none among the most recent 24 operations. Souttar, who had done his single operation in 1925, was present.

Also in 1951, the British Medical Association held a "Festival year conference on tuberculosis and diseases of the chest." Brock presented his results on mitral and pulmonary stenosis in 160 intracardiac operations. Clement

Price Thomas described surgery for coarctation. Oswald Tubbs presented his work on persistent ductus arteriosus in 93 cases, and Holmes Sellors described surgery for constrictive pericarditis.[53]. Cardiac surgery dominated the programme.

In 1952, Brock went to press, 18 months after his first report, with his first 100 operations for mitral stenosis. He adhered to his custom of giving the authors in alphabetical order, also including Paul Wood along with his two colleagues at Guy's.[54]

In 1953 and 1954, there were several reports of large series of mitral valvotomy with modest mortality. Thomas Holmes Sellors, best known for skilled application rather than innovation,[55] described a series of 150 cases from the Middlesex, Harefield, and the London Chest Hospitals with a 4% mortality.[56] Andrew Logan from Edinburgh reported a total of 200 cases performed in just over two years.[57]

The *British Medical Journal* accompanied Holmes Sellors's 1953 report with an editorial "Surgical treatment of mitral stenosis." The editorial stated that "The results obtained by Brock, Holmes Sellors, and other thoracic surgeons are so promising that the operation should be considered for every patients that is severely disabled by mitral disease."

The relief of mitral stenosis was applied in pregnancy in the 16th and 18th weeks by Logan of Edinburgh,[58] and at full term by O'Connell of Dublin.[59] Even after the development of cardiopulmonary bypass, this remained an indication for the closed transatrial operation. Logan also devised and reported on the valve dilator, introduced through the ventricular apex to make the valvotomy more controlled.[60]

The 1954 meeting of the British Medical Association in Glasgow had a session devoted to mitral stenosis. Smiley reported 121 cases from Ulster with a 5% mortality, Mackay of Glasgow had undertaken 146 operations, and Allison from Leeds reported his series.[61] Mitral stenosis had taken over the thoracic units.

There was a further editorial in the *British Medical Journal* in 1954 stressing the commonness of rheumatism as a cause of heart disease.[62] "The value of mitral valvotomy for the relief of mitral stenosis is now well established and the operation is being carried out in many centres in this country and abroad with excellent results."

In his 1954 Strickland Goodall Lecture entitled "An appreciation of mitral stenosis," Paul Wood clearly saw the heart as a pump amenable to mechanical correction.[63] The mechanistic view was in the ascendancy and British cardiac surgery was on a high. Within those few years from Brock's first three mitral valvotomies in the Autumn of 1948, the whole concept of the heart, and its amenability to surgery, had changed.

Impact of hypothermia and stopping the circulation

In 1925, when Henry Souttar performed a mitral valvotomy at the London Hospital, he wrote:

> In animals ... the circulation has been clamped for as long as two minutes. This, however, would never be justified in an human being in view of the extreme danger to the brain from even the shortest check to its blood supply. Any manipulations which are carried out must therefore be executed in the full flow of the blood stream, and they must not perceptibly interfere with the contractions of the heart.[20]

Written 75 years ago, Souttar's paper reveals a stark appreciation of the problems that had to be overcome before open cardiac surgery could be performed. His preoccupation with the vulnerability of the human brain is still shared by the modern cardiovascular surgeon but Souttar did not foresee the use of hypothermia to protect the brain nor cardiopulmonary bypass to support the circulation.

The operations close to but outside the heart could be performed with the heart beating and largely undisturbed. Mitral and pulmonary valvotomy were successfully achieved within the beating heart. Aortic valvotomy as a closed procedure was much less successful and was abandoned. Percutaneous balloon dilatation of the aortic valve has not succeeded either.[64]

There was a clear limit to what could be done on an unsupported circulation. From where they stood in 1950, there were several ways forward. One was to be ever more inventive in operating within the beating heart, another was to support the circulation with cross circulation. This was achieved by mother-to-child support in a few cases in Minnesota (said to be the only operation with a potential for 200% mortality). Perhaps the possibility of circulating the whole of the patient's blood through series of plastic tubes and boxes (which is what we do and call it cardiopulmonary bypass) seemed the least likely.

Using cooling to extend the period that the brain would tolerate the lack of a blood supply was the one explored next, and to most effect in the short term. The limit of the brain's tolerance to circulatory arrest is about three minutes, but it has often been observed that children who have cooled rapidly by falling into icy water have survived long periods of cerebral ischaemia without evident brain damage. The protective effect of cooling is largely due to a reduction in the oxygen requirement of the brain. This knowledge was used to permit the earliest successful open heart surgery.[65]

Ross's work on oxygen consumption

Oxygen consumption during hypothermia was studied at Guy's by the young South African surgeon, Donald Ross.[66] The use of a planned period of total circulatory arrest played an important part in the operative strategy before cardiopulmonary bypass was developed and refined. Moderate hypothermia to about 30°C, induced by surface cooling, was used to provide a few minutes of protection, just long enough to suture a fossa ovalis atrial septal defect.

Repairing simple atrial septal defects

The master of this technique was Holmes Sellors at the Middlesex Hospital.[67] He relied heavily on the diagnostic skill of Evan Bedford, his cardiologist colleague, because only a simple fossa ovalis defect could be sutured in the time available. The more difficult primum defect took too long. Holmes Sellors also relied on the skill of his anaesthetist, Brian Sellick, to judge the cooling to a nicety so that the heart would not fibrillate.

Having cooled the patient in a domestic bath, afloat with ice, the patient was put on the operating table and the chest opened through bilateral anterior thoracotomy. The superior and inferior caval veins were snared, a large clamp was then put through the transverse sinus and the aorta and pulmonary artery were clamped. Holmes Sellors had a few minutes to complete his entry to the right atrium, suture the defect, exclude the air, and close the heart so that the circulation could be restored. Other surgeons used this technique but Holmes Sellors – and Sellick – were the acknowledged masters.[68]

Profound hypothermia

The repair of more complex congenital heart disease required much more time. Donald Ross worked with Brock at Guy's determining what the tolerance to circulatory arrest was at lower temperature. From this he developed veno-venous cooling which he used in completing repairs of tetralogy of Fallot. However, his results in this era were not good.

Profound hypothermia was the logical extension of the method. It emerged empirically with uncertain time limits; sometimes an hour or more of circulatory arrest was used. More rigorous evaluation of clinical experience and laboratory experiments indicate that the technique allows up to about 40 minutes at a below 20°C.[65]

Total body cooling was used by Charles Drew at the Westminster and St George's Hospitals. He devised a technique of bypassing the right and left sides separately still using the lungs before the development of a reliable oxygenator.[69] At 12°C he turned off his pumps, drained out the patient's blood, and operated under post mortem room conditions. Drew persisted in using the technique long after oxygenators were available . . . and probably too late and for too long. The two strategies of cardiopulmonary bypass and of total body cooling are now used in combination.[70]

Belsey in Bristol was probably as advanced as any in the use of these techniques.[71] Donald Ross worked with him as well as with Brock and went on to make many contributions to cardiac surgery. Congenital heart surgery developed from those times, predominately in the United States and Canada. Magdi Yacoub has become the most innovative of British cardiac surgeons, and deserves credit for making the arterial switch operation for transposition a practical proposition.[72]

Cardiopulmonary bypass

Cardiopulmonary bypass became routine for virtually all cardiac surgery and was a necessary part of the equipment and skill needed to "stay in business" as a cardiac surgical unit. Cardiopulmonary bypass was developed predominantly at the Mayo Clinic in Rochester, Minnesota. At the Hammersmith Hospital in London, Dennis Melrose devised a disc oxygenator.[73] The work of Ken Taylor, British Heart Foundation professor at the Royal Postgraduate Medical School, has continued this tradition of applied research in cardiopulmonary bypass.

Myocardial protection

The next big hurdle was to protect the myocardium. All too often, the end result of intraoperative ischaemia was a heart that would not sustain the circulation. Dennis Melrose at the Hammersmith Hospital suggested using potassium to arrest the heart, to reduce its metabolism, and increase its tolerance to surgery.[74] The concentration of potassium citrate was high, the results were not consistently good, and the method was abandoned. For years surgeons relied on speed and intermittent restoration of coronary flow by releasing the aortic cross clamp or cannulating the coronary arteries.

In the 1970s, Mark Braimbridge of St Thomas's Hospital teamed up with a young biochemist, David Hearse, and they began a series of a laboratory experiments. They devised a solution with a potassium content of 20 mmol/l and magnesium of 16 mmol/l which was otherwise similar to the extracelluar electrolyte composition. When delivered cold, this provided myocardial protection by arresting the heart in asystole and maintaining cooling to minimise metabolic activity of the heart. Termed cardioplegia, the mixture was dubbed "St Thomas's solution." There were similar approaches in other countries but Braimbridge's approach was used by many surgeons worldwide and was associated with a striking improvement in results for the whole spectrum of cardiac operations.[75]

Further developments in valve surgery

Wooler and the mitral valve

Mitral stenosis had been very successfully dealt with by valvotomy, but before cardiopulmonary bypass, and the development of prosthetic valves, there was little to offer for mitral regurgitation. Leeds surgeon, Geoffrey Wooler, devised a way of making regurgitant mitral valves competent. The Wooler annuloplasty bears his name, but conservative operations on the mitral valve had variable results. Much later, Alain Carpentier in Paris developed a range of reconstructive techniques. Posterior annulopasty, much as conceived by Wooler, is part of the repertoire of most surgeons who now successfully repair the mitral valve.

Aortic valve replacement

Aortic valve replacement with a human cadaveric valve was first done by Donald Ross.[76] This quickly became an established technique and was soon followed by mechanical valve replacement. Seeking a biological solution, Ross first performed the pulmonary autograft operation in 1967, when he took the patient's own, healthy pulmonary valve and used it in the aortic position, replacing the pulmonary outflow tract with a homograft or some other substitute.[77] For years he alone did this operation, but nearly 30 years later, it has gained popularity and is now used throughout the world as the "ideal" tissue valve. Ross was the best known international figure of British cardiac surgery for many years. The British seem reluctant to give credit to our own inventors. This is now known belatedly as the "Ross operation."

Other living tissues solutions were sought. Marion Ionescu, working in Leeds, proposed using fascia lata taken from the patient's own thigh in the hope of creating a living valve that would survive with the patient.[78] The fascia lata was a disaster; mitral valves made of this material failed with alarming rapidity.[79] But tissue valves spare the patient the need for lifelong anticoagulation treatment. Marion Ionescu promulgated the use of pericardium from cattle, fixed with glutaraldehyde. These valves functioned extremely well and were widely used. They failed, as do all tissue valves, but probably a little earlier, and more suddenly, than other tissue valves and they fell into disrepute. The pig valves were the tissue standard, but in the 1980s the pendulum swung steadily towards mechanical valves, predominantly manufactured in America.

From the 1960s there remained a minority preference for tailoring an unfixed and unmounted human tissue valve to the patient's aortic root (a homograft) with the hope that the valve would be incorporated and live as long as the patient. Donald Ross was a pioneer and champion of the use of tissue valves and as the century closed we are seeing the pendulum swing back towards his views.[80] It became evident that cadaveric human valves, whether antibiotic sterilised or cryopreserved, were dead. Magdi Yacoub has dubbed the valves he salvaged and used fresh from the explanted hearts of transplant recipients "homovital," and the use of the patient's own pulmonary valve to replace the aortic valve in the Ross operation is the epitome of this aspiration. One of only two trials of tissue versus mechanical valves was started in Edinburgh by David Wheatley, later to be professor in Glasgow. The trial showed little survival difference, even beyond 10 years.[81]

Bentall and the aortic root replacement

British cardiac surgery deserves credit for another important valve operation. The dilated aortic root in the fragile tissue of Marfan's syndrome was a major problem. Valve replacement alone left the aortic root at risk of rupture. A composite replacement of the valve and ascending aorta, with reimplantation of the coronary arteries was described by Hugh Bentall of the Hammersmith. It was an "inclusion" technique and is now largely obsolete but the operation of root replacement is still known generically as the Bentall procedure in America and Europe but ungenerously, as with the Ross operation, the British have rarely used this eponym.[82]

Transplantation

Soon after the first human heart transplant was performed by Christiaan Barnard in Capetown, South Africa on 3 December 1967, there was a worldwide flurry of transplant activity, with many surgeons trying their hand at one or two. London's three transplants in this era were performed by Donald Ross and his team – first at the National Heart Hospital on 3 May 1968 and then at Guy's on 16 May 1969.[83]

The mood of the 1960s was very much "anything can be done," which was perhaps the extreme swing of the pendulum towards mechanistic solutions. However, the immunological implications of transplantation were insurmountable. This episode is described in detail in a "Witness seminar" from the Wellcome Institute.[83] In the memories of those closest to these operations, the surgical teams, this was an unhappy episode. They received a great deal of publicity and some of it was harshly critical, including being featured on the front cover of the satirical magazine, *Private Eye*.[84] This came as a rude shock to cardiac surgeons. They had been used to adulation – to be pilloried was a new experience. *Private Eye* has considered itself to have a role in bringing heart surgeons to account; 30 years later it publicised the mortality figures for the switch operation in Bristol.

Resumption after moratorium

A 10 year moratorium was placed on transplantation. This was explicit in Britain, and in a number of other countries, but implicit in the mood adopted throughout the world.[85] In 1980, Terence English at Papworth resumed transplantation.[83] Again, there was much publicity but this was cautiously handled. English ran a well organised unit, but still experienced very great difficulties. He even received letters of criticism from cardiologists within his own unit.

Yacoub started transplantation at Harefield, which he developed to become the biggest transplantation unit in the world. One of the strengths of the control exercised by the NHS was that proliferation of small units was obstructed, at this time by a supraregional funding mechanism, later by the National Services Commissioning Advisory Group. In addition to Papworth and Harefield, transplantation was started and continues in Newcastle, Birmingham, Sheffield, Glasgow, St George's, and the Hospital for Sick Children at Great Ormond Street in London. It was started temporarily

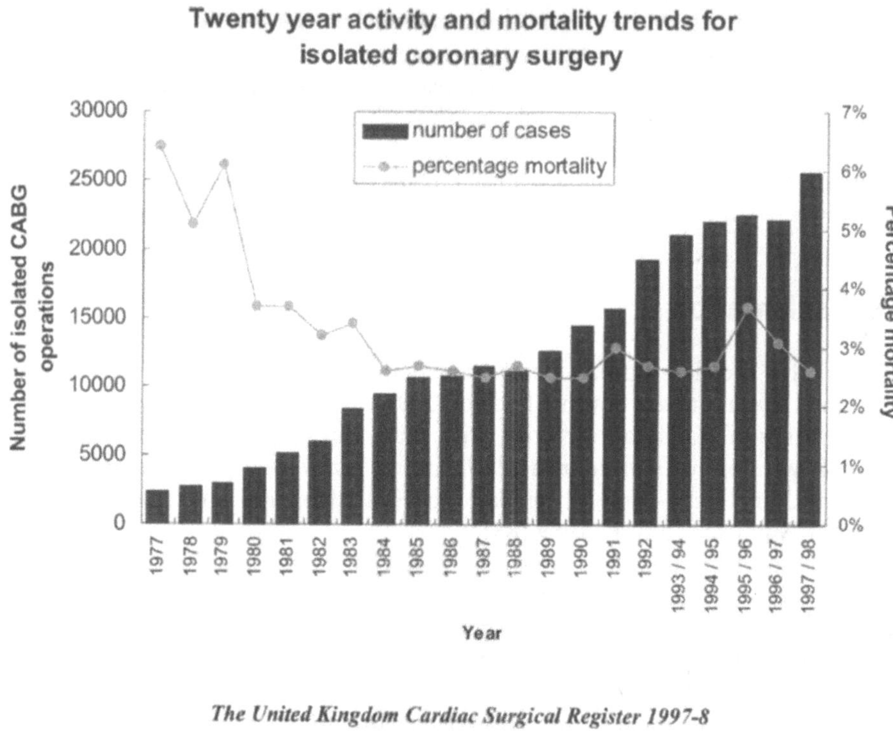

Figure 2 The United Kingdom Cardiac Register 1997–8. The graph represents the first level of analysis but hides the relatively comprehensive nature of procedural data that is collected.

in Leeds and unofficially for a brief period at St Bartholomew's. At a time when the United States had a very large number of units performing, on average, fewer than 10 transplant operations a year, the 300 transplants carried out in the United Kingdom each year were centralised on eight or nine units and were monitored by a special health authority – the United Kingdom Transplantation Service Special Authority.

Coronary artery surgery

O'Shaugnessy suggested the use of the greater omentum (an operation which he thought could be called omentopexy) to bring a blood supply to the ischaemic myocardium.[34] This was a blind alley and no further work was done. The Canadian, Vineberg, did extensive work on the coronary circulation and devised a means of relieving angina by tunnelling the mammary artery into the myocardium about 10 years before direct coronary artery surgery was developed and popularised at the Cleveland Clinic in Ohio. The operation that became established was the vein graft – that is, anastomosis of the saphenous vein as a bypass graft, conducting arterial blood between the aorta and the coronary artery beyond the stenosis. This reliably relieved angina.

Like mitral valvotomy for mitral stenosis, it was quickly evident that there was an effective and achievable solution for a very common affliction. It was taken up by a few surgeons in Britain, possibly by 1969, and certainly by 1970. The data for the number of cases performed in the NHS units is available from the inception of the United Kingdom Cardiac Surgery Register (figure 2). British surgeons played their part in a European trial of surgery compared with medical management (ECS),[86] and later in the RITA (randomised intervention in the treatment of angina) trial between surgery and angioplasty.[87]

Issues of conflict and quality

From the 1970s, throughout the 1980s, and into the 1990s patients came in very large numbers from other European countries to Britain, particularly to London to private clinics and to the private wings of NHS hospitals. There were contracts with German and Dutch organisations and from small well organised countries such as Norway and Iceland. The entirely private hospitals in the West End of London had notices in Greek and Arabic, while British surgeons and their cardiological colleagues travelled abroad to see patients. The paradox is that most European countries increased their capacity to perform surgery while Britain now is behind France, Germany, Holland, Belgium, and all of the Scandinavian countries in cardiac surgical provision.

The context of this "hidden export" of cardiac surgical expertise was driven by the opportunity for NHS surgeons to greatly increase their income. Fees for private cases were already well over £1000 rising to over £2000 per case while NHS salaries were standardised for all consultants at around £45 000 per annum. A cardiac surgeon doing as few as two private cases in a month would earn more for his private than his NHS work, and the economic pressure resulted in fewer innovations and developments in British cardiac surgery. The difference between the comfortable, money-no-object environment of the private clinics and the threadbare NHS was evident. No wonder research and innovation took a back seat in British cardiac surgery in this era compared with the immediate postwar years, and was left to the Americans.

The impression that cardiac surgeons were spending a disproportionate amount of time in private practice was resented to varying degrees, and the standing of cardiac surgeons was low in academic circles. There were suspensions of surgeons on matters related to absenteeism, often with a flavour of jealousy in the background. It was drawn to the attention of the public as the subject of Sunday paper and television exposées. A generation earlier, the novelist AJ Cronin had illustrated the corrupting effect of private practice.[88] Cardiac surgeons were not the only group under criticism as will be obvious from the title of the 1995 book, *Private eye, heart and hip,* but they attracted the most notoriety.[89]

The UK registers

In 1977, the Society of Thoracic and Cardiovascular Surgeon of Great Britain and Ireland (later to rename itself the Society of Cardiothoracic Surgeons of Great Britain and Ireland) asked all its members and all the units performing heart surgery in the United Kingdom and Ireland to submit annual figures for all cases operated on and the mortality at 30 days.[10] This became a very valuable resource for planning the size and distribution of units and for monitoring results, as judged by mortality figures. It was anonymous. Individual surgeons were not identified and then when the unit results were centralised the data were pooled so that no unit could be identified. Anonymity was the culture of the times. In cardiac surgery, death is the most evident deleterious effect and can be counted.

Years later the data were sent for by the lawyers leading the Bristol enquiry in 1999 in an attempt to retrieve information of 10 and 20 years ago from the boxes of anonymised papers. The press and lawyers of the late 1990s cannot understand why it was ever anonymous when instigated in the 1970s.

In 1986, Professor Ken Taylor and his team at the Hammersmith Hospital began collecting data at source for all valves implanted in the United Kingdom. In 1988, and every year since, the "Valve register" has provided us with information about valve practice, tissue versus mechanical valve implants, age of patients, and deaths.[90]

Public attitudes

The public attitude to the register – why was it anonymous – is instructive. Cardiac surgery in the postwar years seemed an impossible ambition. By the 1960s, in the boom of "can do" technology, everything seemed soluble. Surgeons were expected to be responsible, but this included being valued and respected by patients and colleagues. "Accountable" is a term of the 1990s. It is an essential concept but in cardiac surgery has attached to it fear of blame, guilt, and criticism.

The last months of the century end with the Royal Brompton Hospital in disarray because of an anonymous letter from a whistleblower, which in other times might well have been discarded as no more than a poison pen letter. The letter was sent to the satirical magazine *Private Eye* and to the barrister at the Bristol enquiry.

The climate of opinion surrounding Souttar was unaccepting of heart surgery, but then because they thought it was impossible – an unrealistic surgical ambition. In 1925, Souttar wrote on the subject of mitral stenosis:

> the problem is to a large extent mechanical, and as such should already be within the scope of surgery, were it not for the extraordinary nature of the conditions under

which the problem must be attacked . . . and that apart from them the heart is as amenable to surgery as any other organ.

The problem confronting surgeons now is that the heart is amenable to surgery so why do they still sometimes fail to achieve success? Complex cardiac surgery has become routine at the end of a century which began with even the simplest heart operation an impossibility.

References and notes

1. Obituary Lord Brock. *BMJ* 1980;281:814.
2. Cornelius EH, Taylor SF. *Lives of the fellows of the Royal College of Surgeons of England 1974–82.* London: Royal College of Surgeon of England, 1988.
3. Layle I, Taylor SF. *Lives of the fellows of the Royal College of Surgeons of England 1983–1990.* London: Royal College of Surgeon of England, 1995:13–15.
4. Harland JC, d'Abreu F. Lumbo-dorsal sympathectomy in severe hypertension. *BMJ* 1949;1:1019–24.
5. McMichael J. The management of hypertension. *BMJ* 1952;1:932–8.
6. Price FW. *A textbook of the practice of medicine.* 7th ed. London: Oxford University Press, 1946:979.
7. Lewis T. *Diseases of the heart.* 4th ed. London: Macmillan and Co, 1946:159.
8. Keogh BE, Kinsman R. *National adult cardiac surgery database report 1998.* London: Society of Cardiothoracic Surgeons of Great Britain and Ireland, May 1999.
9. Society of Cardiothoracic Surgeons of Great Britain and Ireland. *UK cardiac surgery register.* An annual record of operation numbers and mortality rates by category of operation, form 1977 to the present.
10. English TAH, Bailey AR, Dark JF, Williams WG. The UK Cardiac Surgical Register, 1977–82. *BMJ* 1984;289:1205–8.
11. Anonymous. Surgical operation for mitral stenosis. [Editorial] *Lancet* 1902;i:461–2.
12. Treasure T. Lessons from the Bristol case. *BMJ* 1998;316:1685–6.
13. Dyer C. Compensation claims expected to follow GMC's findings. *BMJ* 1998;316:1691.
14. Brunton L. Preliminary note on the possibility of treating mitrals stenosis by surgical methods. *Lancet* 1902;i:352.
15. Lane WA. Surgical operation for mitral stenosis. [Letter] *Lancet* 1902;1:547.
16. Fisher T. Surgical operation for mitral stenosis. [Letter] *Lancet* 1902;i:547–8.
17. Samways DW. Surgical operation for mitral stenosis. [Letter] *Lancet* 1902;i:548.
18. Pratt JH. Recollections and letter of Sir James Mackenzie. *N Engl J Med* 1941;224:1–10.
19. Robinson RHOB, Le Fanu WR. Lives of the fellows of the Royal College of Surgeons of England 1952–64. London: Royal College of Surgeon of England, 1988:390–2.
20. Souttar HS. The surgical treatment of mitral stenosis. *BMJ* 1925;2:603–7.
21. Ellis RH. Henry Souttar and surgery of the mitral valve. Part I: the surgeon and his patient. *J Med Biog* 1997;5:8–13.
22. Ellis RH. Henry Souttar and surgery of the mitral valve. Part II: the operation and its aftermath. *J Med Biog* 1997;5:63–9.
23. Cutler EC, Levine SA. Cardiotomy and valulotomy for mitral stenosis. Experimental observations and clinical notes concerning and operated case with recovery. *Boston Med Surg J* 1923;188:1023–7.
24. Cutler EC, Beck CS. The present state of the surgical procedures in chronic valvular disease of the heart. A final report of all surgical cases. *Arch Surg* 1929;18:403–16.
25. Treasure T, Hollman H. The surgery of mitral stenosis 1898–1948: why did it take 50 years to establish mitral valvotomy? *Ann R Coll Surg* 1995;77:145–51.
26. Harken DE. The emergence of cardiac surgery I Personal recollections of the 1940s and 1950s. *J Thoracic Cardiovasc Surg* 1989;98:805–13.
27. *Sir John Josias Conybeare 1888–1967.* Textbook of medicine 1st ed. Edinburgh: E and S Livingstone, 1929:389–90.
28. O'Shaugnessy L. An experimental method of suipplying a collateral circulation to the heart. *Br J Surg* 1936;23:665–70.
29. Davies DT, Mansell HE, O'Shaugnessy L. Surgical treatment of angina pectoris and allied conditions. *Lancet* 1938;i:1–10, 76–82.
30. Ribet M. Surgical treatment of carcinoma of the oesophagus and Laurence O'Shaugnessy. *Thorax* 1992;47:842.

31. Souttar H. *A surgeon in Belgium.* London: Arnold, 1915.
32. Harken DE. Foreign bodies in, and in relation to, the thoracic blood vessels and heart. I. Techniques for approaching and removing foreign bodies from the chambers of the heart. *Surg Gynecol Obstet* 1946;83:117–25.
33. Hurt R. The history of cardiothoracic surgery from early times. New York, London: Parthenon, 1996.
34. Bourne G, Keele K, Tubbs OS. Ligation and chemotherapy for infection of patent ductus arteriosus. *Lancet* 1940;ii:444–6.
35. Discussion on the treatment of fractures: with special reference to its organisation and teaching. *BMJ* 1925;2:317–31.
36. Cooter R. The politics of a spatial innovation: fracture clinics in inter-war Britain. In: Pickstone JV, ed. *Medical innovations in historical perspective.* New York: St Martin's Press, 1992: 146–64.
37. The minutes of the Guys Hospital medical committee, and of the house committee, and the operating books referred to were studied by TT during a sabbatical as research fellow at the Wellcome Institute for the History of Medicine in London.
38. Shumacker HB. *The evolution of cardiac surgery.* Bloomington, IN: Indiana University Press, 1992.
39. Blalock A, Taussig HB. The surgical treatment of malformations of the heart in which there is pulmonary stenosis or atresia. *JAMA* 1945;128:189–202.
40. The Minutes of the Peacock Club. The contemporaneous account. Tom Treasure's personal collection.
41. Abbot ME. *Atlas of congenital cardiac disease.* New York: American Heart Association, 1936.
42. Holmes Sellors (1902–87), later Sir Thomas, became president of the Royal College of Surgeons of England (1969–72) as did Russell Brock (1963–66). Holmes Sellors's main base was the Middlesex Hospital where he was appointed in 1947, seven years after his appointment at Harefield. He was held in admiration and respect by his fellow surgeons, and his kindly character, unfailing courtesy, and good humour led to him being always known simply as "Uncle Tom."
43. Layle I, Taylor SF. Lives of the fellows of the Royal College of Surgeons of England 1983–1990. London: Royal College of Surgeons of England 1995, 333–6.
44. Holmes Sellors P. Personal communication to author.
45. Holmes Sellors T. Surgery of pulmonary stenosis. A case in which the pulmonary valve was successfully divided. *Lancet* 1948;i:988–9.
46. Brock RC. Pulmonary valvotomy for the relief of congenital pulmonary stenosis. Report of three cases. *BMJ* 1948;1:1121–6.
47. Conybeare Sir John, ed. *Textbook of medicine.* 8th ed. Edinburgh: E & S Livingstone, 1947:531–4. (Authors include Baker, Brock and Campbell.) The following is included under "Mitral disease": "Although mitral disease is usually described under the headings of regurgitation and stenosis, it is very doubtful whether these two processes are not always concurrent, but in the more severe and chronic cases stenosis is the predominating clinical feature" and "No specific symptoms are associated with mitral stenosis unless the heart muscle is failing."
48. Price FW. *A textbook of the practice of medicine.* 7th ed, 1946. Frederick W Price MD FRS (Edin) was senior physician to the Royal Northern Hospital and Physician to the National Hospital for Diseases of the Heart.
49. Lewis T. *Diseases of the heart.* 4th ed. London: MacMillan and Co, 1946.
50. Editorial. Surgery of congenital heart disease. *BMJ* 1948;1:1192–3.
51. Baker C, Brock RC, Campbell M. Valvulotomy for mitral stenosis. Report of six successful cases. *BMJ* 1950;1:1283–93.
52. Brock RC. One of the cited authors in a report of the Royal Society of Medicine, surgical section 4.4.51. Surgery of the heart and great vessels. *BMJ* 1951;1:946–7.
53. Meeting report. Festival year conference on tuberculosis and diseases of the chest. *BMJ* 1951;2:296–8.
54. Baker C, Brock RC, Campbell M, Wood P. Valvotomy for mitral stenosis. A further report on 100 cases. *BMJ* 1952;1:1043–55.
55. Treasure T. Surgery for mitral stenosis in Guy's and the Middlesex Hospitals 1948–1953. *J R Soc Med* 1996;89:19–22.
56. Holmes Sellors T, Evan Bedford D, Somerville W. Valvotomy in the treatment of mitral stenosis. *BMJ* 1953;2:1059–67.
57. Logan A, Turner R. Mitral stenosis. Diagnosis and treatment. *Lancet* 1953;i:1007–18, 1057–64.
58. Logan A, Turner R. Mitral valvulotomy in pregnancy. *Lancet* 1952;i:1286.
59. O'Connell TCJ, Mulcahy R. Emergency mitral valvotomy at full term. *BMJ* 1955;1:1191–1.
60. Logan A, Turner R. Surgical treatment of mitral stenosis with particular reference to the transventricular approach with a mechanical dilator. *Lancet* 1959;ii:874–80.
61. British Medical Association. Mitral Stenosis. Thursday July 8th. Annual Meeting, Glasgow 1954. *BMJ* 1954;ii:151, 161–2.

62. Anonymous. Mitral stenosis. [Editorial] *BMJ* 1954;1:1138–9.
63. Wood P. An appreciation of mitral stenosis. *BMJ* 1954;1:1051–63, 1113–24.
64. Treasure T. Balloon dilatation of the aortic valve in adults: a surgeon's view. *Br Heart J* 1990;63:205–6.
65. Treasure T. The safe duration of total circulatory arrest with profound hypothermia. *Ann R Coll Surg Engl* 1984;66:235–40.
66. Ross DN. Hypothermia. *Guy's Hosp Rep* 1954;103:116–38.
67. Bedford DE, Sellors TH, Somerville W, Belcher JR. Atrial septal defect and its surgical treatment. *Lancet* 1957;i:255.
68. Sellors TH. Atrial septal defects. *Minerva Cardioangiol Eur* 1960;8:172–83.
69. Drew CE, Keene G, Benazon DB. Profound hypothermia. *Lancet* 1959;i:745.
70. Tan PSK, Aveling W, Pugsley WB, Newman SP, Treasure T. Experience with circulatory arrest and hypothermia to facilitate thoracic aortic surgery. *Ann R Coll Surg Engl* 1989;71:81–6.
71. Belsey RHR, Dowlatshahi K, Keen G, Skinner DB. Profound hypothermia in cardiac surgery. *J Thoracic Cardiovasc Surg* 1968;56:497–509.
72. Yacoub MY, Radley-Smith R, Hilton CJ. Anatomical correction of complete transposition of the great arteries and ventricular septal defect in infancy. *BMJ* 1976;1:1112.
73. Cleland WP. The evolution of cardiac surgery in the United Kingdom. *Thorax* 1983;38:887–96.
74. Melrose DG, Dreyer B, Bentall HH, Baker JBE. Elective cardiac arrest. *Lancet* 1955;ii:21–2.
75. Hearse DJ, Stewart DA, Braimbridge MV. Cellular protection during myocardial ischemia: The development of a procedure for the induction of reversible ischemic arrest. *Circulation* 1976;54:193.
76. Ross DN. Homograft replacement of the aortic valve. *Lancet* 1962;ii:487.
77. Ross DN. Replacement of aortic a mitral valve with a pulmonary autograft. *Lancet* 1967;ii:956.
78. Ionescu MI, Ross DN. Heart-valve replacement with autologous fascia lata. *Lancet* 1969;ii:335.
79. McEnany MT, Ross DN, Yates AK. Cusp degeneration in frame-supported autologous fascia lata mitral valves. *Thorax* 1972;27:23.
80. Treasure T. Rethink on biological aortic valves for the elderly. *Lancet* 1999;354:964–5.
81. Bloomfield P, Wheatley DJ, Prescott RJ, Miller HC. Twelve-year comparison of a Bjork-Shiley mechanical with porcine bioprostheses. *N Engl J Med* 1991;324:573–79.
82. Bentall HH, de Bono A. A technique for complete replacement of the ascending aorta. *Thorax* 1968;48:443.
83. Early heart transplant surgery in the UK. Witness seminar transcript. In: Tansy EM, Reynolds LA eds. *Witnesses to twentieth century medicine.* Vol 3. London: Wellcome Institute, 1999.
84. Front cover. *Private Eye* 5 July 1968. (The surgeons were pictured on the front above the caption '"O.K. So we goofed" say Heart Men')
85. Fox R, Swazey J. The heart transplant moratorium. In: *The courage to fail. A social view of organs transplants and dialysis.* Chicago, London: University of Chicago Press, 1974.
86. European Coronary Surgery Study Group. Long term results of prospective randomised study of coronary artery surgery in stable angina pectoris. *Lancet* 1982;ii:1173–8.
87. Pocock SJ, Henderson RA, Seed P, Treasure T, Hampton JR. Quality of Life, employment status and anginal symptoms after coronary angioplasty or bypass surgery: three years follow-up in the randomised intervention treatment of angina (RITA) trial. *Circulation* 1996;94:135–42.
88. Cronin AJ. *The citadel.* London: Victor Gollancz, 1937.
89. Yates J. *Private eye, heart and hip. Surgical consultants, the National Health Service and private medicine.* Edinburgh: Churchill Livingstone, 1995.
90. Medical Devices Agency. *The United Kingdom Heart Valve Registry report 1996.* London: Department of Health. Crown Copyright, 1998.

Chapter 17

Cardiac Pacing

Aubrey Leatham, Anthony Rickards, and Ronald Gold

Early Days of Pacing at St George's Hospital, London

Aubrey Leatham

In 1954, I left the post of assistant director to Paul Wood at the Institute of Cardiology, the National Heart Hospital to take up a position at St George's Hospital, then at Hyde Park Corner. There was no cardiac department and I was the first cardiologist to be appointed. However, I brought with me Geoff Davies, one of the first cardiac technicians trained in physics, who had been working with Sheila Howarth on pressure manometers.

One of the last patients I had investigated at the National Heart Hospital had died during cardiac catheterisation – of cardiac standstill caused by catheter induced right bundle branch block on pre-existing left bundle branch block. I realised that an external pacemaker, as had recently been described by Zoll, might have enabled her to be successfully resuscitated. Then, a few months later, a patient on quinidine treatment died unexpectedly. Geoff Davies, now attached to the physics department at St George's, began to construct an external pacemaker. Zoll had not described any circuitry, and Geoff had to start from first principles. He added a circuit to prevent an R on T sequence, which was already well known to be a trigger for ventricular fibrillation; his was probably the first demand pacemaker. By the end of 1955, Geoff had finished the pacemaker and had also prepared some emergency apparatus consisting of a high voltage battery, a condenser, and a Morse key to activate the impulses.

The external pacemaker

In November 1955, a lightly built 60 year old woman with almost continuous Stokes-Adams attacks was admitted to St George's.[1] Although she was almost moribund, each impulse at 150 V across the chest wall was followed by an arterial pulse (figure 1), and she immediately regained consciousness. The problem was the pain from the unwanted contraction

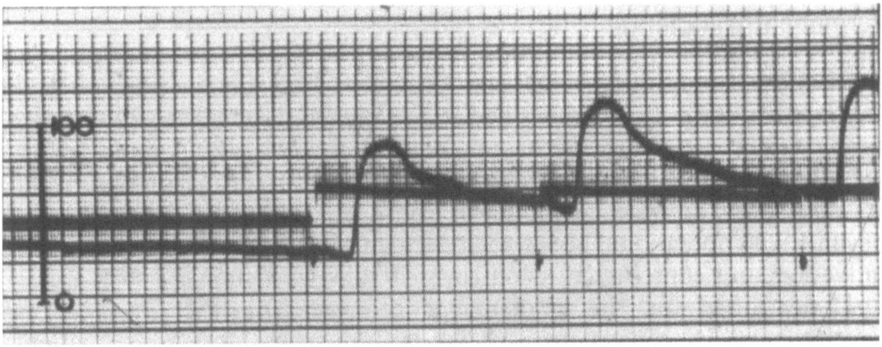

Figure 1 The first patient to be paced in the United Kingdom (1955). The tracing shows arterial pressure which is flat until the pacemaker spikes restart the heart.

of chest wall muscles; it was unaffected by local anaesthesia and the woman needed a light general anaesthetic or very heavy analgesia to tolerate it. A lower voltage was ineffective. After three days of periodic stimulation, spontaneous idioventricular rhythm returned, and for four days the woman was comfortable and free of cerebral damage. She then experienced further cardiac standstills and needed additional electrical stimulation, which was invariably effective. The woman eventually died at a time when the stimulator was not available. At the post mortem examination, Professor Sir Theo Crawford and Dr (later Professor) Michael Davies showed, to our surprise, that the only cardiac abnormality was localised fibrosis of the conducting tissue peripheral to the atrioventricular node.

This unexpected finding, later confirmed in 26 of our first 65 consecutive post mortem examinations,[2] spurred us to continue our investigations. In another more heavily built patient, stimulated contraction at 150 V was not continuously successful. Higher voltages with the emergency apparatus using a high tension battery and a Morse key were successful, but impractical for continued use. Unfortunately, permission for necropsy was not obtained in this patient. The external pacemaker was used most successfully in a patient on quinidine treatment who collapsed and was found to be asystolic; he was paced for 2 hours and made a good recovery.

It was obvious that much lower voltages must be applied directly to the ventricular wall in patients with disease of the conducting tissue. Cardiac catheters with an indwelling wire had been used in animals and were being used by electrophysiologists for experimental mapping via the venous system; we tried this in 1959.[3] Temporary stimulation, using 9 V with the tip of the electrode in the right atrium, was successful in three cases, and this was probably the first attempt at endocardial pacing. We hesitated to place the electrode in the right ventricle because we believed that this might provoke ventricular tachycardia or fibrillation from ventricular irritation or that perforation might occur, and we were worried about the possibility of thromboembolism.

Permanently implantable devices

Around the same time (1958), Leon Abrams and his engineering colleague Ray Lightwood in Birmingham had built external pacemakers for use after surgery to repair ventricular septal defect, and were talking about permanently implantable devices. Because a pacemaker circuit needed to include at least seven discrete components whose life could not be guaranteed beyond 1000 operational hours, they decided to use simple electromagnetic induction, and constructed nylon covered coils with stainless steel epicardial electrodes for the implantable components.[4][5] The external generators were constructed by Lucas Industries, and some patients continued to be paced for 20 years after their first surgical intervention using this system.

Like Abrams and others in the United States and in Sweden, we felt that the way forward was via thoracotomy, suturing of an electrode to the left ventricle (the right ventricle being too thin), and bringing lead wires through the skin to an external source of power. Fortunately, Harold Siddons of St George's, an experienced thoracic surgeon, was interested in joining us. He proved to be a very important part of our pacing team, not only in relation to operative procedures but because he kept detailed records of our results and later joined with Edgar Sowton to write an early book on pacemaking.[6] Infection was, of course, a problem, but we reduced this by having a long subcutaneous course for the stimulating wires.

Eventually, Elmquist and Senning in Sweden devised an entirely subcutaneous epicardial system with a battery operated miniaturised pacemaker in the abdomen. We imitated their developments, and Geoff Davies made the pacemakers and wires at St George's. However, we found that thoracotomy for placement of the electrode carried an appreciable mortality in elderly people. In addition, the threshold frequently increased over a period of months, so that the power of the pacemaker had to be increased. We presumed that this was secondary to the induction of fibrosis or to infection by unknown micro-organisms, but we were unable to establish the cause.

In the meantime, temporary endocardial pacing for acute infarction block was being used at the Montefiore Hospital in the United States, and because of our rejection problems we decided to develop a long term endocardial system.[7] In 1965, we published our results in a series of 65 patients paced for up to 3 years.[8]

Geoff Davies developed miniaturised pacemakers and long lasting endocardial wires at St George's, and Devices later marketed these. Early difficulties with the reliability of the pacemaker meant that we had to exteriorise the unit, but the incidence of septicaemia was not as high as expected, provided that there was a long subcutaneous course for the insertion of the wire into the vein. Compared with the epicardial wires, Davies' endocardial wires rarely caused problems. This was probably because of the relative immobility of the wire in the superior vena cava compared with epicardial wires attached to the apex.

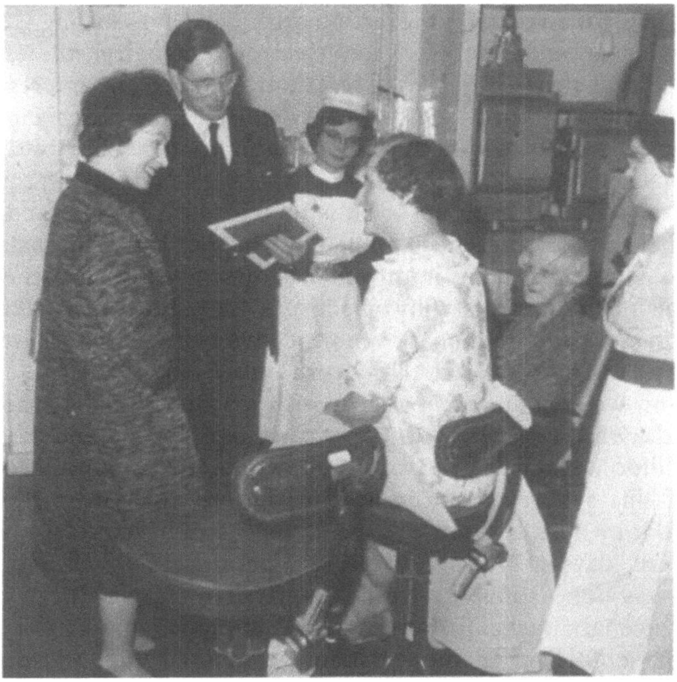

Figure 2 The Queen's visit to see pacing in the cardiac unit at St George's Hospital in 1962. The patient in the foreground, who was paced for Stokes-Adams attacks, was still alive and well 18 years later.

Pacing rate

Our early indwelling pacemakers were used for patients with chronic heart block (not acute coronary disease). They ran at a fixed rate of 70, and we were worried by the possibility of pacemaker induced ventricular fibrillation. However, a statistical analysis of mortality by Harold Siddons, in which the early fixed rate and later demand systems were compared, showed no difference in mortality.[9]

The aetiology of the disease of the conducting tissue in our patients who presented with recurrent syncope was largely idiopathic fibrosis. It was often isolated (as pointed out earlier), and ventricular fibrillation did not usually occur once a satisfactory pacing rate had been established. We were puzzled at first by the massive T wave inversion and ST depression seen in these patients, but there was nothing to suggest myocardial ischaemia. These findings were secondary to the artificial depolarisation, but the mechanism remains unexplained.[10]

At that time we were not dealing with acute infarction block, and no longer used epicardial pacing with its risk of chest complications, anoxia, and arrhythmia. Most of our patients had a fairly good myocardium, and Edgar Sowton in our laboratory showed that there was a satisfactory increase in stroke volume on exertion with fixed rate pacing.[11] Sowton put an immense amount of work into electrophysiological studies in pacing in his doctoral thesis.[12] His dissertation included the interesting point that the optimum pacing rate could be deduced from observing the atrial rate which increased with a fall in cardiac output induced by a less than optimal pacemaker rate.

We also looked at a group of patients with heart failure and complete block who had slow heart rates but no syncope.[13] While patients with exertional dyspnoea alone improved with pacing, this happened in only about half of the patients with objective evidence of heart failure (raised venous pressure and pulmonary venous congestion) – in those whose heart block was caused by an underlying cardiomyopathy.

Early on we encountered patients with isolated sinoatrial disease who presented with less severe symptoms from bradycardia and often experienced additional attacks of paroxysmal tachycardia or flutter. We were well aware of this syndrome since Short at the National Heart Hospital had described it in 1954, and some of the patients had been under my care.[14] In the early days of pacing, inserting a pacemaker in these bradycardic patients was not justifiable – years would often lapse between clusters of minor syncopal attacks. However, we did notice an appreciable incidence of thromboembolism in these patients compared with those with atrioventricular block[15], and we gave them anticoagulants. In the relatively rare patient with sinoatrial disease who was paced, we set the pacemaker at low rates (for example, 50) with hysteresis, so that pacing took place when only required. Thus, we seldom encountered the "pacemaker syndrome." We were rather critical of some establishments where 40% of all patients paced had isolated sinoatrial disease with excellent long term prognosis, though we appreciated fully that some of these patients would develop atrioventricular disease later.

We soon had more than 1000 patients attending our pacemaker clinic and were attracting many patients with acute infarction block from other hospitals. Some of these patients with large infarcts (usually anterior) had low output and heart failure. Our routine was to measure endocardial thresholds daily. We wanted to test the stability of the electrode and to avoid inappropriate pacing and competition in patients with coronary disease, who (unlike patients with isolated fibrosis of the conducting tissue) were prone to ventricular fibrillation.

Kanu Chatterjee (now at the University of California in San Francisco), who almost lived in the cardiac wards in those days, soon noticed the external pacemaker working away in post infarction patients who had returned to sinus rhythm. He found that there was an association between cardiac dilatation and endocardial potentials so low that they could not abolish inappropriate pacing.[16] There is then a great danger of inducing ventricular fibrillation – something that is probably not fully appreciated nowadays. Indeed our awareness of the danger of pacing in patients with coronary disease and cardiac dilatation (usually anterior infarction block) led us to withdraw pacing systems as soon as sinus rhythm returned, and long term follow up supported this conclusion since recurrence of block was rare.[17]

Good outcomes

With the rapid collection of a large number of patients treated for syncope from slow heart rates we soon became very aware, like others, that pacing not only prevented syncope from standstill, it also prevented ventricular fibrillation secondary to a slow heart rate. It seemed logical, therefore, to try pacing at fast rates to prevent recurrent ventricular fibrillation in patients with an acute myocardial infarction, and we reported some success[18]. In 1979, we analysed the prognosis of 839 patients who underwent pacing for chronic atrioventricular block between 1960 and 1974.[19] We excluded patients with acute infarction block (because of its bad prognosis when due to anterior infarction) and those with sinoatrial disease without atrioventricular block (because this was known to have a good prognosis whether paced or not). Once endocardial pacing had been established, the long term results were extremely good. In the older age groups, the outlook for patients was little different from that of the general population, but results were poorer in the 90 patients aged 50–59 years, probably because of a higher incidence of coronary disease as the cause of the problems encountered. Septicaemia was the most worrying possibility with an endocardial pacing system. Fortunately, however, septicaemia was rare, since it meant withdrawing the endocardial system and replacing it with an epicardial system.[20]

From St George's to the National Heart Hospital

Anthony Rickards

I started my postgraduate training at the National Heart Hospital in 1969. At that time Aubrey Leatham and Edgar Sowton were on the consultant staff and John Norman was the chief cardiac technician. Interest in electrical stimulation of the heart was strong. Edgar Sowton had published his doctoral thesis on the haemodynamic consequences of heart block and the effects of cardiac pacing while working as a cardiac registrar to Aubrey Leatham at St George's.[12] He had recently returned from the Karolinska Institute in Sweden where he had collaborated with the team that started clinical pacing. Like St George's, the National Heart Hospital was one of the few tertiary cardiac centres with expertise in pacing, and it attracted both patients and physicians alike.

At the time, pacing for symptomatic heart block was well established. We tended to implant fixed rate devices in patients with stable complete block and demand pacemakers in those with intermittent block. Generators were supplied by Devices, Elema-Schonander, Cordis, and Medtronic. Demand devices were more expensive, and clinical problems were created by undersensing and oversensing. Furthermore, implanting an endocardial lead was straightforward but tedious. This was because of poor screening and lack of tube intensifier angulation and rolling tables, which enabled us to rotate patients into oblique views in order to "drop" floppy electrodes across the tricuspid valve. Because of unpredictable failure modes and unreliable electrodes, pacing systems lasted 2–3 years at best. Programming and interrogation of pacemakers were unknown, and the diagnosis of system failure from external analysis of the pacing pulse became a well developed but imprecise science carried out by a team of very able and highly trained technicians under the tutelage of John Norman.

Research themes

The National Heart Hospital team was pursuing several research themes. The first was the temporary use of pacing for therapy and diagnosis. Edgar Sowton had shown that temporary, fast ventricular pacing could reduce the incidence of ventricular arrhythmias in post infarction patients, and this work was soon extended to the use of temporary atrial pacing for suppressing atrial and ventricular arrhythmias.[21][22]

The diagnostic theme revolved around the investigation of angina. The β blocking drugs had only recently been developed by Imperial Chemical Industries, and a succession of post propranolol derivatives were being actively investigated. These compounds worked in angina by blocking the heart rate response to exercise and reducing the resting heart rate, so it seemed logical to investigate their haemodynamic effects in an environment in which the heart rate was controlled. Heikki Frick and Raphael Balcon described the use of incremental, temporary atrial pacing for the induction of angina.[23] This technique allowed the haemodynamic consequences of ischaemia to be investigated in a resting supine patient in whom measurements of outputs and pressures were unaffected by exercise. Atrial pacing in patients with coronary disease became widely adopted as a standard technique for diagnosing angina and investigating of the effects of ischaemia and candidate drugs for angina.[24]

Improving the interaction between the pulse generator and the patient was another major interest. We realised that demand pacemakers would eventually replace fixed rate devices because they avoided the practical and theoretical problems of asynchronous pacing. Demand pacemakers which stimulated the right ventricle produced a contraction that was not synchronised to atrial activity. There was a wide left bundle branch block QRS complex, which had been shown by Derek Gibson (then a registrar at the National Heart Hospital) to be less effective in terms of ventricular ejection than a narrow QRS complex produced by pacing both ventricles simultaneously.[25]

Edgar Sowton stimulated a whole series of research activities that laid much of the groundwork for improved therapeutic pacing. The most important of these activities are shown in the box (see p. 221).

Further research at the National Heart Hospital

- The invention of rate hysteresis where demand pacemakers had dual escape intervals depending on whether the preceding beat was sensed or paced. Thus, after a sensed intrinsic QRS complex, the escape interval for the pulse generator would be longer (preserving sinus rhythm to a lower heart rate) than after a paced beat (maintaining a reasonable heart rate when pacing)
- Showing that the function of a demand pacemaker could be affected by various external electrical noise generators (such as electric razors, car engines, radios) and that pacemaker function was frequently inhibited by electromyograhic noise produced by pectoral muscle contraction in unipolar configurations[26]
- Work imported from St George's Hospital showing that the intrinsic endocardial QRS complex could be defined in terms of amplitude and frequency content, and that both were important in designing a demand pacemaker able to sense properly in situations such as myocardial infarction[27]
- Research showing the phenomenon of T wave sensing in demand pacemakers. The QRS sensing circuit could be fooled into believing that a ventricular ectopic had occurred if a large amplitude evoked T wave occurred at the end of the post ventricular stimulus refractory period. This meant that the escape interval was reset and the pacemaker rate fell to below the preset pacing rate
- Further work comparing dual chamber and single chamber pacing in AV block showed that the atrial contribution to cardiac output tended to lessen as heart rate increased at rest[28]

Improvement of demand pacemakers

All these research activities and interactions between physicians and technicians working closely together led to three important long term effects on therapeutic pacing. The first was to improve demand pacemakers. The earliest devices (arguably developed at St George's by Geoff Davies) had relatively unsophisticated sensing circuits triggered by intrinsic QRS complexes to reset the pacing escape interval. Work done at St George's and the National Heart Hospital allowed device manufacturers to tune their sensing circuits much more precisely to intrinsic complexes and to reject interference from T waves, electromyographic activity, and external electromagnets. Thus, they were able to develop fail safe systems such as interference pacing when the pulse generator was swamped by electrical noise.

Dual chamber pacing

The second effect was the premature development of dual chamber demand pacing. We were aware of American and Swedish work in which pacemakers with atrial sensing capability had been implanted. Devices which implemented atrial triggered pacing were available from Elema and Cordis. With these devices, electrodes were implanted on the atrium and ventricle at thoracotomy. Electrodes were then connected to a generator, which paced the ventricle either on sensing an atrial impulse (with a suitable AV delay) or at the end of a ventricular post pacing escape interval. These pacemakers had no non-competitive function and tended to be used in young patients (where a heart rate response to exercise was considered important) who were undergoing thoracotomy for other reasons, such as the repair of a congenital cardiac defect.

In 1970, Edgar Sowton was looking after a young man with a cardiomyopathy, sinus bradycardia, and heart block who could accomplish little exercise when paced with a conventional demand pacemaker. We devised a pacing system based on a Cordis Ectocor (a demand pacemaker which emitted a stimulus on sensing rather than inhibition) and a Cordis Atricor (an atrial triggered pacemaker). I constructed a set of wiring in which the output of the Ectocor was connected directly to an atrial lead and also, via a resistor array, to the atrial input channel of the Atricor. This device and its associated wiring were implanted epicardially and the effect was of dual chamber pacing with demand triggered pacing in the atrium (figure 3).

This was probably the first example of dual chamber demand pacing (but with no ventricular demand function), although we subsequently became aware that Nicholas Smyth in the USA had done something similar at the same time. In 1975, Irnich first published his seminal article on the logical requirements for a dual chamber demand pacing system,[29] and Funke later published his experience with the Medtronic Optimized Sequential Stimulator.[30] At the end of the millennium some 50% of the 500 000 pacemakers implanted worldwide are dual chamber demand devices.

Non-atrial responsive generators

The third contribution to the future of pacing was the development of non-atrial rate responsive generators. Edgar Sowton had now become a consultant at Guy's Hospital in London, but he had left a strong legacy of research in pacing. In 1978, we tried to improve the sensing characteristics of ventricular demand pacemakers. In doing this, we were building external pacing devices modified to minimise the polarisation and after discharge effects of the stimulus so that we could observe the pacing evoked response from the pacing electrode lead. Until that time, all pacemakers started a refractory period after emitting a pacing pulse, because it was thought that any intrinsic activity would be of very small amplitude when compared with the after effects of the pacing pulse and was not therefore worth trying

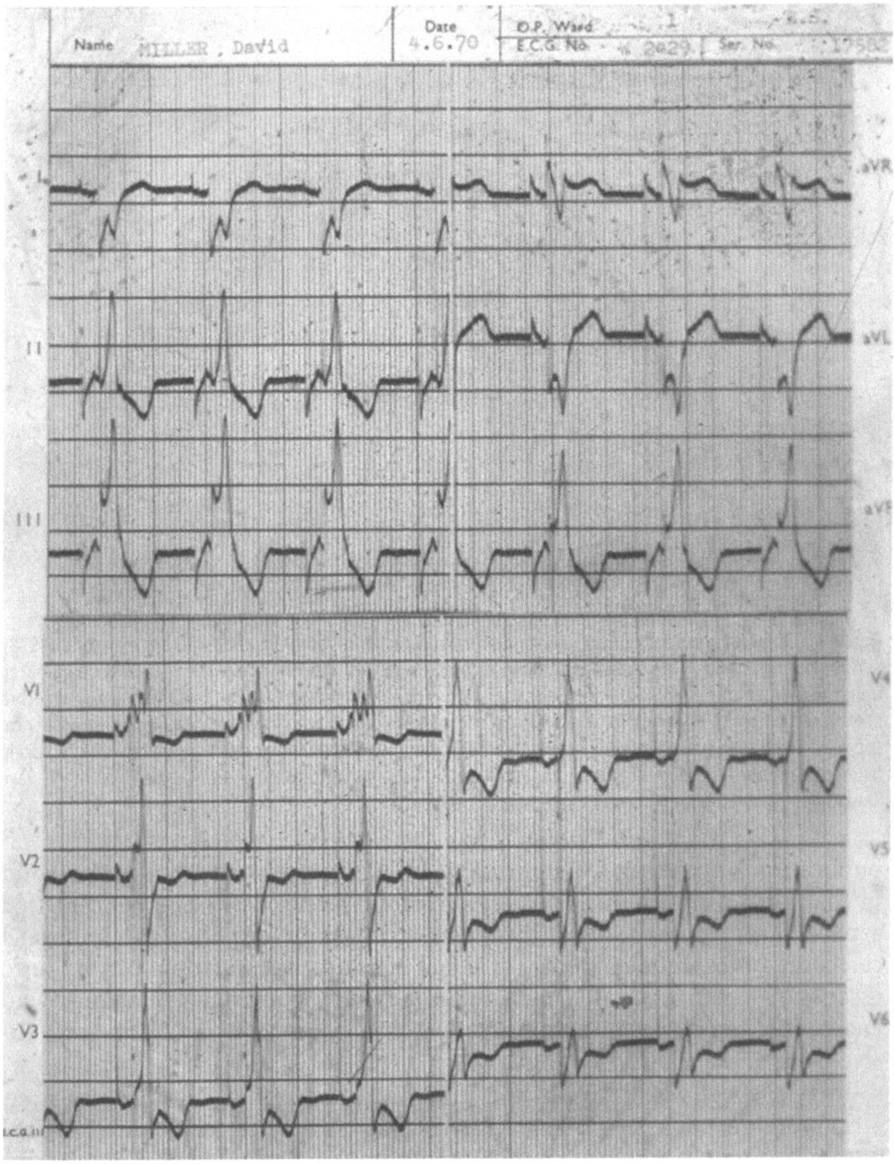

Figure 3 A 12 lead electrocardiogram recorded in 1970 showing dual chamber pacing (left atrium/left ventricle epicardial) with an atrial demand function.

to sense. We built an external generator which could be tuned to an individual electrode lead in an individual patient and which, for the first time, allowed us to see the intrinsic activity that followed pacing (figure 4).

The primary object of this work was to measure the amplitude and frequency content of evoked T waves to improve the discrimination of QRS sense amplifiers in demand pacemakers. I realised that active sensing of the evoked T wave might actually be put to good use; the original Bazett

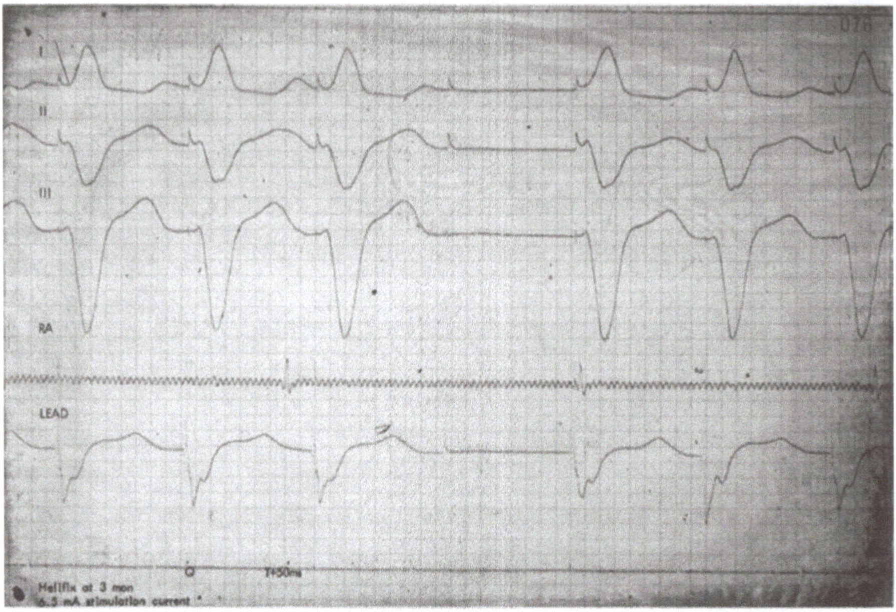

Figure 4 The first recording of an endocardial evoked response from an active pacing electrode (1978). Surface leads I, II, and III are shown with an intracardiac right atrial electrogram. The patient is being paced from the right ventricle with a unipolar electrode and is in complete heart block. "LEAD" is a unipolar record taken directly from the pacing electrode. A sharp pacing spike can be seen followed by a local QRS and T wave complex. The fourth pacing spike is below threshold and shows that electrical activity purely due to pacing (without capture) has been effectively abolished within 10 ms. The recording is not scaled but the T wave amplitude measured approximately 7 mV.

publication on linking QT interval to heart rate seemed to miss the point in that both were a function of sympathetic activity.[31] The concept that a pacemaker could be built to alter heart rate in response to circulating catecholamines, independently of atrial activity, was startling.[32] It led to discussions with a small Dutch manufacturing company (Vitatron), who engineered the device and thus promoted the whole concept of rate responsive pacing.

In retrospect, we were not the first to consider the possibility of non-atrial rate response. In 1966, Krasner had suggested using an external pacemaker whose rate was modulated by impedance changes due to respiration,[33] and Gianni Plicchi in Italy had used this idea to design a device first implanted in 1982.[34] Another eminent Italian, Cammilli, had actually constructed and implanted a ventricular demand pacemaker which had a subcutaneous pH sensor to sense the acidosis related to exercise and increased heart rate.[35] One of these devices was implanted and worked for a short time, producing a rate response to exercise before the first QT sensing pacemaker implant in April 1981. We were, however, the first to conceive, implant, and investigate the haemodynamic consequences of the first practical rate responsive system, and to popularise the concept around the world.[36–39] Around 50% of the 500 000 pacemakers now implanted annually worldwide are rate responsive devices, many of which use the principle of sensing the evoked response.

Quality assurance and coding systems

Finally there are two other small but important areas in which the National Heart Hospital contributed to the practice of pacing. The first was in the establishment of what has become a worldwide system for quality assurance in pacing.[39] In 1974, we started collecting relevant information about the patients and their implanted devices, and in 1978 developed a coding system which defined why patients were paced, what was done, and what were the clinical and technical outcomes. This coding system, the associated databases, and the identification cards carried by patients is now a worldwide standard and has been used by many countries as the basis for quality assurance. More is known about the practice and outcomes of pacing than any other large scale intervention in medicine through the regular world pacing surveys.

The second was the development of the current generator function coding system. As pacemakers became more complex, a simple code to describe the capability of an implanted device became necessary. The current five letter coding system (usually abbreviated to four letters is known as the NBG code (North American Society of Pacing and Electrophysiology, British Pacing and Electrophysiology Group, Generator) and was developed by professional groups in the United States and the United Kingdom with input from the National Heart Hospital.[40]

Acknowledgements

We thank the Editor of *The St George's Hospital Gazette* for permission to reproduce some of the text and also figure 1 from a paper entitled "The development of cardiology at St George's" (1995).

Recollections of Pacing from a Regional Centre

Ronald Gold

During my 30 years of active participation in cardiac pacing, the technological developments have been enormous. Just how great these changes have been, and their effect on patient management, is difficult to comprehend by those not involved in the early days. What follows is, of necessity, a personal and largely anecdotal account of some of my most vivid memories of those 30 years.

Early pacemakers

The first pacemakers I recall as a senior registrar at the Brompton Hospital in the early 1960s were those designed by Geoff Davies and described earlier in this chapter. The first models, produced by Devices Ltd, were for epicardial use only and used a loop electrode connected at both ends to the pacemaker. The later models, both fixed rate and demand, could also be used for endocardial pacing, and were still being implanted in considerable numbers in 1967, when I moved to a consultant post in Newcastle. The latter units were encapsulated in epoxy resin and coated with Silastic. They were commendably small, but had a pacing lifetime of 18 months to 2 years. The discrete components used in the circuits were not always reliable, and on several occasions this produced the phenomenon of "runaway pacemaker," where the pacing rate rose exponentially, sometimes over a few hours. Such an occurrence called for emergency action to remove the pacemaker. One patient I witnessed at the Brompton Hospital presented with a heart rate of 100 beats per minute, and on surgical removal of the pacemaker an hour or so later this had risen to 130. The next morning when I tested the unit on an oscilloscope the rate was over 1000. A lethal situation had thus been avoided.

The Lucas inductively coupled pacemaker referred to earlier had several advantages. The patient could renew the battery and adjust the rate, and the hospital could adjust the power setting. It also had important disadvantages. The external coil could become displaced, with loss of pacing, and the unit could not be taken into the bath. The fact that the patient could alter the rate also produced problems. One unfortunate patient died while in the Brompton Hospital because, being an engineer, it had occurred to him that he could save on batteries by turning the rate down at night, which he did without telling the hospital staff. By turning the rate too low he produced fatal ventricular fibrillation.

Batteries

Most implantable pacemakers available during the 1960s were powered by mercury-zinc Mallory cells. Because of the low voltage generated by these, several had to be used in each pacemaker. The more cells used, the longer the life of the pacemaker, but the consequent increase in the bulk and weight made extrusion of the device more likely. Implantation of these large pacemakers posed severe problems in thin patients, and particularly in young children, in whom the pacemaker had to be implanted in the abdominal wall or even in the extrapleural space. A further drawback of the mercury-zinc cell was that it produced hydrogen, which accumulated inside the encapsulating layer of the pacemaker and diffused out slowly through the capsule. For this reason pacemakers could not be hermetically sealed. Some ingress of body fluids was thus unavoidable, and this sometimes led to malfunction of the electronic circuits.

As the Mallory cells approached the end of their life, the amount of hydrogen they produced increased, causing a build up of pressure of the gas within the pacemaker. This could occasionally lead to disruption of the encapsulation. On one occasion, a pacemaker removed from a patient of mine who presented with the usual signs of battery depletion (slowing

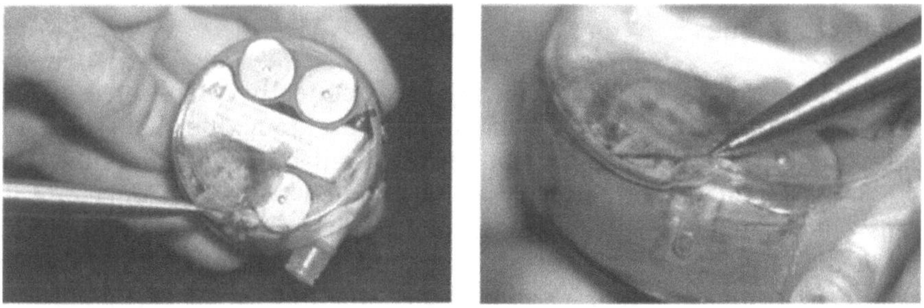

Figure 5 Disrupted pacemaker capsule showing the crack in the epoxy resin (pointer) and staining of one of the Mallory cells.

of the pacemaker rate and reduced amplitude and increased duration of the pacemaker impulse), showed an obvious crack in its encapsulation (figure 5). When I questioned him later, he recollected having experienced "a bit of a thump over the pacemaker a few weeks ago."

A major advance in pacemaker technology during the 1970s was the introduction of the lithium-iodine battery. This was smaller and lighter than the Mallory cell and produced a higher voltage so that only one cell was needed to produce an appropriate pacing stimulus. Furthermore, its lifetime was much greater, so that the hitherto Utopian concept of a pacemaker that would last 10 years or more became a reality. The reduction in size of the pacemaker was particularly advantageous in young children.

Development of the service

In the 1960s and 1970s, few theatres were dedicated to pacing or even to cardiac catheterisation, and the needs of a pacemaker implantation service had to vie with those of a busy radiology department. This made emergency temporary pacing very difficult.

In 1961, when I was a senior registrar at Papworth Hospital, I recall vividly admitting a patient from the Cambridgeshire Fens to the cardiac unit in the middle of the night. The patient had an acute myocardial infarction and was in complete heart block, but he was still conscious despite a heart rate of 10 beats per minute. Transfer to the *x* ray department, which doubled as our catheter laboratory, was not an option. My surgical senior registrar colleague, Mr Findlay Kerr and I introduced a surgical temporary pacing wire percutaneously into the right ventricle via a left ventricular puncture needle, completing the pacing circuit with a stainless steel suture in the skin as the indifferent electrode. The patient returned to sinus rhythm after a few days and was discharged from hospital after 10 days. This must have been one of the earliest examples of emergency pacing via that route, long before the advent of the Elecath needle, specifically designed for this purpose.

Pacing techniques

In the early 1960s, transvenous pacing was frequently complicated by lead displacement during the first 24–48 hours, but seldom after that. Tined and active fixation pacing leads did not become available until some time later. This led Mr Matt Paneth and myself to devise a two-stage procedure for transvenous pacing. The lead was introduced in the catheter laboratory via the medial antecubital vein, as was standard procedure in those days for right heart catheterisation. If the lead position and pacing threshold were satisfactory after 48 hours, the patient was taken to theatre. There the lead and insertion site were sterilised with povidone iodine, the lead was cut off at the point of insertion and brought out through a purse string incision which had been made in the axillary vein, and it was connected to the pacemaker which was then implanted subcutaneously in the axilla.[41] This seemingly primitive technique worked surprisingly well and continued to be used until the advent of better lead designs rendered it obsolete. When I moved to a consultant post in Newcastle in 1967, I found that the technique was still in use there, albeit partly for a different reason. Pressure on the *x* ray room which doubled as a catheter laboratory was such that the short time taken to insert a pacing lead into the right ventricle could be accommodated, but not the longer time required for a complete pacemaker implantation.

Managing a regional service

Managing a regional pacing service in the provinces in the 1960s and 1970s posed a number of problems not often encountered in London. Not the least of these was the wide geographical area that had to be covered by such a service, particularly in the more sparsely populated areas of the north of England and Scotland. For example, the Newcastle Regional Pacing Service embraced the whole of Northumberland, Cumbria,and County Durham, and because of local transport problems, especially in winter, spread beyond these into parts of North Yorkshire and the Borders. The pacing centres in Glasgow had to cover the entire west coast and Western Isles of Scotland.

The low population density coupled with the then low rate of pacemaker implantation meant that it was not economically feasible to establish pacing facilities in every district general hospital. Pacemaker implantation was therefore confined to those centres already equipped to perform cardiac catheterisation, where the medical and technical expertise was also centred.

For the same reasons, follow up of the pacemaker patient was fraught with difficulties. Patients had to travel long distances, often on poor roads and in poor weather conditions to attend the nearest regional centre. In Scotland, the journey even involved air travel. This often meant considerable patient hardship and a large bill in ambulance charges for the local health authority. One remedy for this was to establish pacemaker clinics in the district general hospitals. In early days this meant regular visits from the regional centre by a cardiologist and an experienced technician. This imposed a heavy workload on both and reduced the presence of staff at the regional centre often by the best part of a day.

Another solution, which was evaluated by the Newcastle region for the Department of Health, was the use of telephone transmission of pacemaker data. This was accomplished by means of an acoustically coupled signal (derived by holding a small device on the patient's chest), which produced an audio tone whose pitch varied in proportion to the detected amplitude of the pacemaker artefact and electrocardiogram. At the regional centre this acoustic signal was fed via the telephone receiver into a decoder. This produced a digital read out of the pacemaker pulse duration and pacing interval, as well as an analogue electrocardiographic record. The system, which featured on the BBC's *Tomorrow's World* programme, worked well where the physician and technician in the outlying hospital had some cardiological experience, and for several years linked the outpatient clinic at Carlisle with Newcastle. Elsewhere in the region where such expertise was lacking it was not technically a success and had to be abandoned. There was a considerable saving in patient transportation costs with the system, but a major drawback was the lack of personal contact between cardiologist and patient.

With the appointment of trained cardiologists to district general hospitals, and the increased availability of more "user friendly" pacemaker function analysers and programmers, the implantation and follow up of pacemakers became much more widespread, although those with the more complicated pacing systems still had to attend the regional centre.

The increasing population of fully trained cardiologists with their own facilities for pacemaker implantation has brought about a welcome easing of the case load for regional pacing centres. One possible disadvantage of the dispersal of the pacing population among a greater number of hospitals is that junior staff will have less exposure during training to the various techniques of cardiac pacing, and may therefore take longer to reach the required level of competence and experience. Recruitment to clinical trials in individual centres will be slower and will need to be offset by an increase in multicentre participation in such research activities. It is to be hoped that a happy balance will result, and that the pendulum does not swing too far the other way from the position of 30 years ago.

References and notes

1. Leatham A, Cook P, Davies JG. External electric stimulator for treatment of ventricular standstill. *Lancet* 1956;ii:1185–9.
2. Harris A, Davies M, Redwood D, Leatham A, Siddons H. Aetiology of chronic heart block. A clinico-pathological correlation in 65 cases. *Br Heart J* 1969;31:206–18.
3. Davies JG, Leatham A, Robinson BF. Ventricular stimulation by catheter electrode. *Lancet* 1 1959;i:583–4.
4. Abrams LD, Hudson WA, Lightwood R. A surgical approach to the management of heart-block using an inductive coupled artificial cardiac pacemaker. Lancet 1960;i:1372–4.
5. Abrams LD. Induction pacing. *Ann N Y Acad Sci* 1969;167:964–7.

6. Siddons H, Sowton EG. *Cardiac pacemakers*. Springfield, IL: Charles C Thomas, 1967.
7. Portal R, Davies JG, Leatham A, Siddons H. Artificial pacing for heart block. *Lancet* 1962;ii:1369.
8. Bluestone R, Davies JG, Harris A, Leatham A, Siddons H. Long term endocardial pacing for heart block. *Lancet* 1965;ii:307.
9. Siddons H. Deaths in long-term paced patients. *Br Heart J* 1974;36;1201–9.
10. Chatterjee K, Davies JG, Harris A, Leatham A. T-wave changes after artificial pacing. *Lancet* 1969;ii:759.
11. Sowton E. Haemodynamic studies in patients with artificial pacemakers. *Br Heart J* 1964;26:737–46.
12. Sowton GE. Artificial cardiac pacemaking with particular reference to cardiac physiology. Cambridge: University of Cambridge, 1963. (Doctoral thesis.)
13. Hetzel MR, Ginks WR, Pickersgill Al, Leatham A. Value of pacing in cardiac failure associated with chronic atrioventricular block. *Br Heart J* 1978;40:864–9.
14. Short DS. The syndrome of alternating bradycardia and tachycardia. Br Heart J 1954;16;202–14.
15. Fairfax Al, Lambert CD, Leatham A. Systemic embolism in chronic sinoatrial disorder. *N Engl J Med* 1976;295:190–2.
16. Chatterjee K, Harris A, Leatham A. Fall of endocardial potentials after acute myocardial infarction. *Lancet* 1969;i:760;1308–9.
17. Ginks WR, Sutton R, Oh W, Leatham A. Long term prognosis after acute anterior infarction with atrioventricular block. *Br Heart J* 1977;39:186–9.
18. Sowton E, Leatham A, Carson P. The suppression of arrhythmias by artificial pacemaking. *Lancet* 1964;ii:1098.
19. Ginks W, Leatham A, Siddons H. Prognosis of patients paced for chronic atrioventricular block. *Br Heart J* 1979;42:633–6.
20. Morgan G, Ginks W, Siddons H, Leatham A. Septicaemia in patients with an endocardial pacemaker. *Am J Cardiol* 1979;44:221–4.
21. Lopez L, Sowton E. Overdriving by pacing to suppress ventricular ectopic activity. *J Electrocardiol* 1972:5:65–73.
22. Sowton E, Balcon R, Preston T, Leaver D, Yacoub M. Long-term control of intractable supraventricular tachycardia by ventricular pacing. *Br Heart J* 1969:3l:700–6.
23. Sowton E, Balcon R, Cross D, Frick MH. Measurement of the angina threshold using atrial pacing. A new technique for the study of angina pectoris. *Cardiovasc Res* 1967;1:301–9.
24. Balcon R., Maloy W., Sowton E. Clinical use of atrial pacing test in angina pectoris. *BMJ* 1968;3:91–4.
25. Gibson DG, Chamberlain DA, Coltart DJ, Mercer J. Effect of changes in ventricular activation on cardiac haemodynamics in man. Comparison of right ventricular, left ventricular, and simultaneous pacing of both ventricles. *Br Heart J* 1971:33:397–400.
26. Sowton E, Gray K, Preston T . Electrical interference in non-competitive pacemakers. *Br Heart J* 1970:32:626–32.
27. Chatterjee K, Sutton R, Davies JG. Low intracardiac potentials in myocardial infarction as a cause of failure of inhibition of demand pacemakers. *Lancet* 1968;i:511–12.
28. Rickards AF. The haemodynamics of atrio-ventricular sequential pacing. In: Norman J, Rickards AF, eds. *Proceedings of a pacemaker colloquium*. Arnhem: Tamminga, 1975.
29. Irnich W. Technical considerations in the design of the ideal pacemaker. In: Norman J, Rickards AF, eds. *Proceedings of a pacemaker colloquium*. Arnhem: Taminga, 1975.
30. Funke HD. Eighteen months of clinical experience with the implantable optimized sequential stimulator (OSS). In: Meere C, ed. *Proceedings of the VIth world symposium on cardiac pacing*. Montreal: 1979.
31. Bazett HC. An analysis of the time-relations of electrocardiograms. *Heart* 1920;7:353–70.
32. Rickards AF, Norman J. Relation between QT interval and heart rate. New design of physiologically adaptive cardiac pacemaker. *Br Heart J* 1981;45:56–61.
33. Krasner JL, Noukydis PV, Nardella PC. A physiologically controlled cardiac pacemaker. *J Assoc Adv Med Instrum* 1966;1:14.
34. Rossi P, Plicchi G, Canducci G, Rognoni G, Aina F. Respiratory rate as a determinant of optimal pacing rate. *Pacing Clin Electrophysiol* 1983:6:502–10.
35. Cammilli L, Alcidi L, Papeschi G, Padeletti L, Grassi G. Clinical and biological aspects in patient with pH-triggered implanted pacemaker. *G Ital Cardiol* 1978:8(Suppl 1):252–8.
36. Rickards AF, Donaldson RM, Thalen H J Th. The use of QT interval to determine pacing rate. Early clinical experience. *PACE* 1983:6:346–54.
37. Donaldson RM, Fox K, Rickards AF. Initial experience with a physiological rate responsive pacemaker. *BMJ* 1983:286:677–1.
38. Donaldson RM, Rickards AF. Rate responsive pacing using the evoked QT principle. A physiological alternative to atrial synchronous pacemakers. *PACE* 1983;6:1344–9.
39. Rickards AF. Computer storage of pacemaker data. In: Thalen H, Hawthorne J, eds. *To pace or not to pace*. The Hague: Martinus Nijhoff, 1978.

40. Bernstein A, Camm AJ, Fisher JD, Fletcher R, Mead R, Nathan A, et al. The NASPE/BPEG defibrillator code. *PACE* 1993;16:1776–80.
41. Gold RG, Paneth M, Gibson RV. A new technique for long-term endocardial pacing. *Lancet* 1966;i:908–11.

Chapter 18

Cardiac Rehabilitation

Helen Stokes

For cardiac rehabilitation, as with most evolving specialties, it would be difficult to identify the exact moment of conception. All one can do is trace a series of events and processes which may or may not be obviously linked but have provided an impetus for development. Many have referred to William Heberden, working in London in 1768, as the pioneer of exercise as a treatment for heart disease. Others point to William Stokes in Dublin in 1854, who encouraged graduated exercise for patients with a variety of cardiac problems. However, cardiac rehabilitation as a multifactorial intervention is really a development of the 20th century. Although Wilson identifies the roots of modern cardiac rehabilitation in Sjostrand's work to develop a cardiac work tolerance laboratory in Sweden in the early 1930s,[1] some of the earliest contributions originated in the United States.

Moving on from bed rest

During the 1940s, there was growing awareness of the problems associated with prolonged bed rest in relation to a variety of illnesses, including cardiac disease. In 1944, a symposium entitled "The abuse of rest in the treatment of disease" was held at the Annual Meeting of the American Medical Association in Chicago. Two papers of relevance to the future development of cardiac rehabilitation were presented. One, entitled "The evil sequelae of bed rest" by William Dock, has been widely quoted, although it is not specific to heart patients.[2] The other lesser known paper was presented by Tinsley Harrison and was called "The abuse of rest as a therapeutic measure for patients with cardiovascular disease."[3] In his paper, Harrison describes black patients with congestive heart failure who were treated as outpatients and seemed to recover better than white patients admitted to hospital and treated with bed rest. The hospitalised patients subsequently suffered from "infarction of the lungs, pneumonia and uremia." In exploring the advantages of mobilisation as opposed to bed rest, Harrison found that there were psychological as well as physical benefits in reducing "cardiac neurosis."

In the United Kingdom, the approach adopted during the 1940s to mobilising patients with heart disease was distinctly restrictive. Pearce, discussing nursing care, stated that "all articles must be handed to him (the patient) and he should not be permitted to reach anything from his locker or from a distant part of the bed."[4] In relation to bed rest, she goes on to say that "in addition to the actual rest of lying in bed, all worry and anxiety must be avoided; and since the whole body requires rest, in that no organ must be working more than the barest minimum, the diet will be carefully regulated and the action of the bowel attended to so that all will work quietly and easily." However, Boas and Boas suggested that the physician "in an endeavor to protect himself from blame in case a cardiac accident causes unexpected death . . . unnecessarily restricts the patient's activities."[5] They recommended that "any moderate activity is permissible that does not give rise to symptoms," and suggested that return to work and normal daily activities would help the patient to maintain an interest in life and some self esteem.

Early mobilisation

In the early 1950s, Levine and Lown presented a paper on "Armchair treatment of acute coronary thrombosis" at a meeting of the Association of American Physicians in Atlantic City.[6] They concluded that physiological and clinical studies showed that strict bed rest was harmful to patients with congestive heart failure. This was acknowledged as a major step forward in the development of cardiac rehabilitation, in that a definite shift from total bed rest to early mobilisation (at least allowing patients out of bed for variable periods) was strongly recommended. At the same time, Newman and colleagues were developing a walking programme for patients who had sustained acute myocardial infarction,[7] and Hellerstein and Ford described "an orderly plan for the rehabilitation of the patient with heart disease from the initial illness through convalescence to the return to the world of work."[8] Other similar initiatives based on a graduated increase in physical activity followed.[9–14]

Cardiac rehabilitation as a developing specialty

It is important to place the development of cardiac rehabilitation in a broader perspective. For both physicians and nurses, the development of coronary care units was the first step towards specialisation in cardiac care. Much of this specialisation was led by an increased ability to provide highly technical interventions, such as defibrillation, rather than by a recognition of the holistic needs of the patient. In the 1960s, less was known about the psychological impact of cardiac problems on the patient's quality of life. Thus, the focus of care was primarily on clinical treatment, prevention of pulmonary emboli, and physical aspects of mobilisation. However, in 1969 the World Health Organization, in a definition of cardiac rehabilitation, referred to "physical, mental and social conditions" as well as the importance of individuals taking responsibility for their own health needs.[15] This definition acknowledged the increasingly multifaceted nature of cardiac rehabilitation.

UK services in the 1970s

Cardiac rehabilitation developed relatively late and slowly in the United Kingdom. An early exploration of rehabilitation services took place in 1970, when Groden, Semple, and Shaw sent a questionnaire to members of the British Cardiac Society.[16] The responses showed that 90 centres had no special cardiac rehabilitation facilities, while 11 centres used an advisory pamphlet, 13 had a work advisory clinic, and 9 claimed some form of exercise programme, ranging from early mobilisation to physiotherapy during the patient's stay in hospital. Although 84 cardiologists were in favour of developing special services, 29 saw no need. By the mid to late 1970s, only a handful of programmes had begun. These were mainly hospital based and mostly consisted of an exercise programme with some formal or informal patient education. Dennis Boyle in Belfast set up one of the earliest programmes in 1972.

By the mid 1970s, the Royal College of Physicians and the British Cardiac Society had formed a joint working party to explore these issues further.[17] They concluded that conventional medical treatment was insufficient to ensure a return to a full and active life after myocardial infarction, and that the same principles applied to other forms of heart disease. They acknowledged that ignorance of the condition, together with anxiety, depression, and social difficulties impeded recovery, and that the principle of rehabilitation should be active right from the beginning. Physical conditioning was recommended, as was a further assessment of those who had not returned to work after three months. Further education and research were needed, together with more resources to put the recommendations into practice.

Differences with continental Europe

In 1976, Wenger commented that this report agreed with one from the Task Force on Cardiovascular Rehabilitation of the National Heart and Lung Institute on the fact that psychosocial factors are as important as the amount of cardiac damage in contributing to invalidism.[18] She also pointed out that the British and American approaches to cardiac rehabilitation were very different from that in continental Europe, where rehabilitation using sanatorium or spa facilities was routine.

Cardiology and rehabilitation

In the early 1980s in the United Kingdom, attitudes to mobilisation after myocardial infarction were influenced by a study by Chamberlain and colleagues.[19] This showed that most of the complications preventing an early discharge home could be identified on the first day of admission to hospital. More accurate assessment could be made after 48 hours, and most major complications had emerged by 4 days after admission. Thus, low risk patients could be safely discharged home after 4 days. Technological and pharmacological advances mean that more people are diagnosed with cardiac disease and more survive cardiac events and are therefore eligible for rehabilitation services. However, early discharge means that the healthcare team has less contact time with the patient, and this has reduced the impact of their educational input or motivational effect. As Wood and colleagues showed in the ASPIRE (action on secondary prevention through intervention to reduce events) study in 1996, the recording of risk factor profiles and subsequent treatment varies, and thus the potential to reduce the risk of further events by effective lifestyle intervention is not being achieved.[20] This evidence increases the importance of early and accurate assessment of the individual's needs, effective communication between the hospital and the primary healthcare team, and a flexible rehabilitation service that is designed to address the patient's needs at different times and in different locations.

Psychosocial factors in cardiac rehabilitation

During the 1970s, Cay and Mayou contributed to the understanding of the impact of psychological as well as physical factors on recovery after myocardial infarction by identifying the impact of emotional disturbance such as anxiety and depression on the patient's return to work and attitudes to rehabilitation.[21][22] Mayou discussed three important issues: alerting the physician to the identification of complications and "at risk" patients; offering routine rehabilitation, including systematic, precise advice and the encouragement of coping behaviours; and the use of quantitative psychosocial criteria to evaluate the effectiveness of treatment. Dr Cay represented the United Kingdom on the Scientific Council of the International Society and Federation of Cardiology in relation to the rehabilitation of cardiac patients. She later worked with the World Health Organization, and collaborated on key reports such as *Psychologic and social aspects of coronary heart disease: information for the clinician* and *Rehabilitation after myocardial infarction: the European experience.*[23][24]

Safety and effectiveness of rehabilitation services

By the early to mid 1980s, cardiology was developing rapidly in pharmacological and interventional terms, but relatively little was happening in cardiac rehabilitation. In 1982, Carson et al. published the results of the first randomised controlled trial of cardiac rehabilitation in the United Kingdom concerning the safety of supervised exercise training after myocardial infarction.[25] The report helped to allay fears about the safety of such interventions and encouraged the development of other similar programmes. Subsequently, Bethell et al. published the results of a 5 year trial of exercise based rehabilitation based in a sports centre.[26] This programme remains one of the few truly community based programmes in the United Kingdom.[26]

Widening the focus

The major focus had been on middle aged men post myocardial infarction. During the late 1980s, cardiac rehabilitation began to widen its remit to include, for example, patients recovering from surgery. Recognition was growing that other patients, such as those with angina or heart failure, might also benefit. Coats's pioneering work in the late 1980s challenged long standing beliefs about the value of rest in the treatment of heart failure, by showing that physical training was beneficial in chronic heart failure.[27] Other groups whose needs remained unmet included not only women, elderly people, and ethnic minorities but also the patient's partner and other family members.[28]

Meta-analyses

In the late 1980s, two meta-analyses had an important impact on attitudes to exercise based rehabilitation. Oldridge in 1988 and O'Connor in 1989 showed that rehabilitation with exercise after myocardial infarction achieved significant reductions in overall mortality, cardiovascular mortality, and re-infarction mortality.[29][30] These studies provided more convincing evidence of the benefits of cardiac rehabilitation than had previously been available, and they continue to be widely quoted in support of the provision of such services.

Expansion of services

Although a survey in 1985–6 showed that 46 health districts acknowledged active cardiac rehabilitation programmes,[31] it was not until the early 1990s that cardiac rehabilitation services in the United Kingdom began to expand appreciably. Expansion was affected by two factors. The first was a joint initiative set up in 1988–9 by the Chest, Heart & Stroke Association and the British Heart Foundation to provide "pump priming" grants. The second factor was the launch in 1992 of the British Association for Cardiac Rehabilitation. The pump priming initiative – led by Professor Desmond Julian, medical director at the British Heart Foundation and supported by Brigadier Ian Crawford, chairman of the British Heart Foundation Rehabilitation Committee – provided start-up grants of £25 000 over a two year period. Although some hospitals reneged on the deal after this period, some were persuaded by the British Heart Foundation to continue funding.

But not all the programmes have been able to continue, due to withdrawal of funding. Data obtained from a survey of cardiac rehabilitation programmes in the United Kingdom, show that more than one third of these programmes began between 1990 and 1994, illustrating the recent development of the specialty in this country (unpublished data, British Association for Cardiac Rehabilitation Database, 1998).

British Association for Cardiac Rehabilitation

The British Association for Cardiac Rehabilitation was formed in 1992. It aimed to link healthcare professionals from different disciplines who work in cardiac rehabilitation but did not have a means of networking and sharing their expertise and knowledge. The first elected committee included Hugh Bethell (as president) and Helen Stokes (president elect) with a number of others who had worked on the steering committee, including Jane Flint (subsequent president). In 1994, the association became affiliated to the British Cardiac Society, thus enabling it to participate in combined symposiums at British Cardiac Society meetings and to be represented at council level.

Programmes and self help packages

The early 1990s saw a number of other initiatives. As an advisor to the World Health Organization, Dr Cay was involved in producing a report published on the *Need and action priorities in cardiac rehabilitation and secondary prevention in patients with coronary heart disease.*[32] With the growing awareness of the importance of psychological factors on recovery, Lewin et al. in Scotland developed the *Heart Manual* – a six week, self help package, supported by a manual with audio tapes and a trained facilitator providing telephone follow up.[33] This provided a useful means of helping patients in more rural areas with limited access to the traditional, hospital based cardiac rehabilitation programme. Many of these programmes were set up on a "package" basis, lasting from 6 to 12 weeks and including one to three sessions per week with a varying mixture of patient education, exercise, and stress management.

National audit

An important report published in 1992 stressed that large areas of the United Kingdom had inadequate cardiac rehabilitation facilities, not least because of "a divergence of opinion among cardiologists and physicians about the physical and psychological benefits of rehabilitation."[34] This prompted the NHS Executive, in 1993, to fund a national survey of cardiac rehabilitation supervised by David Thompson.[35] Altogether 199 of 244 centres providing acute cardiac care offered some form of cardiac rehabilitation. An in-depth survey of 25 of these centres showed that although "there was a commitment to cardiac rehabilitation, the range and content of services varied enormously, few programmes kept accurate records of the numbers of patients, staff or costs and none audited its activities."

Key elements

It was becoming clear that although the need for rehabilitation could not be denied, the process by which it should be achieved was a matter for debate. As a result, a consensus workshop was held in October 1994 to develop guidelines and audit standards for cardiac rehabilitation. These guidelines used a "broad brush" approach to outline the key elements considered necessary for rehabilitation services that were emerging from an evidence basis. These elements were described as spanning the four phases mentioned earlier and included:

- Explanation and understanding of diagnosis and management
- Specific rehabilitation interventions
- Long term readaptation
- Re-education.

There was a strong emphasis on individually tailored, appropriate interventions rather than the "blunderbuss" approach used in the past.

Reviewing service provision

An update of survey information published by the British Cardiac Society in 1995 acknowledged the increase in service provision, but still outlined concerns.[36] These included the lack of audit data available, the drop out rate, the selection of patients, and the need to ensure the inclusion of cardiac rehabilitation as a core service in the future. Between 1995 and 1997, there were several key publications, including the national guidelines,[37] the full report of the consensus workshop,[38] guidelines from the British Association for Cardiac Rehabilitation with a more practical "how to do it" approach,[39] a collection of contributions by key individuals highlighting different aspects of cardiac rehabilitation,[40] and a review of evidence from the NHS Centre for Reviews and Dissemination at York.[41]

Education and training

Despite attempts to provide evidence based practical guidance, studies by Stokes[42] and Lewin[43] showed that adoption of guidelines was poor and staff training and resources were inadequate. By this time, the British Association for Cardiac Rehabilitation had initiated two education and training projects. One project, funded by the Department of Health, aimed to develop a learning resource for healthcare professionals in this area. The other, funded by the British Heart Foundation, was to develop a training programme for fitness experts in the community, who are involved in the "phase four" or long term maintenance phase of cardiac rehabilitation.

During the 1990s, with increasing recognition of cardiac rehabilitation services as an integral part of cardiac care, the function of the British Heart Foundation committee has evolved from its original role of facilitating start up funding to include reviewing applications for funding for innovative projects. Other activities include the development of an information pack concerned with business planning, and a software programme to encourage the collection of audit data. In another project, British Heart Foundation liaison nurses provided a link between the hospital and the community. A further 30 posts were funded in 1999, after a 2 year pilot and evaluation of 15 of these posts had been carried out.

Consumer involvement

Many cardiac rehabilitation programmes have facilitated the formation of patient support groups to provide peer support and some continuity after discharge from the supervised component of a programme. The British Heart Foundation has formed an extensive network of such groups. Some, such as the Zipper Club for patients who have undergone cardiac surgery and their families, provide support for specific conditions. Others give more general support such as regular meetings, with speakers or opportunities to continue exercising in a group. Although consumers were represented at the consensus workshop for the national guidelines, the role of the consumer as an active participant in the development of healthcare services is still evolving in the United Kingdom. For example, many clinical guidelines are not published in a format such as a specific patient leaflet (similar to those published by the Agency for Health Care Policy and Research in the United States) that is easily accessible to lay people.

Where are we now?

Looking back over the past few decades, cardiac rehabilitation has evolved from a physical training programme for men who have had a heart attack to a multifactorial, holistic approach to a wide range of individual patients, their partners, and their families. A new understanding about the role of secondary prevention in heart disease changed the definition of cardiac rehabilitation. The aim is no longer simply to return people to previous activities or to work, it also includes "the sum of activities required to influence favourably the underlying cause of the disease."[32]

Some scepticism remains about the outcomes and effectiveness of cardiac rehabilitation services. The national guidelines identified the fact that the uptake of cardiac rehabilitation is often lowest among those who might benefit the most – people with heart failure, valvular heart disease, angina, and hypertension – and higher in patients who have had myocardial infarction and cardiac surgery.[37] There are currently around 300 cardiac rehabilitation programmes in the United Kingdom. Most are hospital based, but the trend is towards a more community based approach, which should facilitate the integration of both the concepts and practice of cardiac rehabilitation and secondary prevention.

Formal standards and accreditation criteria for programmes have not yet been developed in the United Kingdom. Almost quarter of a century ago, in 1976, Wenger stated that "educational programs – public, patient, professional, employer, governmental – are seen as major unmet needs in the field of rehabilitation of the cardiac patient. Research efforts should delineate the most efficient, safest and most attractive means of implementing programs for rehabilitation." Looking back, it is evident that most of the emphasis during the evolution of services has been devoted to justifying their need rather than developing their potential. Looking forward, the emphasis should change from "why" to "how" – that is, to issues of flexibility, effectiveness, efficiency, and, most importantly, to quality.

References and notes

1. Wilson PK. Cardiac rehabilitation: then and now. *Phys Sports Med* 1988;16:75–9, 82, 84.
2. Dock W. The evil sequelae of bed rest. *JAMA* 1944;125:1083–5.
3. Harrison TR. The abuse of rest as a therapeutic measure for patients with cardiovascular disease. *JAMA* 1944;125:1075–7.
4. Pearce E. *Medical and nursing dictionary.* 6th ed. London: Faber & Faber Ltd. 1943:290.
5. Boas EP, Boas NF. *Coronary artery disease.* 1st ed. Chicago: Year Book Publishers, 1949:310, 315.
6. Levine SA, Lown B. "Armchair" treatment of acute coronary thrombosis. *JAMA* 1952;148:1365–9.
7. Newman LB, Andrews MF, Koblish MO, Baker LA. Physical medicine and rehabilitation in acute myocardial infarction. *Arch Intern Med* 1952;89:552–61.
8. Hellerstein H, Ford AB. Rehabilitation of the cardiac patient. *JAMA* 1957;164:225–31.
9. Gottheiner V. Long-range strenuous sports training for cardiac reconditioning and rehabilitation. *Am J Cardiol* 1968;22:426–35.
10. Kellermann JJ, Levy M, Feldman S, Kariv I. Rehabilitation of coronary patients. *J Chronic Dis* 1967;20:815–21.
11. Goble AJ, Adey GM, Bullen JF. Rehabilitation of the cardiac patient. *Med J Aust* 1963;2:975–82.
12. Shephard RJ. Proceedings of the international symposium on physical activity and cardiovascular health: introduction. *J Can Med Assoc* 1967;96:695–6.
13. Sanne H. Exercise tolerance and physical training of non-selected patients after myocardial infarction. *Acta Med Scand* 1973;551(suppl):1–124.
14. Wenger NK. Rehabilitation after myocardial infarction. *JAMA* 1979;242:2879–81.
15. World Health Organization. *Rehabilitation of patients with cardiovascular disease: report on a seminar.* Copenhagen: WHO Regional Office for Europe. 1969.
16. Groden B, Semple T, Shaw GB. Cardiac rehabilitation in Britain (1970). *Br Heart J* 1971;33:756–8.
17. Royal College of Physicians and British Cardiac Society Joint Working Party. Cardiac rehabilitation 1975. *J R Coll Physicians* 1975;9:281–346.
18. Wenger NK. Cardiac rehabilitation: the United Kingdom and the United States. *Ann Intern Med* 1976;84:214–6.
19. Lau YK, Smith J, Morrison SL, Chamberlain DA. Policy for early discharge after acute myocardial infarction. *BMJ* 1980;280:1489–92.
20. ASPIRE Steering Group. A British Cardiac Society survey of the potential for the secondary prevention of coronary disease: ASPIRE (action on secondary prevention through intervention to reduce events). *Heart* 1996;75:334–42.
21. Cay EL, Vetter N, Philip A, Dugard P. Return to work after a heart attack. *J Psychosom Res* 1973;17:231–43.
22. Mayou R. The course and determinants of reactions to myocardial infarction. *Br J Psychiatry* 1979;134:588–94.

23. Sanne H, Wenger NK, eds. *Psychologic and social aspects of coronary heart disease: information for the clinician. A publication of the Scientific Council on the Rehabilitation of Cardiac Patients of the International Society and Federation of Cardiology.* Greenwich: Le Jacq Communications, 1992.
24. Kallio V, Cay E. *Rehabilitation after myocardial infarction: the European experience.* Copenhagen: World Health Organization, 1985. (Public Health in Europe no 24.)
25. Carson P, Phillips R, Lloyd M, Tucker H, Neophytou M, Buch NJ, et al. Exercise after myocardial infarction: a controlled trial. *J R Coll Physicians* 1982;16:147–51.
26. Bethell HJN, Larvan A, Turner SC. Coronary rehabilitation in the community. *J R Coll Gen Pract* 1983;33:285–91.
27. Coats AJS, Adamopoulos S, Meyer TE, Conway J, Sleight P. Effects of physical training in chronic heart failure. *Lancet* 1990;355:63–6.
28. Thompson DR, Cordle CJ. Support of wives of myocardial infarction patients. *J Advanced Nurs* 1988;13:223–8.
29. Oldridge NB, Guyatt GH, Fischer ME, Rimm AA. Cardiac rehabilitation after myocardial infarction: combined experience of randomised clinical trials. *JAMA* 1988;260:945–50.
30. O'Connor GT, Buring JE, Yusuf S, Goldhaber SZ, Olmsterad EM, Paffenbarger RS, et al. An overview of randomised trials of rehabilitation with exercise after myocardial infarction. *Circulation* 1989;80:234–44.
31. Green V, Stansfield BJ, Davidson C. Cardiac rehabilitation in the United Kingdom 1985/86: a questionnaire survey. *Physiotherapy* 1988;74:363–5.
32. World Health Organization. *Needs and action priorities in cardiac rehabilitation and secondary prevention in patients with CHD: report on two consultations.* Copenhagen: World Health Organisation. 1993
33. Lewin B, Robertson IH, Cay EL, Irving JB, Campbell M. Effects of self-help post-myocardial-infarction rehabilitation on psychological adjustment and use of health services. *Lancet* 1992;339:1036–40.
34. Horgan J, Bethell H, Carson P, Davidson C, Julian D, Mayou RA, Nagle R. Working party report on cardiac rehabilitation. *Br Heart J* 1992;67:412–8.
35. Thompson DR, Bowman GS, Kitson AL, de Bono DP, Hopkins A. Cardiac rehabilitation services in England and Wales: a national survey. *Int J Cardiol* 1997;59:299–304.
36. Davidson C, Reval K, Chamberlain DA, Pentecost B, Parker J. A report of a working group of the British Cardiac Society: cardiac rehabilitation services in the United Kingdom 1992. *Br Heart J* 1995;73:210–2.
37. Thompson DR, Bowman GS, Kitson ALK, de Bono DP, Hopkins A. Cardiac rehabilitation in the United Kingdom: guidelines and audit standards. *Heart* 1996;75:89–93.
38. Thompson DR, Bowman GS, de Bono DP, Hopkins A, eds. *Cardiac rehabilitation: guidelines and audit standards.* London: Royal College of Physicians of London, 1997.
39. Coats AJS, McGee HM, Stokes HC, Thompson DR, eds. *British Association for Cardiac Rehabilitation guidelines for cardiac rehabilitation.* 1st ed. Oxford: Blackwell Science, 1995.
40. Jones D, West R, eds. *Cardiac rehabilitation.* London: BMJ Publishing Group, 1995.
41. NHS Centre for Reviews and Dissemination. *Cardiac rehabilitation.* York: University of York, 1998. (Effective Health Care Bulletin 4.)
42. Stokes HC, Thompson DR, Seers K. The implementation of multiprofessional guidelines for cardiac rehabilitation: a pilot study. *Coronary Health Care* 1998;2:60–71.
43. Lewin RJP, Ingleton R, Newens AJ, Thompson DR. Adherence to cardiac rehabilitation guidelines: a survey of rehabilitation programmes in the United Kingdom. *BMJ* 1998;316:1354–5.

Chapter 19

Clinical Trials

Desmond G Julian and Stuart Pocock

British interest in randomised controlled trials started shortly after the second world war. Indeed, the study of streptomycin in tuberculosis carried out by the Medical Research Council (MRC) is generally credited with being the first clinical trial in the world with a properly randomised control group. The MRC trials of antihistaminic drugs for the treatment of the common cold – possibly the first placebo controlled trials – followed shortly thereafter. Randomised trials of treatment for heart disease did not start until several years later, and Cochrane, the arch proponent of evidence based medicine, was particularly critical of cardiologists for not basing their practice on good science. However, cardiology, perhaps more than any other, is now firmly established as a discipline in which most clinical decision making is rooted in well conducted clinical trials. In this chapter we discuss the British contribution to evidence based advances in various clinical contexts and consider how British experience has advanced the principles and practice of the clinical trial.

Prevention and treatment of thrombosis

Anticoagulant therapy

In the 1940s, non-randomised studies of anticoagulant therapy in the United States and elsewhere had convinced many of its value in the short-term management of myocardial infarction. Donald Reid of the MRC wrote in 1960, "The use of anticoagulant drugs in the acute phase of myocardial infarction is now widely accepted as sound practice; and it would be difficult on ethical grounds to attempt at this stage the conduct of a rigorously controlled trial of its value."[1] Notwithstanding this view, the MRC carried out a trial of short-term anticoagulant therapy and published the results in 1969.[2] It was not until the review of Chalmers et al. in 1977 that a more sceptical assessment of the anticoagulant trials was undertaken.[3] Chalmers pointed out that few trials had been correctly randomised, and that most of those which had been were small. However, in three trials of adequate size carried out between 1969 and 1973, anticoagulant therapy had reduced mortality by 21% (from 19.6% to 15.4%, $p = 0.001$). Unfortunately, this information came too late in the day to be of much practical use. By the time the paper was published, mortality from myocardial infarction had fallen dramatically, and the need to prevent venous thromboembolic events (the main reason for giving anticoagulants) had been largely eliminated by early ambulation.

Long term anticoagulant therapy after infarction was also the subject of numerous studies over 30 years, but many of the results were inconclusive. Sir George Pickering presented the first of the MRC studies in 1960.[4] This study was not placebo controlled. Altogether 383 patients were randomly assigned to receive either the dose of phenindione that could maintain their prothrombin time at 2–2.5 times normal or 1 mg phenindione (which was assumed, perhaps wrongly, to have no effect). There were 31 deaths in the group given a low dose of phenindione and 22 in the higher dose group. No statistical tests were applied.

In the MRC's second report on long term anticoagulation after myocardial infarction, mortality was 21.3% in the control group compared with 14.9% in the intervention group during a mean follow up period of 25 months ($p = 0.13$).[5] The question of long term anticoagulation remained controversial until reports from the Netherlands and Norway provided conclusive evidence that this treatment was beneficial.

Platelet active agents

The role of platelet active agents in the management of acute myocardial infarction remained uncertain until the publication of the ISIS-2 study (the second International Study of Infarct Survival).[6] Under the auspices of the Royal College of General Practitioners, Elwood and Williams from the MRC Epidemiology Unit in Cardiff had undertaken a randomised controlled study of aspirin (300 mg daily) in 1705 patients with suspected myocardial infarction.[7] No benefit was observed at 28 days.

The ISIS-2 trial was based on the Clinical Trials Service Unit in Oxford.[6] Altogether 17 187 patients with suspected acute myocardial infarction were randomised, in a factorial design, to one of the following – aspirin, aspirin plus streptokinase, streptokinase, or neither. The most impressive results were observed in patients given both drugs. In this group, mortality from vascular causes was 8%, while in patients given placebo it was 13.2%. Mortality from vascular causes was 9.4% in those given aspirin compared with 11.8% in the group given placebo aspirin. Although this was only a single trial, it convinced the profession (rather surprisingly) that aspirin was indicated routinely in the context of acute myocardial infarction.

By contrast, the value of long term aspirin therapy after infarction has been established in many trials, although few have been large enough by themselves to provide conventionally significant results. Elwood's group in Cardiff was again a pioneer in this field.[8] The two trials of 1239 and 1682 patients respectively failed to show a significant benefit, although consistent with a reduction of about 26% and 17% in mortality. When these findings were pooled with other, later, studies in the Antiplatelet Trialists' Collaboration (coordinated by the Clinical Trials Study Unit), a 25% reduction in odds risk was observed.[9] This result has led to the almost universal acceptance of the value of aspirin in the secondary prevention after myocardial infarction.

Thrombolytic drugs

Many small trials of thrombolysis with fibrinolytic drugs in myocardial infarction were undertaken in Europe and the United States after the first reported use of this treatment in 1958. In 1985, Yusuf et al. were able to review 33 trials of intravenous and intracoronary fibrinolytic drugs therapy.[10] Conventional statistical significance was achieved in few trials, but a 22% reduction in mortality was observed overall. These encouraging reports led to two large trials of streptokinase - GISSI-I (Gruppo Italiano per lo Studio della Streptokinase nell'Infarto Miocardico)[11] based in Italy and ISIS-2[6] described above. In the latter trial, streptokinase alone achieved a 25% reduction in mortality, and the combined streptokinase/aspirin regimen achieved a 42% reduction in mortality at 35 days compared with double placebo. Other major trials in which British centres played a leading role at this time included the Anistreplase Intervention Mortality Study (AIMS)[12] and the Anglo-Scandinavian Study of Early Thrombolysis (ASSET),[13] in which tissue type plasminogen activator (alteplase) was the test thrombolytic agent. These and other trials convincingly showed the effectiveness of thrombolytic treatment, and this was confirmed by the work of the Fibrinolytic Therapy Trialists' Collaborative Group.[14] Furthermore, this large systematic review was able to confirm that some subgroups of patients benefited particularly from thrombolytic treatment - notably those with ST elevation or bundle branch block. Because relatively few patients had been entered into these trials more than 6 hours after the onset of symptoms, the Late Assessment of Thrombolytic Efficacy (LATE) study, based in Nottingham, was undertaken.[15] This showed a worthwhile improvement in prognosis in those receiving therapy 6–12 hours after the onset, but little thereafter.

Controversy over the rival merits of the various thrombolytic agents persisted, and ISIS-3,[16] GISSI-2 (Gruppo Italiano per lo Studio della Sopravivenza nell'Infarto Miocardico),[17] and the trials of the associated International Study Group[18] were set up to address this. In neither case was any difference observed between the agents tested. However, theoretical and experimental evidence suggested that genetically engineered tissue type plasminogen activator was more effective than streptokinase in achieving early patency of the artery occluded by thrombosis. This led to the GUSTO trial, which was based in the United States but included British participants.[19] This trial showed that a new "front-loaded" regimen of tissue type plasminogen activator reduced mortality more than streptokinase but at a somewhat higher risk of cerebral haemorrhage and at considerably greater expense.

β adrenergic blocking drugs, calcium antagonists, nitrates, and magnesium in and after myocardial infarction

There has been a long standing interest in β blocking drugs in the United Kingdom, deriving initially from the pioneering work of Sir James Black and of the ICI company with which he was associated. Indeed, it was the prospect of a beneficial effect in myocardial infarction that provided the main motive for the development of pronethalol. This drug was abandoned shortly after the initial published reports in 1962 because of suspected oncogenic effects. It was promptly replaced by propranolol, and the first favourable findings of this drug's oral use in acute myocardial infarction were soon published. In 1965, Snow of Manchester reported mortality rates of 13% in treated patients and 29% in controls in a trial of 107 patients.[20] The design of the study was severely criticised, and subsequent studies of oral β blockers in myocardial infarction in Britain and abroad failed to substantiate these findings.

Renewed interest in the potential of β blockade in this context followed the work of Braunwald et al. on the limitation of infarct size. However, it was not until the ISIS-1 trial and the subsequent meta-analysis that the effectiveness and safety of intravenous administration of these drugs was firmly established.[21] This trial was a landmark, as it was the first of the mega-trials in myocardial infarction. Rather to the surprise of researchers, the beneficial effect of β blockers in acute myocardial infarction seemed to be due largely to the prevention of cardiac rupture rather than to a reduction in the infarct size.[22]

The use of β blockade as secondary prophylaxis after myocardial infarction is now firmly established, largely on the basis of the Norwegian timolol study[23] and the American Beta-blocker Heart Attack Trial (BHAT).[24] British experience in similar studies was rather unfortunate. The multicentre international study group trial started in 1971 and involved 67 hospitals in 10 countries.[25] Patients were randomised to receive practolol or placebo in the weeks after myocardial infarction. The study was terminated after only 3053 of the planned 4000 patients had been entered because serious side efects (an oculocutaneous syndrome and plastic peritonitis) had been encountered. Although the reduction in mortality in the treated group was non-significant, there seemed to be a substantial reduction in sudden death and myocardial infarction, and the findings were interpreted as promising. This led to a propranolol trial of 720 patients which showed no difference in mortality between the active and control groups.[26] Other British trials which failed to show benefit from β blockers were those of Taylor of Leeds (with oxprenolol)[27] and of Julian et al. in the north east of England (with sotalol).[28] Whether these negative results were due to chance, the choice of drug, or the drug dosage is unclear. In the analysis of the pooled data undertaken by Baber and Lewis referred to above,[29] there was a clear benefit from the long term use of β blockers after myocardial infarction. This has been confirmed by more recent systematic reviews.[30]

Calcium antagonists

Calcium antagonists have been embraced much less enthusiastically in the United Kingdom than elsewhere, perhaps because British scientists and pharmaceutical companies have had little involvement in their development. However, the largest trial (TRENT) of a calcium antagonist in acute myocardial infarction was based on Nottingham.[31] This 4491 patient study had results similar to those of the other calcium antagonist trials in this context in failing to show any benefit.

Nitrates

A meta-analysis of nitrate (and nitroprusside) trials in acute myocardial infarction suggested that these drugs reduced mortality substantially.[32] Concern about the quality and size of the trials and the possibility of publication bias contributed to the decision to test nitrates in two large trials – ISIS-4 (based in Oxford)[23] and GISSI-3 (based in Italy).[24] Both these trials were factorial. In ISIS-4, captopril and magnesium were also studied, while lisinopril was included in the Italian study. Neither study showed that nitrates reduced mortality, but in both cases the frequent usage of nitrate in the control group reduced the possibility of showing a benefit.

Intravenous magnesium

Meta-analysis of several small trials on intravenous magnesium in acute myocardial infarction had suggested that this treatment reduced mortality by at least 50%.[33] In Leicester, the single centre trial (LIMIT-2) of 2316 patients reported a significant reduction in mortality at 28 days – from 10.3% in the placebo group to 7.8% in the magnesium treated patients.[34] However, the subsequent ISIS-4 trial of 58 000 patients failed to confirm this benefit.[23] The explanation for these discrepancies is still a matter of controversy.

Hypertension

Hypertension, including the relevant clinical trials, is addressed fully in chapter 25. Here we mention only four British clinical trials of particular interest. The clinical trial of Hamilton (Chelmsford) is worthy of mention because it was a pioneering effort in the field, although the therapy was not randomised.[35] Patients with severe hypertension were assigned alternately to control or to antihypertensive drug therapy. Five of 30 treated patients had complications compared with 16 of 31 controls. Subsequently, two American randomised studies confirmed the value of antihypertensive treatment in severe hypertension.

The study of Coope and Warrender is interesting because it was conducted in elderly patients in a primary care setting.[36] Altogether 10 718 people aged 60–79 years were screened for hypertension; 884 patients with persistently high systolic and diastolic blood pressures (> 169 mmHg and/or 104 mmHg respectively) were recruited. They were randomised to no treatment or to open active drug therapy. There was no significant difference in mortality or myocardial infarction rates, but stroke was reduced by 70% (from 15 cases to four).

The first MRC trial was designed to determine the effect of antihypertensive treatment of mild hypertension on deaths, strokes, and coronary events in men and women aged 35–64.[37] This trial of 17 354 patients is the largest undertaken in the field of hypertension. Patients, who had to be free of overt heart disease, were enrolled if their blood pressure was persistently in the range of 90–109 mmHg, with a systolic pressure less than 200 mmHg. They were randomised, single-blind initially, to placebo, bendrofluazide, or propranolol, but other drugs could be added to the active arms if necessary to maintain the diastolic blood pressure below 90 mmHg. No difference was seen in the incidence of death or myocardial infarction, but there was a very substantial reduction in stroke in the treated groups.

The second MRC trial was designed to determine the effectiveness of diuretics and β blockers in preventing stroke, coronary heart disease, or death.[38] Altogether 4396 subjects aged 65–74 years, with systolic blood pressures persistently in the range 160–209 mmHg and diastolic pressures less than 115 mmHg, were randomised to a diuretic, atenolol, or placebo. Mortality was similar in the active and placebo groups, but cardiovascular events were reduced by treatment. The benefit seemed to be confined to those receiving a diuretic.

Heart failure

There have been relatively few British studies on heart failure, but British cardiac centres have played an important part in many international studies. However, some British trials are of particular interest.

The xamoterol study involved 516 patients with New York Heart Association (NYHA) classification III and IV heart failure.[39] The drug had both β blocking and β adrenergic properties, which were thought to be potentially beneficial. The primary end point of the study was exercise tolerance. This was not affected, although symptoms improved in patients taking the drug. The study was stopped when the safety committee found that there was a 139% excessive mortality in the active group.

The AIRE study, based in Leeds, involved 2006 patients with left ventricular failure 2–9 days after the onset of myocardial infarction.[40] They were treated with the angiotensin converting enzyme inhibitor, ramipril, or placebo and were followed for 15 months. There was a highly significant reduction in mortality in the treated group, from 22% to 17%. This study was important in establishing the benefit of angiotensin converting enzyme inhibitor drugs in patients with heart failure after myocardial infarction.

As described above, the ISIS-4 trial involved 54 000 patients in the early phase after myocardial infarction who were randomised to captopril or placebo as a component of this factorial study.[23] At 35 days, there was a significant 6%-7% reduction in mortality in the treated group. These results, when taken with those of the GISSI-3 study,[24] are considered by some to indicate that, in the absence of contraindications, angiotensin converting enzyme inhibitor treatment should be used routinely in early myocardial infarction. Others believe that this treatment should be reserved for patients at high risk, because many patients with overt failure in the placebo group had not received optimal treatment for this complication.

The coronary care unit

The coronary care unit is an organisational modality rather than a specific treatment modality. In discussing the various ways in which coronary care units could be assessed, Oliver, Julian, and Donald from the Royal Infirmary, Edinburgh concluded in 1967 that it was difficult to conduct randomised trials of their efficacy.[41] This was because of the evident success of coronary care units in treating the common and otherwise fatal condition of ventricular fibrillation (the prime reason for their existence) when cardiac arrest was seldom effectively corrected in general wards. Furthermore, as with other strategies such as surgery, the efficiency of a unit depends on the experience and skill of the doctors and nurses so that the mere provision of a building and equipment does not guarantee high quality management. In spite of these problems, epidemiologists such as Cochrane and Rose urged the implementation of these trials and, in the event, two were undertaken. One of these centred on Bristol and the south west of England[42] and the other on Nottingham.[43] In both cases, hospital treatment was not significantly better than treatment at home. In retrospect, it is easy to see the flaws in these studies. Patients were often randomised many hours after the onset of symptoms, and only apparently "good risk" cases were included. The wide confidence intervals in the trials precluded valid conclusions so that they could not even show, as was claimed, that there were low risk patients who did not benefit from coronary care. Nonetheless, as these were the only randomised studies in the world of the coronary care concept, they had a considerable effect in discouraging health authorities in the United Kingdom from developing coronary care units.

Coronary artery bypass surgery and angioplasty

Coronary artery bypass surgery and angioplasty are discussed in detail in chapters 11 and 16. British centres played a major role in the European

Coronary Surgery Study, whose principal investigator was Varnauskas of Gothenburg.[44] This trial, together with the Veterans Administration and the Coronary Artery Surgery Studies (CASS) from the United States,[45] established that coronary artery bypass operations not only relieved symptoms but also improved prognosis in patients at high risk, especially those with disease affecting three major coronary arteries.

Although coronary artery surgery was subjected to randomised clinical trials relatively soon after the technique became established, this was not the case with percutaneous transluminal angioplasty. Grüntzig introduced this procedure in 1977, but the first randomised trial was not initiated in the United States until 1987. The British randomised intervention treatment of angina (RITA-1) trial started recruiting patients in March 1988,[46] and the European Coronary Artery Bypass Revascularization Investigation (CABRI) started in July1988.[47] These first trials compared percutaneous transluminal coronary angioplasty with coronary artery bypass surgery. Overall, they showed that there was no apparent difference between the two treatments in terms of the serious complications of myocardial infarction and death. Surgery was somewhat more effective in relieving angina, and angioplasty patients had a higher risk of needing further revascularisation. This latter factor had an important economic influence because it offset the greater initial expense of surgery.

The RITA-2 study was designed to compare percutaneous transluminal coronary angioplasty with conventional medical treatment in patients suitable for either option.[48] Altogether 1018 patients were recruited. The angioplasty group had a better outcome with regard to the relief of angina, but also showed a small but significant excess of the primary combined end point of death and myocardial infarction. The ongoing RITA-3 trial is comparing medical treatment with an "aggressive" programme of cardiac catheterisation followed, if appropriate, by angioplasty or surgery in patients with unstable angina.

Lifestyle, diet, and lipid modifying drugs

These issues are discussed in detail in Chapters 15 and 26. There have been only a small number of randomised trials of lifestyle worldwide, and the United Kingdom has not participated in many of these trials. British factories took part in the World Health Organization (WHO) trial of multifactorial prevention of coronary heart disease.[49] The results of this study in 50 000 workers were inconclusive. This was especially so in the United Kingdom – perhaps because of poor compliance with the low fat, low cholesterol, and non-smoking regimen.

Diet

The United Kingdom MRC trial of 393 individuals involved a dietary regimen of low saturated fat and a supplement of 80 g of soya bean oil daily.[50] No differences between the study and control groups were seen with regard to coronary events or death.

In the Diet And Reinfarction Trial (DART) based in Cardiff, 2033 men who had recovered from a myocardial infarction were randomised to receive or not advice on three dietary regimens – low saturated fat and a high polyunsaturated/saturated fat ratio, high cereal fibre, or increased consumption of fatty fish.[51] A reduction in overall mortality of borderline significance was seen in those given advice about eating fish.

Lipid lowering

The United Kingdom was one of the principal participants in the WHO clofibrate trial.[52] It has been described as "a monumental undertaking at the time it was launched in 1965," and it remains the largest trial of lipid lowering to prevent coronary heart disease.[53] Altogether 10 627 men whose serum cholesterol concentrations were in the upper third of the distribution were recruited in Prague, Budapest, and Edinburgh, and were given clofibrate or placebo. The original reports on this trial included only those patients who continued to take the trial medication – data were not analysed in relation to an "intention-to-treat" – but subsequent publications have not shown material differences. In essence, the study showed a reduction in non-fatal myocardial infarction, but a significant increase in overall mortality, including coronary mortality. The discouraging findings of this study powerfully reinforced scepticism in the United Kingdom about the value of cholesterol reduction; indeed, it resulted in widespread anxiety about the risks of lipid lowering.

Two small studies of clofibrate in patients with manifest ischaemic heart disease were conducted in Newcastle and Edinburgh. Both were encouraging with regard to the reduction in myocardial infarction, but they were too small to allow deductions with regard to the safety of this therapy. The question remained as to whether lipid lowering per se was harmful or the effects were due to the specific drug.

The West of Scotland Coronary Prevention Study (WOSCOPS) established the safety and effectiveness of lipid lowering with pravastatin in high risk, middle aged men who were free of myocardial infarction or electrocardiographic evidence of ischaemic heart disease.[54] The trial recruited 6595 men and followed them for an average of 4.9 years. The primary outcome measure was the combination of non-fatal myocardial infarction and coronary death. This end point occurred in 5.3% of the treatment group and in 7.5% of the placebo group.

Methodology of randomised clinical trials

In addition to the advances in treatment that have arisen from clinical trials research, it is important to recognise from a British perspective the enormous methodological improvements that have been achieved in enhancing the quality and relevance of trials. The single most important feature is the act of randomising patients to alternative treatments (including placebo controls when appropriate) so as to achieve fair (unbiased) comparisons rather than potentially distorted (exaggerated) claims that might arise from uncontrolled or poorly controlled studies. Nowadays, only randomised trials achieve appropriate credibility with journals, regulatory authorities, and the medical community, and it is generally recognised that the pioneering MRC funded trials, initiated by Sir Austin Bradford Hill, were crucial in ensuring this transition to high quality, unbiased evaluation of new treatments in a wide range of therapeutic fields, including cardiology.[55]

Value of large, simple trials

The need to include sufficient patients and a sufficient length of follow up to provide precise estimates of longer term treatment differences has been better recognised in cardiology than in most other areas of treatment research. Also, the focus on major clinical trials with clinical event outcomes, rather than surrogate end points of questionable relevance to patient benefit, has also been increasingly recognised by regulatory authorities, pharmaceutical companies, and other funding bodies. The value of larger, simple, clinical trials of direct relevance to patients has been illustrated particularly by the Oxford Clinical Trials Service Unit directed by Professor Sir Richard Peto. In the ISIS series of trials this group has enrolled tens of thousands of patients.[6][16][21][23] With very limited documentation per patient they have achieved reliable, precise, and pragmatic estimates of treatment effects on patient survival. In the ISIS-2 study, the merits of streptokinase and aspirin treatment after myocardial infarction were a particularly important result in terms of lives saved through simple, practical treatments and an uncomplicated, very large scale trial design.[6] The ISIS trials also illustrate the benefits of a factorial design in enabling more than one treatment factor (for example, streptokinase and aspirin) to be evaluated efficiently within a single simple study.

Systematic reviews

The United Kingdom has also had a major role in recognising that achieving clear results on a treatment often requires an assimilation of evidence from many different but related clinical trials. Thus, the production of quality meta-analyses (sometimes called overviews or systematic reviews) has been a major development. One of the first published meta-analyses by Baber and Lewis provided convincing evidence of the mortality reductions achievable by β blocker therapy after myocardial infarction.[29] The quality of meta-analyses is greatly enhanced if all evidence from all studies, both published and unpublished, is included. In this regard, collaborative efforts to undertake comprehensive meta-analysis in areas such as antiplatelet therapy and percutaneous transluminal coronary angioplasty versus coronary artery bypass grafting have been particularly helpful.

The systematisation of future systematic review has been enhanced by the development of the Cochrane Collaboration, directed by Dr Iain Chalmers. This British initiative, now with collaborative centres worldwide, is enabling the achievement of meta-analyses on all manner of diseases and treatments for which this was not previously possible.

Ethical standards

The ethical standards appropriate for clinical trials in cardiology have also received much attention in the United Kingdom. Particular emphasis has been placed on achieving truly informed patient consent. In addition, many of the procedures and statistical guidelines for data monitoring of interim results in clinical trials have been developed in this country. When to stop a clinical trial for either efficacy, safety (harm), or futility requires a clear interplay of ethical, statistical, scientific, and organisational guidelines.[56] Many major cardiological trials in the United Kingdom have used the concept of "proof beyond reasonable doubt" to prevent trials claiming a treatment advance and stopping too soon. This has often been effective in providing definitive evidence that is sufficiently strong and persuasive to change routine cardiological practice for the better.

Independent funding

British clinical trials in cardiology have also been effective by having: (a) independently funded trial coordinating and statistical centres of high quality and (b) public sector and charity funding bodies such as the British Heart Foundation, MRC, NHS Research and Development, and the Department of Health. These bodies have enabled many important and pragmatic trials of therapeutic issues that could not otherwise have attracted commercial sponsorship. They have thus ensured that a higher proportion of clinical research is devoted to therapeutic and patient management issues that directly relate to the public interest.

Standards of reporting of clinical trials – in medical journals and to regulatory authorities – have improved substantially. This is largely due to British initiatives from the medical journals (for example, the *British Medical Journal* and *Lancet*), the regulators (Medicines Control Agency) and the statistical collaborators in these authorities, and in the trials themselves. Lastly, the cardiological profession is to be congratulated on ensuring higher standards of clinical research and a more productive collaborative spirit than has been possible in some other medical specialties.

References and notes

1. Reid DD. A trial of long-term anticoagulant administration after myocardial infarction. In: Council for International Organizations of Medical Sciences, ed. *Controlled clinical trials*. Oxford: Blackwell, 1960:109–14.
2. Working Party on Anticoagulant Therapy in Coronary Thrombosis. Assessment of short-anti-

coagulant administration after cardiac infarction. Report of the Working Party on Anticoagulant Therapy in Coronary Thrombosis to the Medical Research Council. *BMJ* 1969;1:335–42.
3. Chalmers TC, Matta RJ, Smith H, Kunzler A-M. Evidence favoring the use of anticoagulants in the hospital phase of acute myocardial infarction. *N Engl J Med* 1977;297:1091–6
4. Pickering GW. Clinical problems and results. In: Council for International Organizations of Medical Sciences, ed. *Controlled clinical trials.* Blackwell. Oxford, 1960:115–22.
5. Medical Research Council. Second report of the working party on anticoagulant therapy in coronary thrombosis. *BMJ* 1964;2:837–43.
6. ISIS-2 (Second International Study of Infarct Survival) Collaborative Group. Randomised trial of intravenous streptokinase, oral aspirin, both, or neither among 17 187 cases of suspected acute myocardial infarction: ISIS-2. *Lancet* 1988;ii:349–60.
7. Elwood PC, Williams WO A randomized controlled trial of aspirin in the prevention of early mortality in myocardial infarction. *J R Coll Gen Pract* 1979;204:413–6.
8. Elwood PC, Cochrane AL, Burr ML, et al. A randomized controlled trial of acetyl salicylic acid in the secondary prevention of mortality from myocardial infarction. *BMJ* 1974;95:436–40.
9. Antiplatelet Trialists' Collaboration. Collaborative overview of randomised trials of antiplatelet therapy: 1. prevention of death, myocardial infarction, and stroke by prolonged antiplatelet therapy in various categories of patient. *BMJ* 1994;308:81–106.
10. Yusuf S, Collins R, Peto R, et al. Intravenous and intracoronary fibrinolytic therapy: overview of results on mortality, reinfarction and side-effects from 33 randomized trials. *Eur Heart J* 1985;6:556–85.
11. Gruppo Italiano per lo Studio della Streptokinase nell'Infarto Miocardico (GISSI). Effectiveness of intravenous thrombolytic treatment in acute myocardial infarction. *Lancet* 1986;i:397.
12. AIMS Trial Study Group. Effect of intravenous APSAC on mortality after acute myocardial infarction. *Lancet* 1988;i:545–9.
13. Wilcox RG, von der Lippe G, Ollson CG et al. Trial of tissue plasminogen activation for mortality reduction in acute myocardial infarction. Anglo-Scandinavian study of early thrombolysis (ASSET). *Lancet* 1988;ii:525–30.
14. Fibrinolytic Therapy Trialists' Collaborative Group. Indications for fibrinolytic therapy in suspected myocardial infarction: collaborative overview of early mortality and major morbidity results from all randomised trials of more than 1000 patients. *Lancet* 1994;343:311–22.
15. Late Study Group. Late efficacy of thrombolysis (LATE) study with alteplase 6–24 hours after onset of acute myocardial infarction. *Lancet* 1993;342:759–66.
16. ISIS-3 (Third International Study of Infarct Survival) Collaborative Group. ISIS-3: a randomised comparison of streptokinase vs tissue plasminogen activator vs anistreplase and of aspirin plus heparin vs aspirin alone among 41 299 cases of suspected acute myocardial infarction. *Lancet* 1992;339:753–770.
17. Gruppo Italiano per lo Studio della Sopravvivenza nell'Infarto Miocardico (GISSI-2). A factorial randomised trial of alteplase versus streptokinase and heparin versus no heparin among 12 490 patients with acute myocardial infarction. *Lancet* 1990;336:65–71.
18. The International Study Group. In-hospital mortality and clinical course of 20 891 patients with suspected acute myocardial infarction randomised between alteplase and streptokinase with or without heparin. *Lancet* 1990;336:71–5.
19. The GUSTO Investigators. An international randomized trial comprising four thrombolytic strategies for acute myocardial infarction. *N Engl J Med* 1993;329:673–82.
20. Snow PJD. Effect of propranolol in acute myocardial infarction. *Lancet* 1965;ii:551–3.
21. ISIS-1 (First International Study of Infarct Survival) Study Group. Randomised trial of intravenous atenolol among 16 027 cases of suspected acute myocardial infarction. ISIS-1 *Lancet* 1986;ii:57–66.
22. ISIS-1 (First International Study of Infarct Survival) Collaborative Group. Mechanisms for the early mortality reduction produced by beta-blockade started early in myocardial infarction. ISIS-1. *Lancet* 1988;i:921–3.
23. Norwegian Multicenter Study Group. Timolol-induced reduction in mortality and reinfarction in patients surviving myocardial infarction. *N Engl J Med* 1981;304:801–7.
24. Beta-blocker Heart Attack Study Group (BHAT). A beta-blocker heart attack trial. *JAMA* 1981;246:2073–4.
25. Multicentre International Study. Improvement in prognosis of myocardial infarction by long-term β-adrenoceptor blockade using practolol. *BMJ* 1975;3:735–40.
26. Baber NS, Wainwright Evans D, Howitt G, et al. A multicentre propranolol post-infarction trial in 49 hospitals in the United Kingdom, Italy and Yugoslavia. *Br Heart J* 1980;44:96–100
27. Taylor SH, Silke B, Ebbutt A, et al. A long-term prevention study with oxprenolol in coronary heart disease. *N Engl J Med* 1982;307:1293–301.
28. Julian DG, Prescott RJ, Jackson FS, Szekely P. Controlled trial of sotalol for 1 year after myocardial infarction. *Lancet* 1982;i:1142–7.

29. Baber NS, Lewis JA. Confidence in results of beta-blocker post-infarction trials. *BMJ* 1982;284:1749–50.
30. Held PH, Yusuf S. Effects of β-blockers and calcium channel blockers in acute myocardial infarction. *Eur Heart J* 1993;14 (suppl F):18–25.
31. Wilcox RG. Hampton JR, Banks DC, et al. Trial of early nifedipine in acute myocardial infarction: the TRENT study. *BMJ* 1986;293:1204–8.
32. Yusuf S, Collins R, MacMahon S, Peto R. Effect of intravenous nitrates in acute myocardial infarction. *Lancet* 1988;i:1088–92.
33. Teo KK, Yusuf S, Collins R, Held PH, Peto R. Effects of intravenous magnesium in suspected myocardial infarction: overview of randomised trials. *BMJ* 1991;303:1499–503.
34. Woods KL, Fletcher S, Roffe C, Haider Y. Intravenous magnesium sulphate in suspected myocardial infarction: results of the second Leicester intravenous magnesium intervention trial (LIMIT-2). *Lancet* 1992;339:1553–8.
35. Hamilton M, Thompson EN, Wisniewski TKM. The role of blood pressure control in preventing complications of hypertension. *Lancet* 1964;i:235–8.
36. Coope J, Warrender TS. Randomised trial of treatment of hypertension in elderly patients in primary care. *BMJ* 1986;293:1145–51.
37. Medical Research Council Working Party. MRC trial of treatment of mild hypertension. *BMJ* 1985;291:97–104.
38. Medical Research Council Working Party. Medical Research Council trial of treatment in older adults. *BMJ* 1992;304:405–12.
39. The Xamoterol in Severe Heart Failure Study Group. Xamoterol in severe heart failure. *Lancet* 1990;336:1–6.
40. The Acute Infarction Ramipril Efficacy (AIRE) Study Investigators. Effect of ramipril on mortality and morbidity of survivors of acute myocardial infarction with clinical evidence of heart failure. *Lancet* 1993;342:821–8.
41. Oliver MF, Julian DG, Donald KW. Problems in evaluating coronary care units. *Am J Cardiol* 1967;20:465–74.
42. Mather HG, Morgan DC, Pearson NG, et al. Myocardial infarction: a comparison between home and hospital care for patients. *BMJ* 1976;i:925–9.
43. Hill JD, Hampton JR, Mitchell JRA. A randomised trial of home versus hospital management for patients with suspected myocardial infarction. *Lancet* 1978;i:837–41.
44. European Coronary Surgery Study Group. Coronary artery bypass surgery in stable angina pectoris: survival at two years. *Lancet* 1979;ii:889–93.
45. CASS Principal Investigators and their Associates. Coronary artery surgery study (CASS): a randomized trial of coronary artery bypass surgery. *Circulation* 1983;68:939–50.
46. RITA Trial Participants. Coronary angioplasty versus coronary artery bypass surgery. The randomised intervention treatment of angina. *Lancet* 1993;341:573–80.
47. CABRI Trial Participants. First year results of CABRI (coronary angioplasty vs bypass revascularization). *Lancet* 1995;346:1179–84.
48. The RITA-2 participants. Coronary angioplasty versus medical therapy for angina: the second randomised intervention treatment of angina (RITA-2). *Lancet* 1997;350:461–8.
49. World Health Organisation European Collaborative Group. European collaborative trial of multifactorial prevention of coronary heart disease. *Lancet* 1986;i:869–72.
50. Research Committee of the Medical Research Council. Controlled trial of soya-bean oil in myocardial infarction. *Lancet* 1968;ii:693–700.
51. Burr ML, Fehily AM, Gilbert JF, et al. Effects of changes in fat, fish and fibre intakes on death and myocardial infarction (DART). *Lancet* 1989;ii:757–61
52. Committee of Principal Investigators. A cooperative trial in the primary prevention of ischaemic heart disease using clofibrate. *Br Heart J* 1978;401:1–118.
53. Roussouw JE. Lipid-lowering agents. In: Pitt B, Julian DG, Pocock SJ, eds *Clinical trials in cardiology*. London: Saunders, 1997:88.
54. Shepherd J, Cobbe SM, Ford I, et al. for the West of Scotland Coronary Prevention Study Group. Prevention of coronary heart disease with pravastatin in men with hypercholesterolemia. *N Engl J Med* 1995;333:1301–7.
55. Hill AB. *Statistical methods in clinical and preventive medicine*. Edinburgh: Livingstone, 1962.
56. Pocock SJ. When to stop a clinical trial. *BMJ* 1992:305;235–240.

Chapter 20

Cardiovascular Pathology

Michael J Davies

In a narrow sense, pathology is an observational discipline that describes the macroscopic and microscopic morphology of diseased tissue. Its wider importance lies in the need to understand disease processes and how these produce structural and functional change. Both of these aspects can be found in the evolution of cardiovascular pathology in Britain.

Morphology

In the early part of the 20th century the descriptive aspects of cardiovascular pathology were well developed, based as they were on the 19th century tradition of James Hope and Carswell.[1] Carswell had produced a clear description of aortic valve stenosis caused by a calcified bicuspid valve, and the correlation between valve abnormality and the clinical sequelae was well understood. This was hardly surprising since many clinicians at that time either carried out autopsies or were assiduous attenders at them. However, it was the work of the meticulous morphologists of mainland Europe that dominated, and many eponyms from that time – for example, the giant cell granulomas of acute rheumatic fever (Aschoff bodies), medial calcification in the lower limb arteries (Monckeberg's sclerosis), and, in the heart, the conduction cells of the distal left bundle branch (Purkinje fibres) – are still used today.

British workers

Some British names from this early era of cardiovascular morphology stand out. Keith and Flack in 1907 would have described themselves as physiologists rather than pathologists, but were expert morphologists. When I consider these early workers, I wonder whether the current rather rigid distinctions between specialties and disciplines fostered by the royal colleges actually impede advances in knowledge. Keith and Flack described the sinus node and carried out experimental work that established the principles of atrioventricular conduction.[2] In 1913, Kent described atrioventricular connections at many sites around the mitral and tricuspid rings.[3] At the time, his observations confused the issue over the importance of the atrioventricular (A-V) node and bundle of His as the sole pathway of normal atrioventricular conduction, but they can now be put into context. The conduction system develops from a ring of tissue around each A-V valve orifice which is steadily reduced until only the His bundle and the A-V node remain. In 1974, Anderson et al. described the frequent persistence of remnants of this ring tissue in normal adult hearts.[4] The remnants often have a nodal-like structure, and while they do not usually connect atria to ventricles they may do so in pre-excitation. It is these nodal remnants that Kent was describing and, unknowingly, laying the basis for understanding not normal conduction but the pre-excitation states.

Academic pathology

By the 1930s, most British medical schools had established chairs of pathology whose incumbents had a major role in undergraduate teaching and ranked alongside the professors of medicine, surgery, and obstetrics in influence. Autopsy pathology was a very important part of both undergraduate and postgraduate teaching and was considered vital to the understanding of clinical disease. The tradition of academic pathology was stronger in Scotland, and when I began my career few professors of pathology were English. Although there were no specialist cardiovascular pathologists, the high prevalence of cardiovascular disease ensured that the level of knowledge of cardiac pathology was generally good. By the 1940s, the seeds of specialisation were sprouting – departmental research became orientated toward tumour pathology or cardiovascular disease. Neuropathology became the first discipline to have specialist pathologists, because of the need for very close correlation between clinical features and the detailed anatomy of the brain. From 1940 on, British cardiovascular pathology began to make its mark in new work, particularly in atherosclerosis.

Atherosclerosis research

Pathologists from mainland European made all the early running in atherosclerosis research. In 1856, Virchow suggested in situ fatty degeneration or lipid insudation as mechanisms for the accumulation of lipid in the intima, while, in 1852, Rokitansky had already suggested encrustation of the intima by blood products – an idea that later developed into the thrombogenic theory of atherosclerosis. The term atherosclerosis (from Greek meaning gruel-like hard lesions) is said to have been used first by Marchand in 1904.[5] Reginald Hudson, pathologist at the National Heart Hospital in London, pithily remarked that likening the contents of an atheromatous plaque to gruel or porridge is a loathsome concept even to a Scotsman. There was, at that time, a strong link between cardiovascular pathology and Egyptology. In 1910, Ruffer studied the aortas of Egyptian mummies from the first and second centuries BC and found evidence of extensive atherosclerosis.[6]

Foam cells

In 1913, Anitschow produced experimental atheroma by feeding rabbits a diet rich in cholesterol.[7] This was the first serious attempt to produce animal models of atherosclerosis and to relate the disease to dietary and plasma lipid concentrations. The foam cell – a cell whose cytoplasm is distended by numerous fine vacuoles of lipid – came into prominence as a feature of atherosclerosis. Smooth muscle cells, considered to be the origin of most cells in the intima, were also thought to be the origin of foam cells. Adams, professor of pathology at Guy's Hospital, interpreted the presence of enzyme granules in the cytoplasm of foam cells to suggest that at least some were of monocyte lineage.[8]

Monocytes

Experimental work was also beginning to implicate the monocyte. Although these ideas originated outside the United Kingdom, their proof and validation were established by two decades of work from the Dunn School of Pathology in Oxford.[10][11] Work from Dunn, Poole, French, and Florey showed the structure of the endothelium, using enface preparations stained with silver to show up the "cement lines" marking cell boundaries. Adhesion and migration of monocytes was studied. Before any knowledge of adhesion molecules existed, it was suggested that the endothelium over plaques was altered in some way to cause monocyte adhesion and that an unknown factor attracted the monocyte to enter the intima across the intact endothelial surface. Today we recognise the existence of monocyte chemotactic protein produced by cells within the intima as the stimulus for migration.

In 1984, Mitchinson at Cambridge was the first to use immunohistochemical techniques to resolve the controversy of the origin of foam cells.[12] Using specific antibodies to monocyte antigens, most foam cells were found to be positive. Today, everyone uses immunohistochemistry to identify macrophage lineage cells by their possession of the CD68 antigen and it is difficult to appreciate the problems that histologists had in the past when they were able to identify cell types only by their appearances in haematoxylin and eosin stained sections.

Atherosclerosis Discussion Group

In the autumn of 1957, a young Michael Oliver persuaded John French in Oxford to support the creation of a British society for the interchange of views in atherosclerosis research. Howard Florey, although a Nobel prize winner for his work in penicillin, had been the stimulus for the work on experimental atherosclerosis. He delegated Michael Oliver to find £250 and start an Atherosclerosis Discussion Group. The group had a closed membership and met twice a year – one in Oxford, one in Cambridge. The Atherosclerosis Discussion Group transformed itself only recently into an open membership British Atherosclerosis Society.

The role of the thrombus

One of the great names of cardiovascular pathology in relation to atherosclerosis was JB Duguid, professor of pathology in Cardiff and subsequently in Newcastle. In 1926 he published an article on the importance of mechanical factors, stretching and stress on the arterial wall, in localising the sites of plaque formation.[13] In a series of papers from 1946 onward, Duguid supported the deposition of small thrombi becoming incorporated into the vessel wall as a cause of plaque growth.[14]

Numerous other workers showed that the incorporation of surface thrombus was present in human plaques followed Duguid. Over succeeding years, Crawford, Woolf, and Carstairs at St George's Hospital, London and Walton in Birmingham used the newer techniques of immunohistochemistry to show platelets and fibrin in a banded pattern deep within plaques in the human aorta.[15][16][17][18][19] Elspeth Smith in Aberdeen established the concept that fibrinogen insuded into the intima in a manner similar to that of low density lipoprotein and could be converted to fibrin within the plaque.[20] In experimental pig models of thrombi induced by intimal injury, Woolf showed that lesions became indistinguishable from plaque.[21] However, all this work was related to slow plaque growth rather than to the initiation of acute clinical symptoms.

Lipids versus thrombus

WB Robertson, who became professor of pathology at St.George's Hospital, London carried out his doctorate work on coronary atherosclerosis and myocardial infarction with Duguid in Newcastle. He deduced that "until relatively recently the Americans have been much influenced by lipids and unimpressed by thrombosis other than as a complication, whereas British researchers have been proponents of thrombosis as the most important factor precipitating clinical symptoms."[22]

This dichotomy of views persisted for 20 years. Most workers in Britain believed that thrombosis of the coronary arteries caused infarction, a view enunciated by Herrick in an American journal in 1912.[23] In 1928, Parkinson and Bedford published an article in *Heart* entitled "Successive changes in the ECG after cardiac infarction (coronary thrombosis)," and followed it by a pathology paper describing the thrombi that were found in the coronary arteries.[24][25]

I became interested in cardiovascular disease while an undergraduate on Evan Bedford's "firm" at the Middlesex Hospital, London in 1960. I realised the beautiful correlations that could be drawn between structure and function in cardiac disease. Bedford was a great believer in knowing the pathological basis of disease. He was a gifted teacher of undergraduates . . . but only if they showed interest in cardiac disease, a modicum of intelligence, and a willingness to attend his ward on Saturday.

In 1949, Victor Harrison, professor of pathology at the Postgraduate School at Hammersmith, coauthored with Paul Wood an article published in the *British Heart Journal* describing the use of post mortem coronary arteriography and linking myocardial fibrosis to chronic coronary stenosis as well as highlighting thrombosis as a key element in infarction.[26] The death of Wood from thrombosis in the left anterior descending coronary artery confirmed at autopsy is particularly poignant in this context.[27]

The inconstant thrombus

In the 1950s, however, there emerged the view (a heretical one to those who taught me my pathology) that thrombosis was an inconstant feature of acute myocardial infarction and indeed if present was a secondary phenomenon. The curious idea that infarction caused coronary thrombosis, therefore thrombosis was largely secondary and relatively unimportant, was largely initiated in North America but was resisted in Britain vehemently by most, but not all, pathologists. The main opponents of the thrombotic cause of infarction were Levine and Brown,[28] Ehrlich and Shinohara,[29] Roberts,[30] and Spain and Bradess.[31][32] Spain, a forensic pathologist studying sudden deaths, found that coronary thrombi were present in 16% of patients who died within one hour and in 54% of those who died 24 hours of the onset of symptoms. What is surprising, in retrospect, is that it was assumed that sudden death in ischaemic heart disease must be due to myocardial infarction even if none was visible to the pathologist. This view was only finally squashed by studies of resuscitated subjects who survived out-of-hospital ventricular fibrillation and in whom only about 40% developed infarction.[33]

Explaining discordant results

In Britain, the view that thrombosis was unimportant had aiders and abettors. In Edinburgh in 1957, Branwood and Montgomery studied 108 recent myocardial infarcts and found thrombi in only 39%.[34] When aged by histological criteria, the infarcts were deemed to be older than the thrombi. Yet in 1966, Arthur Harland, a highly skilled cardiovascular pathologist in Glasgow (who was to die suddenly at a relatively young age) found that 91% of patients with acute infarcts had thrombi in the subtending artery and wrote in the *Lancet* that "thrombotic occlusion was the final event always secondary to atheroma and often overlying an atheromatous abscess."[35] This "abscess" is, of course, what we would now call a lipid rich plaque.

Then, as now, Glasgow had a high frequency of coronary artery disease, and Bill Fulton, one of its professors of cardiology, made an immense contribution to the understanding of coronary thrombosis using pathology techniques he had developed.[36][37] Fulton's work was largely described in a book and through oral presentations and is not therefore as well known as it deserves. He gave radiolabelled fibrinogen to patients with chest pain at the time of their admission to hospital, and in those who developed an acute infarction and died, he used autoradiography to make detailed autopsy studies of the coronary arteries. Today, it might be difficult to get ethical approval for such a study. Thrombi were found consistently in the artery supplying the infarct, the most proximal portion of the thrombus was radionegative (it predated hospital admission) and the more distal thrombus was radiopositive (the thrombus had continued to propagate after admission). At a stroke the discordant results reported by pathologists, Branwood and Montgomery,[34] were explained by Fulton, a clinician.

There can be no better example of one of the besetting sins of many pathologists – the belief that what they see at autopsy – at one moment in time – must be the same as the appearances 24 hours earlier or later. Disease processes are dynamic, but recognition of dynamism does not seem to be in the nature of many pathologists.

Increasing incidence

It is interesting, and relevant, that in 1910 Osler confessed that he had not seen a case of angina pectoris before becoming a fellow of the Royal College of Physicians.[38] He considered "coronary artery disease to be a disease for seniors to discuss, since juniors see it but rarely." Writing in the *British Heart Journal* in 1949, Ryle and Russell analysed the Registrar General's report over a 25 year period between the two world wars and showed a 15-fold increase in coronary heart disease mortality in men aged 40–55 that could not be explained by changes in diagnostic criteria.[39] In 1951, Morris studied the pathology records at the London Hospital and compared 1908–13 with 1944–9.[40] He showed an apparent reduction in the extent of atherosclerosis between the two periods, but a sevenfold increase in coronary disease as a cause of death. The fact that this study could be carried out is a mark of the detailed autopsy observations made in the first half of the century in Britain.

Atherosclerosis was the major research theme of Theo Crawford who was appointed professor of pathology at St George's Hospital, London from 1946. The rising incidence of clinically expressed coronary artery disease was one of his interests, and he speculated over whether it resulted from an increase in atherosclerosis per se or of the thrombotic complications of atherosclerosis.

Central Middlesex years

I joined Theo Crawford's department as a registrar in 1964. My career to that point has interesting facets. After preregistration jobs I went back to my undergraduate medical school, the Middlesex Hospital, to seek a post in pathology. On hearing I was interested in cardiovascular disease, the professor of pathology, Robert Scarff, said rather crushingly that I was not the sort of person he wanted in his department. (It is not without interest that he also turned down Valentin Fuster.) By chance, a post came up at the Central Middlesex Hospital, where Roger Drury had a distinguished record in atherosclerosis research. The senior registrars were Ariela Pomerance, who later became pathologist to Magdi Yacoub and a pioneer in transplant pathology, and Sue Rowlett, an expert in animal hearts who became the cardiovascular pathologist for the Chicago Zoo. I still remember carrying a bucket of formalin in my car to collect dead hedgehogs for Sue Rowlett, although I cannot remember what particular curiosity exists in their hearts.

In those days, the Central Middlesex carried out over 1500 autopsies a year and Ariela Pomerance insisted that I looked at every heart with her. It is difficult to see how a young pathologist could gain this amount of experience today with the precipitate decline in autopsy rates over the last 10 years. At that time, Ariela Pomerance was producing a set of classic pathology observations on the ageing heart. She described atrial amyloid deposition[41] and valve calcification[42] in what are still the seminal papers in the area.

Roger Drury recommended me to Theo Crawford at St George's Hospital, London as someone suitable for an academic career in cardiovascular pathology, and for better or worse I am still there as the professor. The British Heart Foundation took over the funding of the post in 1981.

St George's Hospital

Theo Crawford was a highly skilled cardiovascular pathologist who used post mortem coronary arteriography to investigate coronary disease. The technique enabled me to recognise the angiographic appearances of coronary thrombi. I knew the angiographic appearances of the culprit lesions of acute ischaemic events long before the classic descriptions of type I and type II lesions from in vivo angiography appeared in published reports.

In 1953, Theo Crawford had described another phenomenon that was much later taken up as an important concept.[43] He described the medial thinning behind plaques which allowed the lumen to remain unaltered in size, with the result that the angiogram would not detect many plaques. Today the concept of "remodelling" is very fairly ascribed to the Glagov's classic paper from the United States.[44] I must admit, however, that the only reaction to this paper at St George's was, "well everyone knows that."

Writing a paper at the correct time for clinicians to be receptive is crucial. In 1974, Sir Theo Crawford delegated to me to survey the experience of the relation of coronary thrombosis to acute infarction at St George's. At that time deaths in hospital from acute myocardial infarction were far more common than they are now. The department had a triad of pathologists committed to cardiovascular pathology – myself, Neville Woolf, and Bill Robertson. Bill Robertson had worked with Duguid in Newcastle and then became involved with the international atherosclerosis project while working in the West Indies. The international atherosclerosis project was organised by Henry McGill in New Orleans and showed very clearly that in all populations risk factors such as hypertension and diabetes increase the number of plaques present.[45] The results of our study in London were interesting in that we three consistently found over 95% of regional infarcts had thrombi in the supplying artery.[46] A fourth pathologist whose main interest was surgical tumour pathology produced very discordant results and perhaps it was more than a coincidence that he soon obtained a post elsewhere more suited to his very real skills in the histological diagnosis of tumours.

Understanding the controversy

It is difficult now to appreciate the reasons for the controversy over thrombosis when in vivo angiography by De Wood and others in the first hour of infarction showed occlusions which often spontaneously opened over the next few hours and when the introduction of fibrinolytic treatment has been so successful in accelerating the opening of the artery.[47][48] The original controversy over the role of thrombosis resulted from preconceived notions held by pathologists. One notion was that sudden ischaemic death was synonymous with acute myocardial infarction – even if they could not see an infarct it must be there. Another opinion was that high grade stenosis alone could cause infarction. Holding this view obviates the need to look for thrombi. Many clinicians also believed that high grade stenosis was related to infarction and was a prerequisite of a final thrombotic episode. An early presentation I made to the British Cardiac Society meeting on the fact that the stenosis on which thrombosis developed was usually not severe invoked a very courteous, but firm, rebuke from Walter Sommerville to reconsider the data.

Plaque disruption

From 1975–90 my own path of research lay in the discovering why plaques should suddenly develop a major thrombotic episode. I had been introduced by Roger Drury to the concept that intraplaque haemorrhage was a precipitator of coronary thrombus.[49] However, that a large mass of platelets and fibrin within a plaque could come from the capillaries that entered the plaque from the media, seemed illogical to me. As part of my doctoral thesis, I studied the conduction system in chronic heart block, an investigation in which cutting serial histological sections to follow structural change was an established technique.

After Constantinides's paper on plaque fissuring,[50] it seemed natural to test his views by reconstructing a number of coronary thrombi and their associated plaques from serial sections. Such an approach shows that when a thrombus is found within the plaque, there will be connection, upstream or downstream, between the lipid core and the arterial lumen via a break in the plaque cap.[51] Interestingly, Bill Robertson recollects that Duguid's views on organised thrombus and the plaque evolved after he re-examined a series of many histological levels of a plaque prepared for an undergraduate teaching class set. Duguid found that the appearances of the plaque changed in the different sections. A common limitation among pathologists is a belief that a single histological section is representative of the whole. This may be true for the liver but not for coronary arteries with plaques.

Plaque rupture

In 1975, I went to a meeting on the pathogenesis of unstable angina in Amsterdam. I was amazed to find there was uncertainty. We were shown angiograms with appearances that I knew to be ruptured plaques with non-occluding thrombi; yet most of those present did not seem to realise this. I make no claim to the discovery of plaque rupture – but I did point out its clinical importance. The discovery is usually attributed to Constantinides,[50] but "ulceration" of an atheromatous "abscess," the extreme expression of plaque rupture, was well known in the last century. Theo Crawford, in a monograph on the *Pathology of Ischaemic Disease*, records descriptions of plaque rupture by Kock and Kong in 1932, Leary in 1934, and in British publications by Morgan in 1956 and by himself in 1963.[52]

The burgeoning interest in the clinical sequelae of plaque disruption increased my desire to understand its basic mechanisms. In 1989, Peter Richardson in Rhode Island, Gus Born, and I were the first people to study circumferential wall stress across plaques using finite element analysis to show concentrations of stress up to eight times normal occurred on the plaque cap.[53] We also showed the high concentrations of macrophages and the presence of metalloproteinases that characterised ruptured plaques.[54][55][56]. All these aspects were very rapidly expanded by research groups in the United States, particularly brilliantly by Peter Libby in Boston. Today we know that thrombosis over a plaque is initiated by a "self destruct" inflammatory process leading either to breakdown of the connective tissue of the cap (plaque disruption) or loss of the endothelium over the plaque (erosion). It now seems from the work of our own group[57] and from the United States [58] that disruption is the predominant mechanism for thrombosis in men, while in women erosion is as frequent as disruption in causing thrombosis.

Cardiomyopathy and myocarditis

Britain has always been in the forefront of work on hypertrophic cardiomyopathy. In 1958 Donald Teare, the professor of forensic medicine at St George's Hospital in London, described the characteristic pathological features of asymmetric hypertrophy of the interventricular septum in eight cases of sudden death.[59] He described the characteristic histological appearances of myocyte disarray and recognised the familial nature of the condition. The paper was the first to bring the condition into sharp focus, although Brock had earlier reported functional obstruction to the left ventricle, simulating aortic valve stenosis but with no valve abnormality.[60] Wood had worked out the existence of a functional subaortic stenosis from first principles a year earlier.[27] In fact, Reginald Hudson knew of exactly similar cases and had noted the myocyte disarray, but he did not publish his work until 1965.[61] Hypertrophic cardiomyopathy remains a major research interest at St George's and we have "closed the loop" by showing that the living relatives of some of Donald Teare's original cases have mutations in the heavy chain myosin gene.

John Goodwin at the Hammersmith Hospital illustrated the fact that all top class cardiologists are excellent morphologists. He worked with Victor Harrison and Eckhard Olsen to develop the pathophysiological classification of cardiomyopathies which has become adopted worldwide.[62] John Goodwin's work illustrates so well the basic tenet that structure cannot be separated from function . . . and vice versa.

Britain has made contributions in the field of myocarditis, although it must be admitted that this is still a grey area. Eckhardt Olsen who succeeded Reginald Hudson as pathologist to the National Heart Hospital, London was a member of the "Dallas group" of pathologists who interpreted cardiac biopsies and laid down the criteria for the tissue diagnosis of myocarditis.[63] These criteria helped in one way, in that they precluded the use of terms such as healed myocarditis for a scarred myocardium in which there was no actual evidence of a prior myocarditis. However, the Dallas group was not explicit about how many inflammatory cells needed to be present for the diagnosis of acute myocarditis. The criteria continue to be refined by the WHO and European Society of Cardiology working groups, but there are still discrepancies in reported positivity rates in cardiac biopsy specimens from centres in Europe.

Reginald Hudson

No account of cardiovascular pathology in Britain can be complete without a special mention of Reginald Hudson, pathologist to the National Heart Hospital, London and the Institute of Cardiology from 1948 to his retirement. In 1965, he published his tour de force – *Cardiovascular pathology* – a textbook in two volumes that was updated later by adding a third volume.[61] The book served three purposes. Firstly, it was an exhaustive reference source . . . so exhaustive that the sheer number of references inhibited anyone other than those writing a thesis themselves. Reginald Hudson and his meticulous card index served the function of today's Medline. The drawback to this was maintaining the database without Reginald. There was no solution and the book retired with him rather than going into a fourth volume. The second aim was to illustrate very beautifully the full spectrum of cardiovascular pathology, both congenital and acquired, for his clinical and pathological colleagues when confronted with a problem. The book's final purpose was to relate the pathology to the clinical manifestations. Here it was less successful. Face to face, Reginald Hudson was very good at correlating pathology and clinical features; he was regularly invited to the United States to demonstrate this skill. But his talent does not come through in the book, and it was never as popular as other large American textbooks. One reason was that Reginald Hudson's book contained too much. For example, it discussed the mechanism of coagulation, details of fluid balance, and the principles of bacteriology. This was because Reginald Hudson was responsible for all these general pathology aspects at the National Heart Hospital. But one would not usually consult Hudson's book for advice on how to manage electrolyte balance after surgery.

Reginald Hudson was a man of immense humility, integrity, and kindness. He examined my doctoral thesis on the conduction system over tea and biscuits for a whole afternoon in his office. He tolerated listening to my self assured, young man's views, but, characteristically, he seldom gave his own views on theory or reasons. When I showed him a particular piece of pathology, he did not expound on how this could arise, but usually produced several other examples of the same thing from his own collection or published reports. He was, par excellence, an observer, a classifier, and a cataloguer of disease states.

Mystery of the floppy valve

Reginald Hudson introduced the floppy mitral valve to me in 1965. I had taken him surgical specimens of valves from patients with mitral regurgitation in which the changes were clearly not those of rheumatic fever. But what were they? He said at once, "these are parachute deformities," and showed me other examples. Within a year the term "floppy" valve had been applied by Reed,[64] and the National Heart Hospital adopted this terminology because the word parachute had been used by Shone for a totally different entity.[65] I became very interested in the floppy valve with its myxomatous transformation weakening the cusp to allow expansion in area, elongation of chordae tendenae, and chordal rupture and carried out an autopsy study to show its frequency and natural history in the general population.[66]

Even today the pathogenesis of mitral myxomatous change remains uncertain in most cases. A few cases are associated with genetic defects in connective tissue synthesis such as the fibrillin in Marfan's disease, but what of the majority? Will extensive gene analysis in the 21st century reveal many more genetic causes or will the floppy valve remain a mystery?

Isolated aortic regurgitation continues to be another grey area for the pathologists of the 21st century. In the United Kingdom, many cases are a result of idiopathic non-inflammatory aortic root disease, but we do not know whether this is due to genetic defects in some aspect of the metabolism or connective tissue synthesis of the aortic media.

Cardiovascular pathology in the 1990s

It is possible to be optimistic or pessimistic over cardiovascular pathology. On the negative side the interest and expertise in cardiovascular pathology by the vast majority of general pathologists is at an all time low. This is partly because of a decline in the use of the autopsy caused by increasing resistance among relatives to giving consent and the decreasing ability of pathologists to gain sufficient clinical knowledge to carry out correlations that seem worthwhile to clinicians. Clinicians with modern imaging techniques at their disposal are more inclined to feel confident, not necessarily with entire justification, about antemortem diagnosis. The increasing sophistication of the diagnosis of malignancy in surgical material and biopsy specimens is likely to remain the major interest of general pathologists, who generate almost all their income from such work.

On the optimistic side there are now specialist cardiovascular pathologists. The impetus came from cardiac transplantation and the need for expertise in reading cardiac biopsies to detect rejection. British pathologists have made significant contributions to developing criteria for rejection. Ariela Pomerance working with Magdi Yacoub rapidly became highly experienced in the techniques and has taught the rest of us involved in such work. There is now a United Kingdom group of cardiovascular pathologists involved in transplant work who meet regularly to audit their work and run a quality assurance programme. Nat Cary at Papworth Hospital, Cambridge has for many years been on the international panel to lay down criteria and classification of cardiac rejection. A by-product of the transplant programme is that each centre will have a pathologist who will see many explanted hearts, learn their morphology, and have material available for modern research techniques.

References and notes

1. Hollman A. The paintings of pathological anatomy by Sir Robert Carswell (1723–1857). *Br Heart J* 1995;74:566–70.
2. Keith A, Flack M. The form and nature of muscular connections between the primary divisions of the vertebrate heart. *J Anat Physiol* 1907;41:172–89.
3. Kent, AFS. Observations of the auricular-ventricular junction of the mammalian heart. *Q J Exp Physiol* 1913;7:193–5.
4. Anderson R, Davies M, Becker A. Atrioventricular ring specialised tissue in the normal heart. *Eur J Cardiol* 1974;2:19–27.
5. Marchand F. Über Arteriosklerose. *Verhandlung der Kongres für innere Medizine* 1904;21:23–59.
6. Ruffer MA. On arterial lesions found in Egyptian mummies. *J Pathol Bacteriol* 1911;15:453–62.

7. Anitschow N, Chalatow S. Über experimentelle Cholesterinsteatose und ihre Bedentung für die Enstehung einiger pathologische Prozesse. *Centralblatt für Allgemeine Pathologie* 1913;24:1–10.
8. Adams CWM, Bayliss OB. Detection of macrophages in atherosclerotic lesions with cytochrome oxidase. *Br J Exp Pathol* 1976;57:30–6.
9. Leary T. The genesis of atherosclerosis. *Arch Pathol* 1941;32:507–55.
10. French JE. Atherosclerosis. In: Florey H ed. *General pathology.* 2nd ed. London: Lloyd-Luke, 1956.
11. Florey HW, Poole JC, Meek GA. Endothelial cells and "cement" lines. *J Pathol Bacteriol* 1959:77:625–36.
12. Aqel N, Ball R, Waldmann H, Mitchinson M. Monocytic origin of foam cells in human atherosclerotic plaques. *Atherosclerosis* 1984;53:265–71.
13. Duguid JB. Atheroma of the aorta. *J Pathol Bacteriol* 1926;29:371–87.
14. Duguid JB. Thrombosis as a factor in the pathogenesis of coronary atherosclerosis. *J Pathol Bacteriol* 1946;58:207–12.
15. Crawford T, Levene C. The incorporation of fibrin in the aortic intima. *J Pathol Bacteriol* 1952;64:523–6.
16. Woolf N. The distribution of fibrin within the aortic intima: an immunohistochemical study. *Am J Pathol* 1961;39:521–532.
17. Carstairs K. The identification of platelets and platelet antigens in histological sections. *J Pathol Bacteriol* 1965;90:225–31.
18. Woolf N, Carstairs KC. Infiltration and thrombosis in atherogenesis – a study using immunofluorescent techniques. *Am J Pathol* 1967;51:373–86.
19. Walton K, Williamson N. Histological and immunofluorescent studies on the evolution of the human atheromatous plaque. *J Atherosclerosis Res* 1968;8:599–624.
20. Smith E. Fibrinogen and fibrin degradation products in relation to atherosclerosis. *Clin Haematol* 1986;15:355–70.
21. Woolf N, Bradley JWP, Crawford T, Carstairs KC. Experimental mural thrombosis in the pig aorta. The early natural history. *Br Heart J* 1968;49:257–64.
22. Robertson WB. *Coronary atherosclerosis and myocardial infarction.* St Andrews, University of St Andrews, 1959. (Doctoral thesis.)
23. Herrick JB. Concerning thrombosis of the coronary arteries. *Trans Ass Am Physicians* 1912;59:2015–9.
24. Parkinson J, Bedford DE. Successive changes in the ECG after cardiac infarction (coronary thrombosis). *Heart* 1928;14:195–239.
25. Parkinson J, Bedford DE. Cardiac infarction and coronary thrombosis. *Lancet* 1928;1:4–11.
26. Harrison CV, Wood P. Hypertensive and ischaemic heart disease: a comparative clinical and pathological study. *Br Heart J* 1949:11:205–29.
27. Somerville J. Paul Wood lecture – the master's legacy. *Heart* 1998;80:612–8.
28. Levine SA, Brown CL. Coronary thrombosis: its various clinical features. *Medicine* 1929;8:245–8.
29. Ehrlich JC, Shinohara Y. Low incidence of coronary thrombosis in myocardial infarction. *Arch Pathol* 1964;78:432–45.
30. Roberts WC. Coronary arteries in fatal acute myocardial infarction. *Circulation* 1972;45:215–30.
31. Spain D, Bradess V. The relationship of coronary thrombosis to coronary atherosclerosis and ischaemic heart disease. *Am J Med Sci* 1969;240:701–10.
32. Spain D, Bradess V, Mohr C. Coronary atherosclerosis as a cause of unexpected and unexplained death. *JAMA* 1960;174:384–5.
33. Cobb L, Baum R, Alvarex H, Schaffer W. Resuscitation from out-of-hospital ventricular fibrillation 4 year follow-up. *Circulation* 1995;51:111–23.
34. Branwood A, Montgomery G. Observations on the morbid anatomy of coronary disease. *Scott Med J* 1956;1:367–75.
35. Harland WA, Holburn AM. Coronary thrombosis and myocardial infarction. *Lancet* 1966;ii:1158–60.
36. Fulton W, Sumner D. 125 I-labelled fibrinogen, autoradiography and steroarteriography in identification of coronary thrombotic occlusion in fatal myocardial infarction. *Br Heart J* 1976;38:880. (Abstract.)
37. Fulton WFM. *The coronary arteries.* Springfield, IL: Thomas, 1965.
38. Osler W. The Lumleian lectures on angina pectoris. *Lancet* 1910;697:839–844.
39. Ryle JA, Russell WT. The natural history of coronary disease. A clinical and epidemiological study. *Br Heart J* 1949;11:370–89.
40. Morris J. Recent history of coronary disease. *Lancet* 1951;i:69–73.
41. Pomerance A.The pathology of senile cardiac amyloidosis. *J Pathol Bacteriol* 1966;91;357–67.
42. Pomerance A. Ageing changes in human heart valves. *Br Heart J* 1967;29:222–31.
43. Crawford T, Levene C. Medial thinning in atheroma. *J Pathol Bacteriol* 1953;66:19–23.
44. Glagov S, Weisenberd E, Zarins C, Stankunavicius R, Kolettis G. Compensatory enlargement of human atherosclerotic coronary arteries. *N Engl J Med* 1987;316:1371–5.

45. Robertson WB, Strong JP. Atherosclerosis in persons with hypertension and diabetes mellitus. *Lab Invest* 1968;18:538–42.
46. Davies M, Woolf N, Robertson W. Pathology of acute myocardial infarction with particular reference to occlusive coronary thrombi. *Br Heart J* 1976;38:659–64.
47. DeWood M, Spores J, Notske R, Mouser LT, Burroughs R, Golden MS, et al. Prevalence of total coronary occlusion during the early hours of transmural myocardial infarction. *N Engl J Med* 1980;303:897–902.
48. Brosius F, Roberts W. Significance of coronary arterial thrombus in transmural acute myocardial infarction. A study of 54 necropsy patients. *Circulation* 1981;63:810–6.
49. Drury RAB. The role of intimal haemorrhage in coronary occlusion. *J Pathol Bacteriol* 1954;67:207–15.
50. Constantinides P. Plaque fissures in human coronary thrombosis. *J Atherosclerosis Res* 1966;6:1–17.
51. Davies M, Thomas A. Plaque fissuring – the cause of acute myocardial infarction, sudden ischaemic death and crescendo angina. *Br Heart J* 1985;53:363–73.
52. Crawford T. *Pathology of ischaemic heart disease.* London: Butterworths, 1977:47–63.
53. Richardson P, Davies M, Born G. Influence of plaque configuration and stress distribution on fissuring of coronary atherosclerotic plaques. *Lancet* 1989;ii:941–4.
54. Davies MJ. Stability and Instability: Two faces of coronary atherosclerosis: the Paul Dudley White lecture 1995. *Circulation* 1996;94:2013–20.
55. Felton CV, Crook D, Davies MJ, Oliver MF. Relation of plaque lipid composition and morphology to the stability of human aortic plaques. *Arteriosclerosis Thromb Vasc Biol* 1997;17:1337–45.
56. Henney A, Wakeley P, Davies M et al. Localization of stromelysin gene expression in atherosclerotic plaques by in situ hybridization. *Proc Natl Acad Sci USA* 1991;88:8154–8.
57. Davies M. The composition of coronary-artery plaques. *N Engl J Med* 1997;336:1312–3.
58. Arbustini E, Dal Bello P, Morbini P, Burke A, Bocciarelli M, Specchia G, Virmani R. Plaque erosion is an important substrate for coronary thrombosis in acute myocardial infarction. *Heart* 1999;82:20–4.
59. Teare D. Asymmetrical hypertrophy of the heart in young patients. *Br Heart J* 1958;20:1–8.
60. Brock RC. Functional obstruction of the left ventricle (acquired subaortic valvar stenosis). *Guy's Hospital Rep*:106:221–38.
61. Hudson REB. *Cardiovascular pathology.* London: Edward Arnold, 1965.
62. Goodwin J. The frontiers of cardiomyopathy. *Br Heart J* 1982;48:1–18.
63. Aretz H. Myocarditis: the Dallas criteria. *Hum Pathol* 1987;18:619–24.
64. Read RC, Thal AP, Wendt VF. Symptomatic valvular myxomatous transformation (the floppy valve syndrome): a possible forme fruste of the Marfan syndrome. *Circulation* 1965;32:897–910.
65. Shone JD, Sellers RD, Anderson RC, Adams P, Lillehei CW, Edwards JE. The development complex of "parachute" mitral valve, supravalvular ring of left atrium, subaortic stenosis and coarctation of aorta. *Am J Cardiol* 1963;11:714–25.
66. Davies M, Moore B, Braimbridge M. The floppy mitral valve: study of incidence, pathology and complications in surgical, necropsy and forensic material. *Br Heart J* 1978;40:468–81.

Chapter 21

Paediatric Cardiology

Gerald Graham and James Taylor

From the beginning, and over the years, three specialties - paediatrics, cardiology, and cardiac surgery - have made closely intertwined contributions to establishing and developing paediatric cardiology. Before the second world war, the diagnosis and treatment of heart disease in children were largely limited to the effects of infection on the heart, and, in particular, rheumatic heart disease. Congenital heart disease, which eventually became the centre of paediatric cardiology, was generally treated as a genetic condition, simply divided into acyanotic and cyanotic defects. Sir James Mackenzie, in the third edition of his *Diseases of the heart*, devoted less than a page to the "aetiology, symptoms, prognosis, treatment" of "congenital affections of the heart."[1] Until the 1930s, patent (or persistent) ductus arteriosus and (isthmic) coarctation of the aorta were the most commonly diagnosed congenital extracardiac conditions, while ventricular septal defect and Fallot's tetralogy were the most frequently diagnosed intracardiac defect and cyanotic condition respectively. However, the morphological stage for the precise classification of congenital cardiac disease had been established in 1935 by Maude Abbott with her landmark atlas of these defects.[2] In 1939, the first book in Britain devoted entirely to congenital heart disease was written by JW Brown.[3]

Pioneers and pioneering procedures

It was Gross's pioneering 1938 operation to ligate a ductus arteriosus that marked the beginning of a change in the attitude of paediatricians and cardiologists to congenital extracardiac and intracardiac disease (from here on referred to together as congenital heart disease).[4] These disorders began to be viewed as potentially treatable. The next crucial step was taken by Crafoord in Sweden in 1944, who was the first surgeon to resect a coarctation in a 12 year old boy.[5] The third important step was taken by Blalock, on the suggestion of Helen Taussig and after considerable experimental work. He constructed a subclavian artery shunt to the pulmonary artery to increase pulmonary blood flow in Fallot's tetralogy.[6] Although this was an extracardiac procedure, it was the first operation dealing with the palliation of an intracardiac defect.

Angiography

These pioneering achievements were not only significant in themselves, they set the stage and provided the impetus for advances in the precise and detailed diagnosis of congenital heart disease. In 1938, Castellanos and colleagues had taken the first step in Cuba. These workers visualised radiographically "the heart cavities and the large vessels of the heart" by injecting radio-opaque contrast medium through a peripherally inserted small tube into the heart of children with suspected congenital defects.[7] They coined the term "angiography." It was not until nearly 10 years later that Cournand and Richards, building on Forssmann's self experiments in the late 1920s, introduced cardiac catheterisation in humans.[8] This procedure quickly established itself as the central diagnostic tool, as applied first by Cournand et al. and later by Richard Bing, and colleagues.[9][10]

In Britain, the effects of the second world war meant that, although these advances had become known, their fruits were slow to mature. However, McMichael's group at the Hammersmith Hospital soon applied cardiac catheterisation and the Fick principle to the problem of heart failure.

What gave the main impetus (in Britain and elsewhere) to paediatric cardiology as a specialty was the recognition that most of those born with a serious form of heart disease would, without treatment, die in infancy or early childhood, and that early treatment was necessary to prevent serious and lasting secondary effects, not limited to the heart. It had become clear that this required the development of special expertise and techniques, both investigational and surgical, working in tandem.

Roy Astley

Roy Astley in 1949 was the first doctor in Britain to undertake cardiac catheterisation in children with congenital heart disease. In 1948, just before the establishment of the NHS, he had been appointed to the Birmingham Children's Hospital as the first full time consultant paediatric radiologist in Britain. Astley performed the procedures himself, under fluoroscopic control. Some years later, he introduced angiocardiography (as did some other centres at about the same time), first with a home-built, manual, rapid cassette changer which could take 12 pictures in 2 seconds (R Astley, personal communication). In the early 1950s, Astley used the recently developed electronic generator (British General Radiological Company), which gave short radiation pulses (rates of up to 100 per second), to improve the fluoroscopic imaging. Soon afterwards he obtained an image intensifier and attached a motor driven Rolex camera, which, with some additional equipment, enabled him to perform cine-angiography at 32 pictures per second.

Establishing paediatric cardiac units

Liverpool

In Britain, several other paediatric and cardiological units, in conjunction with their respective radiological departments, had begun to establish the diagnosis of congenital heart disease. In 1947, at the Royal Liverpool Children's Hospital, John Hay, professor of paediatrics, set up with Ronald Edwards (surgeon) a heart clinic that included cardiac catheterisation. Interestingly, Hay's father (also named John Hay, professor of medicine in Liverpool) had been a co-founder of the Cardiac Club with Mackenzie. The first cardiac catheterisation in children was performed in 1950, and angiocardiography, with the Elema-Schonander machine, was started in 1960 (R Arnold, personal communication).

Great Ormond Street

In London, the first organisationally joint effort to learn the lessons of both the diagnostic and therapeutic advances in children with congenital heart defects occurred in 1953 at the Hospital for Sick Children, Great Ormond Street (now the Great Ormond Street Children's Hospital). In this year, the thoracic (later cardiothoracic) unit, a combined paediatric and surgical unit devoted to heart disease was opened with Richard Bonham Carter and David Waterston as consultant paediatrician and paediatric surgeon, respectively. Thus, paediatric cardiology with cardiac surgery as a joint specialty was born in Britain. This joint unit became consolidated structurally a few years later when a two-storey annex that included a ward of 20 beds, an intensive care area, and a suite of two operating rooms was built. The unit was complemented by the establishment of routine cardiac catheterisation and angiocardiography from 1955 onwards (some 40 diagnostic cardiac catheterisations had been performed in the preceding two years) by one of us (GG) who then set up the department of clinical physiology, which was responsible for all invasive and non-invasive cardiac diagnosis. It took nearly 10 years for a dedicated catheter-angiography suite to be built, and with the installation of an image intensifier and simultaneous biplane rapid film changer (Elema-Schonander), the full range of diagnostic and interventional procedures could be done. In 1970, single plane cine-angiography supplemented the biplane roll film angiography.

National Heart and Brompton Hospitals

Advances in heart surgery, such as Brock's pulmonary valvotomy in 1948 and the successful introduction of open heart (intracardiac) surgery, had stimulated the drive towards ever more exact preoperative diagnosis of congenital heart disease.[11] At the National Heart Hospital and the Brompton Hospital (originally established for adult patients) these investigations were at first performed by cardiologists and paediatricians, respectively. A children's "ward" – consisting of 15 beds over two floors – had been opened at the Brompton Hospital in 1965 when Michael Joseph, consultant paediatrician at Guy's Hospital, was appointed for two sessions as a paediatrician there. Joseph performed some cardiac catherisations on children in the adult cardiac investigative suite, until Graham Miller, its director, took over. The first consultant paediatric cardiologist, Elliott Shinebourne, was appointed five years later (M Joseph, personal communication).

Birmingham

At the Birmingham Children's Hospital, it was the pioneering work of consultant paediatrician Clifford Parsons, supplemented by Astley's diagnostic work, which was the moving force in establishing a unit for children with congenital heart disease. Two cardiac surgeons, D'Abreu and Abrams, began to operate on children, but Abrams soon became the only surgeon to continue working in this area (L Abrams and E Silove, personal communications). At the end of 1999, the unit has four consultant paediatric cardiologists and two cardiac surgeons who operate only on children, with an emphasis on infants. It is now the second busiest unit in Britain and among the leading British centres with regard to its diagnostic/interventional and surgical results.

Other regional developments

In the late 1950s and 1960s, other teaching hospitals in England, Northern Ireland, Scotland, and Wales established cardiac services – most of them both diagnostic and surgical. The impetus for this development came largely from the need to operate on children with congenital heart disease, as more and more cardiac defects became amenable to at least palliative, if not curative, treatment. Furthermore, as many of the children with more complex defects will die in infancy unless treated, the urgency to diagnose and operate on infants and even the newborn accentuated the need for special facilities, dedicated to the management of ever younger children.

Paediatric cardiology did not lag behind at the Royal Belfast Hospital for Sick Children. In fact, ligation of a ductus arteriosus was first recorded in 1951, and by 1953 more than 100 children had undergone extracardiac surgical procedures of various kinds (C Mulholland, personal communication).

At the other of the five children's hospitals in the United Kingdom (at Bristol, Edinburgh, Glasgow, Liverpool, and London), the 1960s and 1970s saw a rapid expansion of the diagnostic facilities as described for both Birmingham and Great Ormond Street, although the pace of advance may have varied between them.

Scotland

Glasgow and Edinburgh, while only 50 miles apart and with good road and train connections, have maintained separate paediatric cardiological services for many years. Paediatric cardiology had been initiated in Edinburgh by a few adult cardiologists with an interest in congenital heart disease. In particular, it was RM Marquis, encouraged by R Gilchrist, who, soon after his return from service in the second world war, began to see children with suspected congenital heart disease in the adult cardiology department of the Royal Infirmary. By the middle 1960s, cardiac clinics for children were held at the Royal Hospital for Sick Children. In 1967, closed cardiac surgery in children had begun in the adult cardiac unit of the Royal Infirmary, and the children were returned to the Sick Children's Hospital after the immediate postoperative period. Open heart surgery with cardiopulmonary bypass in children began in 1974, and a paediatric cardiac unit was established in the mid-1970s. Michael Godman was later appointed as the hospital's first consultant paediatric cardiologist. He has since been joined by two more consultant paediatric cardiologists. Since the mid 1980s, children with congenital heart disease from further north (Aberdeen, Inverness, Dundee), often diagnosed first by adult cardiologists or paediatricians with cardiac experience, have been referred to the Royal Hospital for Sick Children in Edinburgh for full investigation.

Glasgow's Hospital for Sick Children has played a role similar to that of its Edinburgh counterpart in the development of local and regional paediatric cardiological services and in cardiac surgery. All paediatric cardiac procedures have been undertaken at the Children's Hospital since 1973 (A Houston, personal communication). Its cardiac unit has grown rapidly, especially in the last 15 years. There are now three consultant paediatric cardiologists and a joint surgical unit. It has recently been decided that the Scottish paediatric cardiological units and their corresponding surgical services will soon be combined on the Glasgow site. While this may seem a rational and cost effective solution in relation to the number and geographical distribution of Scottish children with congenital cardiac defects, it will mean increased hardship to the parents and children from north east Scotland, and particularly the Orkneys and Shetland Isles.

Wales

From the early 1960s, a congenital heart clinic had been located at Sully Hospital, initiated and led by Leslie Davies, consultant cardiologist who had been working largely in adult cardiology. Diagnostic procedures such as cardiac catheterisation were also undertaken there. A cardiac surgical service had opened soon after at the hospital, led by Tom Rosser and later by Ian Breckenridge, which also looked after children with congenital heart disease. In 1974, these facilities were transferred to the University Hospital of Wales in Cardiff. On Davies's death in 1986, Richard Kirk and soon after

Graham Stuart were appointed consultant paediatric cardiologists to provide a specialist paediatric cardiac service.

Establishment of consultant posts

It was not until 1966 that the first consultant post (even then only part-time) in paediatric cardiology was created, in Leeds. Olive Scott was the first incumbent. In November of the year of her appointment, she was the first person in Britain to perform a balloon atrial septostomy (having been shown the procedure by William J Rashkind who had invented and developed it) in an infant with transposition of the great arteries. This patient subsequently had a successful Mustard operation (placement of an intra-atrial baffle) at Great Ormond Street. At the time of writing, he is well and running a restaurant in Scarborough. (Olive Scott, personal communication). Soon after that first atrial septostomy for transposition of the great arteries, the procedure became established at Great Ormond Street. There, over the next few years, nearly as many intra-atrial baffle operations were performed as in Toronto, where W Mustard had developed the procedure named after him.

In quick succession, consultant paediatric cardiologists were appointed at all of the hospitals where cardiac surgery was performed in children. As the diagnostic and surgical workloads increased, most centres began to appoint additional paediatric cardiologists. To date, there are nearly 60 cardiologists in 18 centres in England (Birmingham, Bristol, Leeds, Leicester, Liverpool, London (Brompton, Great Ormond Street, Guy's, and Harefield Hospitals), Oxford, Manchester, Newcastle, and Southampton); Northern Ireland (Belfast); Scotland (Edinburgh and Glasgow) and Wales (Cardiff). All but Cardiff and Manchester now have special cardiac surgical services for infants and children.

Professional associations

In 1956, on the initiative of Bonham Carter, Hay, and Parsons, a Paediatric Cardiology Group was formed, which in 1991 became the British Association of Paediatric Cardiologists, now affiliated to the British Cardiac Society. In parallel, Hamish Watson, an adult cardiologist in Dundee with an interest in congenital heart disease founded, together with some of his continental colleagues, the Association for European Paediatric Cardiologists in 1963. From a small group of enthusiasts working in adult or paediatric cardiology, or both, it has flourished, and now has several hundred members from all parts of Europe, meeting annually in a different country.

Investigations

Since the early 1980s, the availability of echocardiography, especially cross-sectional and Doppler techniques, has brought profound change to the diagnostic and interventional procedures performed in children with congenital heart disease. This is not only because it is a non-invasive technique (a consideration of particular significance when diagnosing disorders in neonates and infants) but with rapid advances in equipment, echocardiography now provides moving images of such discrimination that in many instances it is sensitive, accurate, and reliable enough to define the presence, position, and size of all defects in a given child. Thus, invasive techniques that were previously essential for preoperative diagnosis have been obviated. The numbers of primarily diagnostic cardiac catheterisations performed by the various units in Britain has fallen significantly and will probably continue to do so, while interventional catheter techniques are expanding. At the same time, further refinements in magnetic resonance imaging, first developed (as was computed tomography) by Geoffrey Mansfield in Nottingham, will extend the application of non-invasive techniques for both structural and functional assessment of congenital cardiac defects. Most of the specialised paediatric cardiac units now have access to imaging technique.

Development of a paediatric cardiac service

Great Ormond Street

Great Ormond Street remains the only hospital in the United Kingdom where paediatric cardiology and paediatric cardiac surgery have been fully integrated (in terms of both staff and structure) into one unit, associated with a major academic department (supported by the British Heart Foundation) in the same complex (Great Ormond Street/Institute of Child Health). It now has five full time consultant paediatric cardiologists, a clinical professor, and three consultant paediatric cardiac surgeons. The unit has remained the largest in the United Kingdom. As its inception and development illustrate some of the ups and downs of the specialty in Britain, they will be described here at some length, as a paradigm.

The first closed cardiac operations (ligation of a ductus arteriosus) were performed in 1948, but it was not until the early 1950s that other closed cardiac surgical procedures were added (Blalock–Taussig shunt; Blalock–Hanlon atrial septectomy, pulmonary valvotomy, pulmonary artery banding and resection of coarctation of the aorta). At first, there was only one cardiothoracic surgeon, David Waterston. He introduced a new operation, which carries his name, as an alternative to the Blalock–Taussig systemic to pulmonary arterial shunt procedure.[11]

At the end of the 1950s, a few open heart operations (closure of atrial septal defect) were performed using hypothermia. In the meantime, various heart-lung machines had been developed to allow open heart surgery, mainly in adults, by using an extracorporeal circulation. However, it was felt that the size of equipment was not optimal for children.

In 1957, the hospital's board of governors made private funds available to establish a small research unit to develop both a pump and an oxygenator suitable for extracorporeal circulation in children, including infants. A horizontally rotating set of large disks was developed and an industrial pump (for jam and similar items), consisting of a helical stainless steel rotor rotating in a stator was adapted for human use.[12] Unfortunately, both designs proved to be too damaging to human blood. When the department of clinical physiology was established in 1960, its staff (under GG) was given the additional task of designing and building a heart-lung machine, suitable for the full range of infants and children of all sizes. The easily available and well tried de Bakey pump was adapted for smaller volumes, as was the Kay–Cross oxygenator, equally well tried (in older children and in adults). A "family" of heart-lung machines with the lowest possible priming volume was built and all accessories (tubing, heat exchanger, suction assembly) and control console were similarly purpose-built and miniaturised. This assembly was used successfully and without problem for many years (the first intracardiac operation with the heart-lung machine had been performed in December 1961). The oxygenator was first replaced by the Bramson membrane oxygenator (first operation in March 1969), and then by other types of membrane oxygenator, which later were used for extracorporeal membrane oxygenation, mainly in neonates for conditions in which the lungs were not providing adequate oxygenation.

Advances in surgical procedures were made possible only by the parallel progress in diagnostic techniques. These followed very much the course described above under the Birmingham Children's hospital. More or less in step with these developments was an increase in staff. Throughout the early period, Waterston, trained as a paediatric and thoracic surgeon, was the only consultant cardiac surgeon. The increase in the number and complexity of operations in 1962 led to the appointment of a second surgeon, Eoin Aberdeen, an Australian who had been trained as a paediatric and (in the USA) an adult cardiac surgeon. From 1963 onwards, the unit played a leading role in the diagnosis and treatment of children with transposition of the great arteries. This was one of the reasons that the unit attracted young paediatric cardiologists and surgeons from many countries to be trained in diagnostic and early interventional cardiology as well as paediatric cardiac surgery.

Guy's Hospital

At Guy's hospital, despite Brock's pioneering work in cardiac surgery, paediatric cardiology only became established as a specialty with the appointment in 1978 of Michael Tynan as consultant paediatric cardiologist (subsequently professor of paediatric cardiology and head of an academic unit, supported in part by the British Heart Foundation). At about the same time the paediatric cardiac surgical service started with the appointment of Philip Deverall, trained in both adult and paediatric cardiac surgery. But if its beginnings were delayed, it has since expanded rapidly so that there are now five consultant posts in paediatric cardiology and one in fetal cardiology. In 1981, Lindsay Allen had established the division of fetal cardiology within the department. She had pioneered the echocardiographic diagnosis of cardiac abnormalities in the fetus, originating from her work with Darryl Maxwell, obstetrician at Guy's Hospital. Fetal cardiology has become firmly established throughout the world for routine intrauterine diagnosis of congenital heart disease. The treatment of fetal arrhythmias by administering cardioactive drugs to the mother was another original contribution derived from her diagnostic work. The department as a whole has taken a leading part in the application of interventional cardiology in children and was among the first to exploit the technique of magnetic resonance imaging in the diagnosis of congenital heart disease. Much of the unit's research work has been supported by grants from the British Heart Foundation.

Harefield hospital

Special note should be taken of the developments at Harefield Hospital, Middlesex, which had been built as a chest hospital, mainly for tuberculosis. Cardiac surgery was initiated there by Thomas Holmes Sellors, and it was there, in 1947, that he performed the world's first pulmonary valvotomy. In 1969, Magdi Yacoub came to Harefield Hospital as consultant cardiothoracic surgeon and started to operate on children with congenital heart disease. Two years later, the first consultant paediatric cardiologist, Rosemary Radley-Smith, was appointed (there are now three). In 1975, Yacoub, a pioneer of heart and lung transplantation in Britain, was also the first surgeon in Britain to perform the switch operation for transposition of the great arteries (connecting the pulmonary artery to the right ventricle and the aorta to the left ventricle). Initially, this was done after first banding the pulmonary artery soon after birth, but as a primary procedure the first switch operation in a neonate was performed by Yacoub in 1981 (R Radley-Smith, personal communication). Later, in 1987, he was appointed to the British Heart Foundation chair of cardiac surgery at the National Heart and Lung Institute and at the Brompton Hospital, of which Harefield Hospital had become a part. At the institute and Harefield Hospital, the academic unit under Yacoub's leadership has pursued an active research programme incorporating several problem areas in paediatric cardiac surgery as well as in the basic sciences applied to both paediatric and adult cardiology. It is anticipated that most of the medical and surgical services now provided by the staff at Harefield Hospital will ultimately be transferred to the Brompton Hospital. Paediatric cardiology will be among the first units to move.

Academic units

Great Ormond Street

During the 1960s, an impetus grew to diagnose and also to operate on ever younger children with congenital cardiac defects. By 1969, open heart surgery for infants had become fully established at Great Ormond Street. Paediatric cardiological diagnosis and interventional procedures grew apace, and this led directly to the founding of the British Heart Foundation Vandervell chair of paediatric cardiology, whose first incumbent was Fergus Macartney. This appointment, jointly at the hospital and the Institute of Child Health (in the laboratories built up by the department of clinical physiology), began to formalise the academic side of paediatric cardiological research initiated in the thoracic unit. It was later augmented by the appointment of Glennis Haworth as reader; her work, also supported by the British Heart Foundation, led to her being promoted to a personal professorship. Haworth's unit has focused particularly on experimental investigations into morphological changes in the pulmonary circulation that occur in children with some forms of congenital heart disease.

Heart and heart-lung transplantation, begun in the late 1980s, was expanding when the chair fell vacant with the resignation of Fergus Macartney. John Fabre was appointed as professor to continue his own work in transplantation research, particularly the experimental side of xenotransplantation. This complemented the clinical programme of heart and lung transplantation led by Marc de Leval, who was appointed professor of paediatric cardiac surgery in 1999 – the first such chair in the United Kingdom. By the end of 1999, 187 transplantations (heart and heart-lung) had been undertaken.

Brompton Hospital

In 1977 the Brompton Hospital and its Heart and Lung Institute established an academic unit of paediatric morphology within its department of paediatrics, endowed by the Joseph Levy Foundation and supported by the British Heart Foundation. The first director and professor (from 1979) was Robert H Anderson. However, he and some of his staff transferred to the Institute of Child Health at Great Ormond Street in 1999. The wide-ranging research of the department has focused on analysing the morphology and pathology of congenital cardiac defects.

Conclusions and prospects

Paediatric cardiology in Britain, unknown as a specialty in 1950, has, in the second half of the century, become firmly established as both a clinical and an academic entity. Its growth within paediatric and some general teaching hospitals has had many facets within its clinical and academic disciplines.

The outstanding advances made in diagnostic as well as therapeutic (both surgical and non-surgical) aspects and in various areas of research have greatly influenced other fields, for example, various imaging techniques, intensive care, vascular surgical procedures; treatment of cardiac arrhythmias and of renal failure, and extracorporeal circulation.

Looking at the end of the century, at the challenges ahead, paediatric cardiology in Britain has, through the NHS, the great advantage that its services are centred on relatively few units, most of which have successfully integrated their medical and surgical services. The largely uncompetitive financial relationship between hospitals and their staff (except for a period from the late 1980s to the late 1990s when hospitals were not only allowed but often forced to compete against each other) and the regional funding of paediatric cardiac services for more than 30 years or so, will continue to ensure that the various paediatric cardiological units cooperate in the referral or transferral of patients in their best interest. This development is aided by the growing pressure (from government, parents, and the units themselves) to monitor their results so that certain complex cardiac defects may well become the "prerogative" of just a few units.

Ever earlier (even intrauterine) and more precise non-invasive diagnostic facilities, several pioneered in Britain, the rapid growth in interventional cardiology, and the advances in perioperative care and techniques will be of particular value in an organisational milieu which favours planned concentration in a few optimally equipped and staffed centres, in conjunction with other disciplines. This trend, probably inevitable in the context of the NHS, will not only avoid the absence of significant disparity of results between units but also ensure the ability to apply advances quickly wherever and by whomever made. Within a European and international context it will mean that paediatric cardiology in Britain will continue to be in the vanguard of achievements. In parallel with these developments, there will be research in many areas related to cardiac disease. This will include the early recognition of cardiac disease that does not manifest itself until adulthood; myocardial changes at a molecular level; and genetic factors of congenital and other cardiovascular disease – their early recognition, mechanism of effect and, ultimately, their prevention.

Notes and references

1. Mackenzie J. *Diseases of the heart.* London: Oxford University Press, 1918:846.
2. Abbott M.E . *Atlas of Congenital Heart Disease.* New York: American Heart Association, 1936.
3. Brown JW. *Congenital heart disease.* 1939.
4. Gross RE, Hubbard JP. Surgical ligation of a patient with ductus arteriosus: report of the first successful case. *JAMA* 1939;112:729–31.
5. Crafoord C. and Nylin G. Congenital coarctation of the aorta and its surgical treatment . *J Thoracic Surg* 1945; 14: 347–361.
6. Blalock A, Taussig HB. Surgical treatment of malformations of the heart, in which there is pulmonary stenosis or pulmonary atresia. *JAMA* 1945;128:189–202.
7. Castellanos A, Pereiras R, Garcia A. *La angio-cardiografia en el niño.* (Angiocardiography in the child). Proceedings of the 7th Congress Pan American Medical Association, Havana. 1939:75–82, 109–13.

8. Forssmann W Sondierung des rechten Herzens. *Klin Wschr* 1929;89:2085–7.
9. Cournand A, Baldwin JS, Himmelstein A. *Cardiac catheterization in congenital heart disease: A clinical and physiologic study in infants and children.* New York: Commonwealth Fund, 1949.
10. Bing RJ, Vandam LD, Gray FD Jr. Physiologic studies in congenital heart disease: I. Procedures. *Bull Johns Hopkins Hosp* 1947;80:107–20.
11. Waterston DJ. Treatment of Fallot's tetralogy under 1 year of age (in Czech) . *Rozhl Chir* 1962;41:181.
12. Hall JE, James PA, Lucas BGB, Waterston DJ. A pump for extracorporeal circulation *Lancet* 1959;i: 347.

Chapter 22

Grown up Congenital Heart Services for Adolescents and Adults

Jane Somerville

The advent of cardiac surgery changed the lives of patients and transformed medical interest in congenital heart disease. Before the first successful operations on persistent duct and coarctation in 1938 and 1944 respectively, patients with congenital heart disease were, necessarily, regarded mainly as interesting diagnostic problems, often classified in case notes as "CMC" – congenital morbus cordis.

The paper on atrial septal defect by Bedford et al. in 1941 was an important step towards better diagnosis,[1] and in 1949 Cournand's demonstration of physiological measurements by cardiac catheterisation permitted accurate in vivo diagnosis for the first time.[2] This vital understanding of haemodynamics was ably taken up, exploited, and expanded by Paul Wood.[3]

Probably the most important event to stimulate advance in the management of congenital heart disease in the United Kingdom was the visit of Alfred Blalock from Johns Hopkins to Guy's Hospital in 1947. There he demonstrated the Blalock–Taussig operation. The Guy's surgeon, Russell Brock, went on to initiate direct surgery on the heart for pulmonary stenosis (chapter 28). Other thoracic surgeons, such as Thomas Holmes Sellors, who did the world's first pulmonary valvotomy, quickly took up the challenge.

By 1950, cardiology was becoming an established speciality and cardiologists trained in adult medicine were developing a special interest in congenital heart disease. Particularly notable were Maurice Campbell at Guy's, Paul Wood and Evan Bedford at the National Heart Hospital, James Brown in Grimsby, and Bobby Marquis in Edinburgh. However, it soon became clear that the real problem of congenital heart disease occurred in infancy and childhood. It was associated with a mortality of 60% to 70% in infancy, and one that was particularly high in neonates, and only 15% to 20% of untreated children with congenital heart disease reached adult life.

Development of paediatric cardiology and cardiac surgery

During the 1950s, Ronald Edwards, John Hay, and Jackson Rees (of endotracheal tube fame) were performing successful extracardiac surgery with shunts in infants and younger children at Alder Hey Hospital in Liverpool. At the Hospital for Sick Children at Great Ormond Street, London, David Waterston, a technical maestro, and Dick Bonham Carter, together with other hospitals, set the route for the development of paediatric cardiology and cardiac surgery. By the mid-1960s, the decline in cases of rheumatic fever in the developed world meant that congenital heart disease had become (and still is) the commonest form of heart disease in children. Congenital heart disease in adults became a diminishing problem, although for Wood, the master of the subject, about 10% to 15% of his patient population were affected. With parallel and integrated services – surgical, medical and anaesthetics – for children with heart disease, the speciality of paediatric cardiology developed and separated from adult cardiology.

Problems of specialisation

Inevitably, adult cardiologists in training saw fewer cases of congenital heart disease of any type. By the 1970s, and certainly the 1980s, there was little or no expertise in these problems among British cardiologists unless they were of the old school and had been part of the development of both paediatric and adult cardiology. The refinement and success of paediatric cardiac surgery and support disciplines dramatically changed the prognosis of patients born with congenital heart disease. Thus, by the 1980s, at least 70% survived to adulthood, many of whom had had complex surgery and basically serious anomalies. Those in training to be cardiologists knew little or nothing about congenital heart disease, other than the simple, common lesions such as atrial and ventricular septal defect and aortic valve stenosis. The more complex, rare, and repaired lesions were a clinical mystery, often with incomprehensible terminology. Furthermore, paediatric cardiologists usually had no training in adult medicine, limited or no access to adult facilities outside the children's hospital, and no experience with the "toys" and techniques of adult cardiology. Their often-declared life long ownership of their patients caused other doctors and patients some problems.

Establishing a service

By the 1970s, increasing numbers of adults and adolescents with curious and complex congenital problems which had been modified by cardiac surgery in infancy and childhood were being seen at hospitals where there was surgical and medical interest and expertise. I trained as an adult cardiologist with a lifelong interest in the results of surgical treatment of congenital heart disease, and having started with professional training in cardiac surgery, set out to establish optimal services for adolescents and adults with congenital heart disease.

Many patients were anxious to leave the paediatric environment, but adult cardiologists could not provide the necessary specialist care. The gulf between paediatric and adult medicine is a transition period and the need to provide an adolescent cardiac unit was obvious. New surgery for congenital heart disease, pioneered by Donald Ross since 1965 and carried out by Keith Ross and Magdi Yacoub, brought national referrals together. Much support came from Dick Bonham Carter in Great Ormond Street who had always sent his older children and adolescents to Paul Wood at the National Heart Hospital and now referred those who could be helped by the innovative surgery. Close links with the Hospital for Sick Children were beneficial since this was a "factory" of long term survivors of congenital heart disease, thanks to the genius of David Waterston.

Developments at the National Heart Hospital

With support from the surgeons and the radiology department at the National Heart Hospital led by Keith Jefferson, the then chairman of the medical committee, the concept of an adolescent unit was encouraged and a new consultant cardiologist appointment – "consultant physician for congenital heart disease" – was created in 1972. This allowed "seamless" practice of paediatric and adult cardiology. When the new north block of the National Heart Hospital was planned, it included facilities to treat more children and develop a unit for adolescents. Once I had been appointed as a consultant, it was possible, with the support of the house governor, Ron Denney, to establish a separate unit for congenital heart disease instead of a noisy corner of the adult ward. It was made clear that the money must be raised to build a new adolescent unit, an unusual, if not unique, demand on a newly appointed consultant to pay to "build their own patch." It appeared that this was the only way such a service would start. What seemed to be a huge amount of money at the time (£60 000) was needed, and as more young patients were admitted to beds in the adult wards the need became more obvious. Money and support came through a meeting in the coffee shop of Fortnum & Mason with its owner who asked me if I wanted anything to help my work.

The first adolescent unit

In 1975, at the height of surgical success in the National Heart Hospital, the first adolescent cardiac unit was opened, separate but close to cardiac medical and surgical beds where patients who were too mature for a unisex area could be accommodated. Some patients who had been operated on in infancy were being referred and there was a sudden increase in the number of adolescent patients who had had palliative surgery, confirming the need for the service. This was the start of establishing services for grown up patients with congenital heart diseases – "GUCH." It was the first

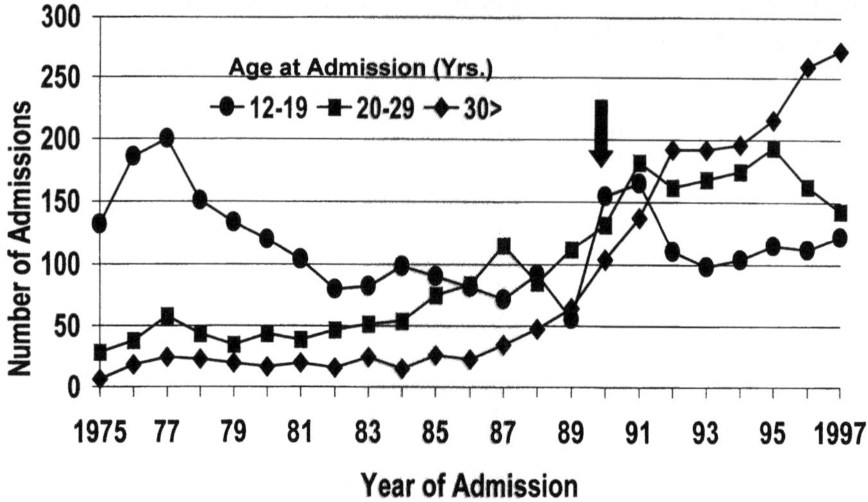

Figure 1 Number and age of grown up congenital heart disease patients admitted to the National Heart Hospital and Royal Brompton GUCH unit in 1975–97. The vertical arrow shows when the two hospitals joined.

adolescent cardiac ward in the United Kingdom, and possibly in the world. John Keith in Toronto had already recognised the need for long term supervision beyond the paediatric department. He had asked the bright, innovative, John Evans to set up a service in the Toronto General Hospital across the road from the Sick Children's Hospital, where Bill Mustard's genius, continued by George Trussler, produced so many successful survivors.

Establishing a database

Between 1975 and 1985, the provision of a service, the new adolescent unit, and the surgical expertise increasingly attracted referrals of patients (figure 1). Adult admissions (over 30 years) increased too, confirming this was not a paediatric problem needing paediatric solutions. To establish, maintain, and expand the service needed data, as it was already clear that many battles would be fought to keep and maintain an optimal service for this increasing group of patients. Neither money nor support for data collection was available, so a system with Hollerith cards was slowly turned into a computerised database. This has been maintained since 1982 by one coordinator, Sue Stone, with a special program designed and updated by Lorne Somerville. We decided not to amalgamate our database with others. These were too complicated and were the subject of continued tedious debates on nomenclature. The "go it alone" principle paid off. The unit was always willing and able to provide data for others to use.

Move to the Brompton Hospital

The adolescent and adult congenital heart services flourished in the 1980s, but the closure of the National Heart Hospital and its move to the Brompton Hospital was a blow to plans for continued growth and development. For the "GUCH service," as it had now been christened, this move could have been an advantage because of the active and supraregionally funded paediatric cardiac service. However, on arriving at the Brompton and on moving to the new hospital, which was opened in 1990, there was no unit. It had been "planned out," because of advice given to the planners that it was "not important."

Re-establishing a service

With the move in 1990 to the new hospital, without a unit but with an enthusiastic though disappointed staff, a four bedded bay in cardiology was assigned to the service. The GUCH unit concept and staff floundered for a while, and the patients came from everywhere except locally. The cardiology department accepted their increase with good grace and much support. After a depressing period, relieved by the pleasures of creating a roof garden outside the new office, the spring flowering provided the inspiration and vigour to create a new unit. This would be part of the Department of Cardiology – where it should be, since the patients are adults. Fortunately, the professor of cardiology, Philip Poole-Wilson, liked the concept of a grown up congenital heart disease unit, recognised its value for teaching, and, as clinical director, pushed the idea. Financial support came from the National Heart Hospital League of Friends, who had been disappointed by the loss of one of their "gems." For the second time, as "times were hard" within the new marketplace of medicine, we had to find the money to pay for the new unit, which opened in 1994 at the Royal Brompton Hospital.

It had what a GUCH unit required – a kitchen for occupational therapy and to satisfy the hunger of the teenagers; a quiet room for study, relatives, and examinations; a noisy room where snooker or music could be played; a seven bedded ward with suitably placed partitions to divide the sexes; and a two bedded high dependency unit for emergency admissions and postoperative or catheter interventions. There was a single room for special needs – such as a young GUCH mother with her baby, infected patients, or mentally disturbed patients.

When patients are admitted to a GUCH unit they cost much more than other cardiac patients. Since these patients comprise only 6% of the total adult cardiac medical and surgery patients, we felt that it was better not to draw attention to this initially. However, the governors of the Royal Brompton Hospital recognised its success and in July 1997 arranged for the opera singer Ms Jessye Norman to name the unit as the "Jane Somerville GUCH Unit."

Other aspects of GUCH

The first World Congress of Paediatric Cardiology was held in London in June 1980. The success of the congress, and support from the world, particularly from Canada, meant that paediatric cardiology had reached maturity. Concerns for the long term care of these patients were voiced in the final session on "the future," which was entitled "Triumphs and disasters – adolescent survivors." Already, many doctors were being confronted with demanding medical problems in adult survivors without any organised services to deal with them.

There were no other established services in the United Kingdom at this time. Paediatricians either held on to their patients in children's hospitals or made no plans for their long term care. Just as adolescents free themselves from parental care and supervision, so the patients left the paediatricians ... but without guidance or knowledge of their disease, medical needs, or even any idea that future surgery was inevitable. This new patient population – the fruits of our labours – was increasing and received poor medicine because of lack of service, lack of expertise, and sometimes lack of interest of some cardiologists.

Failure to consolidate a national service

In the United Kingdom, the child becomes an adult at age 16 years. The adolescent years are really the teenage years – the period of transition from childhood to adulthood and what should be from paediatric to adult medical care. The Department of Health did not recognise adolescent needs as a special entity or the need for specialised care for adolescents and adults with congenital heart disease. Attempts to establish and to consolidate national services for GUCH at supraregional level, based on the original few supraregional services for infant cardiac surgery, failed. Paediatric cardiologists felt it was their territory – combining with adult cardiology seemed out of the question. However, good services were established in Southampton and Newcastle in the 1990s. Excellent national integrated paediatric and adult congenital heart services were established in Toronto, Canada and in Denmark.

A difficult mix

The path for providers of GUCH services never has been easy, nor is it even now in most countries and centres. It requires the paediatric cardiologists to give up their patients to work with an adult cardiologist trained in their discipline. Problems are inevitable in a small, elite, and expensive service. Add to this the difficult to achieve mix of a cardiology department willing to have the service, administrators willing to pay, and cardiac surgeons experienced in congenital disease and adults.

Although it should be the responsibility of adult cardiology, the input and cooperation of paediatric cardiology is most important. Despite difficulties in obtaining this, it is the paediatric cardiologists who have stimulated the establishment of ideal GUCH services in departments of cardiology in France, Austria and Switzerland.

Keeping the name

The 1990s saw the expansion of the interest in grown up congenital heart disease and the "GUCH" name became established. It was not accepted in *Heart*, however, and the British Paediatric Cardiology Association has stopped using it recently. The GUCH Patients' Association want the name, the Department of Health uses it, and the term is established in Europe. In Canada they have CACH (Canadian Adult Congenital Heart) with a CACH Network, Boston has BACH, and Switzerland has Watch. The USA have AACHD (adolescent and adult congenital heart disease), though they have only a few centres namely at the Mayo Clinic with Dr Carole Warnes (British), at Portland, Oregon and Iowa, and at Los Angeles with pioneer Joseph Perloff, influenced by Paul Wood's training.[4]

There were no other GUCH units in London until the Middlesex Hospital opened its own GUCH unit for the large numbers of patients from Great Ormond Street. The unit is headed by Professor Deanfield, and is situated within an active cardiac department with all the necessary technology and facilities.

Needs of a GUCH service

During this period, the needs of a GUCH unit were established. Good cardiac surgery with expert, interested surgeons and anaesthetists is vital. One admission in five to a specialist centre is for cardiac surgery. This is often difficult and complex, with higher morbidity and mortality than other cardiac surgery for adult and paediatric patients. As the patients increased, so did the complexity of their conditions, and the unit was designated in one of the many reports of the time as fulfilling a quaternary service. There was a large group of adults with simple congenital heart disease who needed little or no expert advice and could be regarded as cured, but the patients referred to one of the few designated GUCH units had the worst and most complex conditions (table 1). Many had, and still have, a battle to persuade doctors and health authorities to refer them. Patients with rare and difficult lesions such as Fontan, atresias, malposition, and transposition need expert care, and should not be seen as an occasional patient in a cardiac department. Probably about 20% of GUCH patients need the specialist centre's expertise. Advice is required about life's problems such as pregnancy, contraception, employment, driving, the law and other aspects.[5]

With colleagues in Newcastle, Southampton, and Birmingham, attempts were made to organise five to six supraregional centres for these problems, but official agreement to establish such centres was not obtained. The 1997 view of the NHS is that each of the eleven new regions in the United

Table 1 Cardiac lesions that need expert management

Complex, rare, and difficult cardiac lesions (operated and unoperated)
Aorto-left ventricular fistula
Atrioventricular septal defects
Corrected transposition
Double outlet ventricle
Ebstein's anomaly
Eisenmenger – physiological response to several different congenital cardiac lesions, both simple and complex. Classified as complex because of management difficulties
Fallot's tetralogy
Mitral atresia
One ventricle (also called double inlet, outlet, common, single, primitive)
Pulmonary atresia
Pulmonary atresia with intact ventricular septum
Total anomalous pulmonary venous drainage
Transposition of the great arteries
Tricuspid atresia
Truncus arteriosus/hemi-truncus
Ventricular septal defect with:
Aortic regurgitation
Subaortic stenosis
Mitral valve disease
Absent valves
Straddling tricuspid/mitral valve
Other complex abnormalities of atrioventricular and ventriculoarterial connection not included above, such as criss-cross heart, isomerism
Additional lesions considered to be complex when previous operation under 12 years of age and requiring further surgery
Coarctation of the aorta
Left ventricular outflow tract obstruction (valve, subvalvar, supravalvar, and regurgitation)
Ventricular septal defect with other anomalies
Mitral and tricuspid valve disease
Pulmonary valve needing replacement

Kingdom will have its own regional GUCH centre.[6] It should be understood that for the complex lesions there are not enough patients to give a big enough experience in nine centres but, of more importance, there are not enough medical experts. Thus, in the year 2000, optimal medical treatment for GUCH has not yet been achieved in the United Kingdom.

GUCH information and services across the world

The European Society of Cardiology established a GUCH working group, which serves to unite the GUCH doctors of Europe in relation to education, communication, and sharing experience. An International Society of Adult Cardiology, mostly North American, welcomes and maintains international communication. Organisation for GUCH is needed in Asia, the Far

East, and South America. Australia is aware and active. A thriving national GUCH Patients' Association has been established in the United Kingdom to help them look after each other, share problems, and lobby for their needs.

Wherever there has been good cardiac surgery for infants and children there are plenty of grown up patients with congenital heart disease needing help. GUCH centres should "grow up" near or integrated with the originally supported supraregional centres for infant cardiac surgery.

The future

In 1993 the British Cardiac Society arranged a plenary session on the subject of grown up congenital heart disease at its annual meeting. The president, Douglas Chamberlain, ordered a working party to report on the services for this group of patients. It has not reported but will do so in 2000.

A nationwide survey, carried out by Professor S Hillis, of patients with grown up congenital heart disease admitted to centres with coronary care units confirms that the patients are scattered in the most unlikely places.

GUCH is established in islands. The patients know they are special and require the best and all that goes with it. There is a task force of the European Society of Cardiology to create guidelines for GUCH management.

The problems will be solved with flexibility, putting away the vested interests and with the will to do the best for patients. I hope that the patients will learn to demand what they deserve from the profession. They may have to become a political lobby force in some countries to overcome the problems of the profession and available resources. Already much effort and resource has brought them through childhood to adulthood. GUCH's will be there and need the "superspecialist" care in the 21st century. Let us hope it will be organised throughout the world by the 22nd century.

References and notes

1. Bedford DE, Papp C, Parkinson J. Atrial septal defect. *Br Heart J* 1941;3:37–68.
2. Cournand A, Baldwin JS, Himmelstein A. *Cardiac catheterisation in congenital heart disease: a clinical and physiological study in infants and children*. New York: Commonwealth Fund, 1949.
3. Wood P. Congenital heart disease. A review of its clinical aspects in the light of experience gained by modern techniques. St. Cyres lecture. *Br Med J* 1950;ii:639–45, 693–8.
4. Perloff JK. Congenital heart disease after childhood: an expanding patient population. *J Am Coll Cardiol* 1991;18:311–42.
5. Somerville J. The grown-up congenital hearts: good care is the profession's responsibility. *Br J Cardiol* 1998;5:570–84.
6. Secretary of State for Health. *The new NHS, modern dependable*. London: Department of Health, 1997. (Cmd Paper 3807.)

Chapter 23

Rheumatic Fever

Edwin Besterman

In discussing acute rheumatic fever, I need to acknowledge the work of a few physicians who practised before the 20th century began and who initiated and developed understanding of the disease. The correlation of meticulous clinical observations with post mortem findings, undertaken by the same observers, led to the understanding of diseases in the 18th and 19th centuries.

History

Rheumatic fever was recognised in the 17th century by Sydenham,[1] but its association with carditis was not made until the late 18th century. In 1789, Jenner described valvular heart disease at post mortem examination in patients with rheumatic fever.[2] Wells presented clinical and pathological findings of carditis, and first described subcutaneous nodules in 1812.[3] His pathological findings included "excrescences" on the interior of the left auricle and on the mitral and aortic valves.

The introduction of the stethoscope by Laennec in 1819 was followed by the accurate clinical diagnosis of carditis. In 1829, Latham described pericarditis and murmurs.[4] Several other British physicians, particularly Hope,[5] contributed to the increasing knowledge of the clinical signs of carditis. However, the book by the French physician Bouillaud remains preeminent.[6] Vituperative correspondence ensued between Hope and Bouillaud over the right to claim the distinction of being the first person to describe the clinical signs of acute rheumatic heart disease. According to Hope, "I discovered and published the grand pathognomic signs of acute endocarditis, namely valvular murmurs." While Hope analysed murmurs according to their origins from particular valves, Bouillaud was the first to note changes in systolic murmurs and to describe the development of diastolic murmurs. In 1839, Hope stressed that mitral regurgitation was the most important lesion of acute carditis.[7]

Murmurs

The cause of mitral systolic murmurs was disputed in the early years of this century. In 1918, Poynton and others attributed mitral incompetence to dilatation of the heart.[8] Valvular deformity as a cause was proposed by Carey Coombs of Bristol in 1924.[9] Others were reluctant to accept a systolic murmur alone as evidence of carditis – they required a diastolic murmur or cardiac enlargement as additional proof. Coombs found mitral systolic murmurs in 474 of 669 patients with acute rheumatic endocarditis, and in 90% of those who died from this disorder.[9] In 1952, Bland reported pure mitral incompetence in 22%, mitral systolic and diastolic murmurs in 75%, and mitral stenosis in 3% of 709 children with acute rheumatic endocarditis.[10]

Mitral diastolic murmurs in acute rheumatic carditis are well known and it is agreed that mitral stenosis is rare in children. Valvulitis that produces turbulence in diastole is the accepted explanation.[9] Coombs noted that the soft and localised characteristics of this murmur often caused it to be overlooked, and also described its transient nature in 75% of patients. The disappearance of aortic diastolic murmurs with recovery from rheumatic fever was first noted in 1892 by Sturges.[11] In 1930, Coombs reported the ratio of mitral to aortic valvulitis as 2:1.[12] Wood suggested that this reflected the differences in pressures acting on the two valves.[13]

The clinical difficulty in detecting soft aortic diastolic murmurs is well known. Although Still in 1927 found this murmur in only nine of 250 patients, he noted aortic incompetence in 28 of 36 cases at necropsy examination.[14] The disappearance of both systolic and diastolic murmurs was described in the 19th century and it was concluded that valvulitis could resolve with a return to normal valve function. In 1908, Coombs described the development and disappearance of mitral and aortic diastolic murmurs.[15] Poynton made similar observations in 1918.[16][17] In 1933, Coombs stated that 25% of mitral systolic murmurs resolved with recovery from acute carditis.[18] In our Taplow series (see below), we found that mitral systolic murmurs resolved in 17% of cases, mitral diastolic murmurs resolved in 27% of cases, and aortic diastolic murmurs disappeared in 22% of cases.[19]

Cardiac dilatation

Dilatation of the heart used to be diagnosed by percussion, and whether these findings represented true cardiac enlargement or a pericardial effusion in acute carditis was disputed. Coombs believed that dilatation was rare in first attacks of rheumatic carditis.[9] With the advent of *x* rays, Parkinson supported this view.[20] Keith also believed that early, sudden increases in the size of the heart shadow were a result of pericardial effusions and that true cardiac enlargement took 6 months to develop.[21] Our experience at Taplow (see below) confirmed this.[22]

Chorea

Begbie first described chorea in association with rheumatic fever and carditis in 1847.[23] In 1887, MacKenzie found carditis in 35% of patients with chorea,[24] and in 1894 Osler stated that at post mortem examination, endocarditis was more common in patients with chorea than in those with any other condition.[25] Chorea became less severe early in this century. At Taplow, chorea was seen in patients without carditis and with a normal erythrocyte sedimentation rate.

Aetiology

A throat infection by group A β haemolytic streptococci is a trigger for an attack of acute rheumatic fever. However, this sequel occurs only in a few people with a streptococcal throat infection, and the cause of susceptibility in these few people remains unclear. Suggestions include hyperimmune allergic reaction to the streptococcal antigen or an autoimmune response. Immune complexes have been shown to have a role.[26] Overcrowding, poverty, and malnutrition are further factors provoking susceptibility. A genetic predisposition is widely acknowledged, but again this is poorly understood. After a streptococcal infection there is a rise in the titre of antistreptolysin O, but although higher titres are often found in rheumatic fever, this is not a diagnostic criterion. There are children with rheumatic fever who have no history of a sore throat, and adults with chronic rheumatic heart disease with no history of rheumatic fever. Thus, in the past 50 years we have made no real progress in understanding the causation of rheumatic heart disease.

Changing prevalence

Scarlet fever, like rheumatic fever, is triggered by the group A streptococcus and is also commoner in children than in adults. In the late 19th century, scarlet fever was the most frequent cause of death in children aged over 1 year. Rheumatic fever was also common,[27] and in 1901 Still reported that 25% of the children admitted to Great Ormond Street Hospital had this disease.[28] The mortality and prevalence of both conditions declined dramatically in the early years of this century, long before antibiotics were developed. This change may have resulted from diminished virulence of the streptococcus and improved resistance in the host. In the 1920s, rheumatic fever was still a leading cause of death in the 5–20 year olds living in the House of the Good Samaritan, Boston, but later it abated dramatically.[29] Further details of the reduced incidence were published in 1943 and 1970.[30][31] However, this improvement is more evident in the affluent societies of the west. Rheumatic fever remains common in the tropics and the Indian subcontinent. In 1985, Zabriski estimated that 15–20 million new cases occurred annually in developing countries.[32]

Limited data

As rheumatic fever has never been a notifiable disease in the United Kingdom, we only have data on certain local populations. In London school children, the annual death rate from acute rheumatic fever fell from 67 per million in 1900 to 2 per million in 1965.[31] In 1961, Bywaters reported an annual prevalence of 0.5 per 1000 school children.[33] In a few areas in which the disease was notifiable, the incidence fell from 0.05% of the child population in 1948 to 0.014% in 1961.[34] In the Toronto Hospital for Sick Children, admission rates for rheumatic fever were 23 per 1000 in 1930 and fell to 2 per 1000 in 1953.[35]

Epidemics in army barracks were reported by Dudley in 1926,[36] and the hazards of overcrowding were noted in Bristol by Perry.[37] Other studies stressed dampness and poverty as factors that predisposed to both streptococcal infection and rheumatic fever. The decline in incidence in the West seems to be related to economic improvements in affluent societies; rheumatic fever continues to be common in developing countries with poor economies. As far back as the 1920s, both Hutchison[38] and Coombs[39] had noted the rarity of rheumatic fever among the well to do. Its further decline between 1936 and 1956 was also attributed by Wilson to improving social conditions.[40]

A disease of poverty

I have seen the disappearance of rheumatic fever in British children, and in 22 years (from 1962) as visiting cardiologist to Malta I found a marked decline in prevalence of the disease as social conditions improved. However, in my 15 years in Jamaica I have seen little change. Millard saw 1000 cases between 1975 and 1985 in the Kingston area alone.[41] In 1999, Pierre states that rheumatic fever remains common in impoverished Haiti (Pierre G, personal communication). By contrast in the West Indies, prosperous Martinique has virtually abolished the disease (Donatien Y, personal communication). One geographical difference in clinical presentation that I found in Jamaica is the absence of subcutaneous nodules and the infrequency of chorea. Chorea was present in only two of 100 patients with rheumatic fever.

An exception proving the rule?

To confuse these hypotheses of causality, no-one can explain a local resurgence of rheumatic fever in the Salt Lake City area of the United States in 1987.[42] Studies from the Unites States had reported a 90–99% reduction in the incidence of rheumatic fever over the previous 25 years. This outbreak was comparable to the incidence 30 years earlier. Moreover the victims were

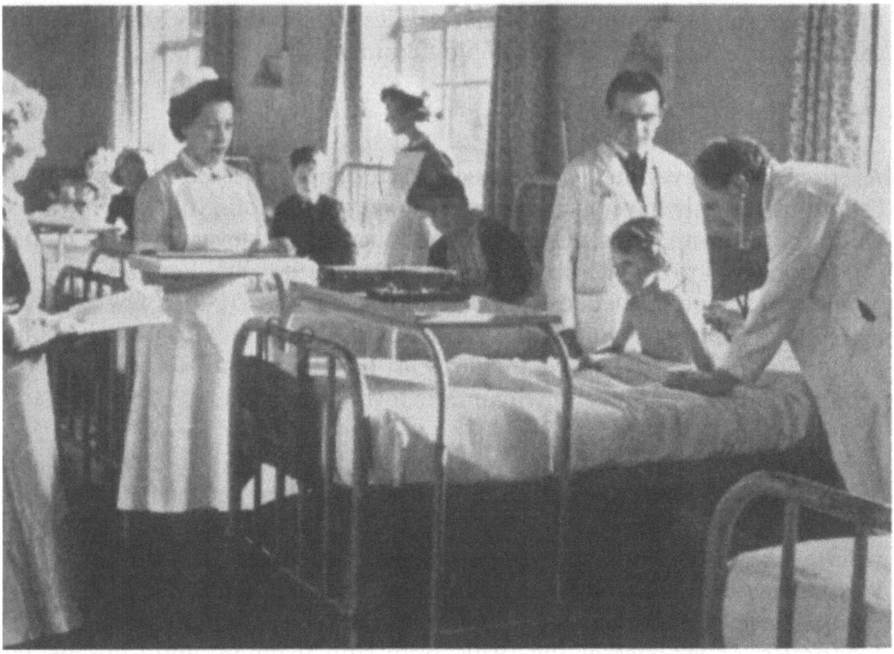

Figure 1 Ward round in the special unit for juvenile rheumatism, at the Canadian Red Cross Memorial hospital.

children from prosperous upper middle class families. A useful diagnostic "spin off" of this report was that carditis was diagnosed clinically in 72% of cases, while Doppler studies increased the figure to 98%. Perhaps a new, more virulent strain of streptococcus is responsible for this unusual outbreak?

Canadian Red Cross Memorial Hospital, Taplow

This hospital was presented to the Ministry of Health by the Canadian government with the wish that a research centre should be established as well as a general hospital. Thus, the Medical Research Council's special unit for juvenile rheumatism was founded in 1947 (figure 1). EGL Bywaters was director and Paul Wood was visiting cardiologist. The unit comprised 100 beds, and patients came from all over the United Kingdom. From 1947–55 more than 1000 patients were admitted with acute rheumatic fever. I spent four years at Taplow from 1949, and we were able to conduct several studies in these long stay patients.

Cardiac enlargement and pericarditis

Apparent cardiac enlargement on the *x* ray was found to be caused by true cardiomegaly only in those patients with chronic valvular disease who were admitted with second or third attacks of acute carditis. In children with first attacks of acute carditis, a sudden increase in heart size seen on *x* ray was shown to be caused by acute pericardial effusion. This was long before the advent of echocardiography, and the Wood technique was used for diagnosis.[13] Contrast medium was injected through a catheter with its tip impacted on the lateral wall of the right atrium.[22] This outlined the atrium, and the shadow beyond it was due to pericardial fluid. Subsequent serial *x* rays showed reduction in the "heart" shadow.

We then studied rheumatic pericarditis, and found a notable difference in outcome between children with "dry" pericarditis (that is, those with a rub alone) and those with effusions.[43] In the former group, there was no influence on prognosis, while half of the 30 cases with effusions died. In a later retrospective study of 441 cases of rheumatic carditis, pericarditis occurred in 14%.[19]

Murmurs

Significant murmurs are the most important diagnostic sign of carditis in acute rheumatic fever. Apical systolic murmurs are common in children and are usually of no importance. However, pansystolic apical murmurs are organic and were first recorded on a phonocardiogram by Schwarzchild in 1934.[44] This murmur of mitral regurgitation was present in 65% of our 441 cases. A Carey Coombs, short mitral diastolic murmur occurred in 82% and an aortic diastolic murmur was heard in 88% of the series.[19]

Phenylephrine

In some children with tachycardia, it is difficult to distinguish pansystolic from ejection murmurs. In the same children, soft diastolic murmurs are also difficult to detect. To try to improve diagnosis in these patients, we used phenylephrine. This drug produces transient hypertension with a reflex bradycardia, both factors that help to enhance murmurs. It was used in 64 patients and proved to be of diagnostic value.[45]

Phonocardiography

Paul Wood suggested the need for objective recording of the murmurs of acute carditis, not only to confirm their presence but to record changing murmurs in serial studies. Conventional phonocardiographs of that era were too insensitive for the purpose. The cathode ray tube has no inertia and seemed the ideal device for a sensitive phonocardiograph. With technical help, we designed and built a multichannel cathode ray phonocardiograph with a photographic recorder.[46] This device proved so sensitive that it had to be housed in a sound proof building. In practice, it was of diagnostic value in illustrating pansystolic murmurs and in distinguishing short mitral diastolic murmurs from third heart sounds. It produced the first record of the Carey Coombs murmur. It was also used in the phenylephrine study. Serial recordings illustrated both the develop-

Table 1 Resolution of heart murmurs in relation to the interval between the onset of symptoms and admission to hospital in 227 patients observed during their first episode of rheumatic fever with carditis

Duration of symptoms before admission	Number of patients	Resolution (%)
1–28 days	116	38
4–8 weeks	48	22
> 9 weeks	63	11

ment and regression of murmurs.[19][47] Regression of mitral and aortic murmurs confirmed valvulitis as the cause of regurgitation, rather than cardiomegaly as had previously been proposed by some authorities.

Changing murmurs

In the series of 441 cases, changing murmurs occurred in 56%; these developed in 163 and disappeared in 73 cases.[24] A separate study was made of 225 patients seen in their first attack of acute rheumatic carditis. Resolution of murmurs in these children was related to the duration of rheumatic fever before admission to hospital (table 1).

Cardiac output studies

The clinical benefits of bed rest in acute carditis have long been known. To seek a cardiovascular justification for rest, we measured cardiac outputs by cardiac catheter. Observations were made at rest, on mild exertion, and subsequent rest in patients with active carditis (without arthritis), and in convalescing cases as controls.[48] The controls showed a normal increase of output on effort, whereas those with active carditis failed to raise their cardiac outputs. This evidence justifies the policy of bed rest in patients with active rheumatic carditis.

Other data

In this series of 441 cases, there was a 20% incidence of chorea. Fifteen per cent of patients had subcutaneous nodules, and the case mortality was 4.5%.

Taplow closes

In the 1960s, the rapid decline in the incidence of rheumatic fever in the United Kingdom led to Taplow becoming a centre for juvenile rheumatoid arthritis. In 1978, there was only one patient admitted with acute rheumatic fever, and that patient had no carditis.[49] The hospital was closed in 1989.

Treating rheumatic fever

Salicylates and steroids

Acute rheumatic fever was a virtually untreatable disease until Thomas Maclagan of Dundee pioneered the use of salicin in 1876.[50] Salicin is extracted from the bark of the willow tree and is converted in the body to salicylic acid. Subsequently, salicylates became the treatment of choice for rheumatic fever. In the early 1950s, very high doses were used - producing tinnitus and, occasionally, frightening hallucinations of green beetles. There was no proof that these high doses were advantageous and a conventional dosage is now used.

Steroids were found to be of short-term benefit in severe exudative cases with florid polyarthritis and pericardial effusions. They may also help when salicylates fail to reduce the erythrocyte sedimentation rate. Steroids are not recommended routinely because of their side effects and the difficulty in weaning patients off this therapy.

Hench and Duckett Jones initiated and supervised a multicentre US–UK (including Taplow) trial of salicylates, adrenocorticotropic hormone, or cortisone in treating rheumatic fever - the first international multicentre study of therapy.[51] After a 10 year follow up, no difference was seen in the development of carditis between the three groups.

Bed rest

Bed rest has long been the accepted treatment in an endeavour to reduce the demands made on the heart and thus, it is hoped, reduce the subsequent development of chronic valular heart disease. At Taplow, bed rest was continued until the erythrocyte sedimentation rate returned to normal - usually 10 to 12 weeks but often longer. Today, patient compliance with prolonged rest is poor. It is of value also in other types of carditis and cardiomyopathies. In the 1950s and 1960s bed rest was accepted by everyone as the treatment for pulmonary tuberculosis. Today's population has no such experience and patients are reluctant to follow this advice. Prophylactic penicillin has proved of value in reducing recurrences of rheumatic fever, which would otherwise occur in 50% of cases (see Chapter 15).

Remaining problems

Erythrocyte sedimentation rate as an index of activity

The erythrocyte sedimentation rate remains our only test of rheumatic activity. This is a non-specific test - the rate is also raised by any infection, anaemia, or pregnancy and is depressed by cardiac failure. It is our sole index of activity when treating acute rheumatism. It is also important in chronic adult rheumatic heart disease. Closed mitral valvotomy is still practised and if it is carried out on a patient with active carditis, restenosis of the valve often ensues. Bromley, at St Mary's Hospital, London, carried out closed mitral valvotomies in 501 of our patients, including 44 with restenosis.[52] In all cases, this implied continued rheumatic activity despite a normal erythrocyte sedimentation rate. The safety of this operation was shown by the reported operative mortality of 0.8%.[57] At open heart surgery, we see acute rheumatic vegetations in 60 year olds with normal erythrocyte sedimentation rates. In 1977, Virmani reported Aschoff bodies in 21% of 191 operative cases.[53] We desperately need a more specific and sensitive index of rheumatic activity.

Identifying those at risk

More important than streptococcal infection in aetiology is the identification of the susceptible child who then develops rheumatic fever. Once immunologists can identify these "at risk" children, preventive antibiotic therapy can be targeted accurately as a primary prevention measure.

In conclusion

It is ironic to recall that in my student days we were taught that streptococcal infections and rheumatic fever never occurred in hot climates such as the tropics. Today, in Jamaica, the rheumatic fever picture resembles that at Taplow in the 1950s. Even if it is no longer a problem in the United Kingdom, rheumatic fever remains a serious childhood health hazard in most tropical, economically deprived countries. This, in turn, leads to the significant adult population with chronic valvular disease that we see in our cardiac clinic.

References and notes

1. Sydenham T. *Processus integri from works*. Translated by Swan J. London, 1742.
2. Keil HA. A note on Edward Jenner's lost manuscript on "Rheumatism and the heart". *Bull Hist Med* 1939;7:409–11.
3. Wells WC. On rheumatism and the heart. *Trans Soc Improvement Med Chir Knowledge* 1812;3:373. Wells was an American who was not in sympathy with the war of independence. He trained in Edinburgh and became physician to St Thomas's Hospital, London.
4. Latham PM. Pathological essay on some diseases of the heart. *London Med Gazette* 1829;3:1–7.
5. Hope J. *A treatise on diseases of the heart and great vessels*. London: William Kidd, 1831.
6. Bouillaud J. *Traité clinique du maladies du coeur*. Paris: JB Baillière, 1835.
7. Hope J. A treatise on diseases of the heart and great vessels. 3rd ed. London:William Kidd, 1839.
8. Poynton FJ. The nature and symptoms of cardiac infection in childhood. *BMJ* 1918;1:417.
9. Coombs CF. Rheumatic heart disease. Bristol: John Wright, 1924.
10. Bland EF, Jones TD. The natural history of rheumatic fever. *Ann Intern Med* 1952;37:1006–26.
11. Sturges O. Some special features in the heart affections of childhood. *Lancet* 1892;i;621–3.
12. Coombs CF. A British Medical Association lecture on the diagnosis and treatment of rheumatic heart disease in its early stages. *BMJ* 1930;1:227–30.
13. Wood P. *Diseases of the heart and circulation*. London: Eyre and Spottiswoode, 1950.
14. Still GF. *Common disorders and diseases of childhood*. London: Oxford University Press, 1927.
15. Coombs CF. Rheumatic myocarditis. *Q J Med* 1908;2:26–49.

16. Poynton FJ. The nature and symptoms of cardiac infection in childhood. *BMJ* 1918;1:417–20.
17. Poynton FJ. Cardiac infection in childhood. *BMJ* 1918;2:305–7.
18. Coombs CF. Cardiac disease from a clinical standpoint: III rheumatic heart disease. *Clin J* 1933;62:54–6.
19. Besterman EMM. *Phonocardiography in rheumatic carditis.* Cambridge: University of Cambridge, 1954. (MD thesis.)
20. Parkinson J. Rheumatic fever and heart disease. *Lancet* 1945;ii:657–62.
21. Keith JD. *Heart disease in infancy and childhood.* New York: McMillan, 1958:617.
22. Besterman EMM, Thomas G. Radiological diagnosis of rheumatic pericardial effusion. *Br Heart J* 1953;15:113–20
23. Begbie JW. Remarks on rheumatism and chorea.- Their relation and treatment. *Monthly J Med Sci Lond Edin* 1847;7:740–54.
24. MacKenzie S. Reports of the Collective Investigation Committee of the British Medical Association. Chorea: cancer of the breast. *BMJ* 1887;1:425–41.
25. Osler W. *On chorea and choreiform affections.* London: H K Lewis, 1894.
26. Williams RC. Infective and postinfective disorders. In: Lessof M, ed. *Immunology of cardiovascular disease.* New York: Dekker, 1981:112–7.
27. Cheadle WE. *Lectures on the practice of medicine and on rheumatism of childhood.* London: Smith Elder, 1900.
28. Still GF. Rheumatism in childhood. *Practitioner* 1901;46:52–63.
29. Bland EF. Rheumatic fever, the way it was. *Circulation* 1987;76:1190–5.
30. Paul JR. *Epidemiology of rheumatic fever and some of its public health aspects.* American Heart Association, 1943.
31. Besterman E. Changing face of acute rheumatic fever. *Br Heart J* 1970;32:579–82.
32. Zabriskie JB. Rheumatic fever, the interplay between host, genetics and microbe. *Circulation* 1985;71:1077–86.
33. Bywaters EGL. *Rheumatic fever, modern practices in infectious fevers.* London: Butterworth, 1951:156–96.
34. Ministry of Health. *Ministry of Health notifications.* London: Ministry of Health, 1961.
35. Keith J. *Heart disease in infancy and childhood.* New York: McMillan, 1958:612.
36. Dudley JF. *Droplet infection.* London: Medical Research Council, 1926. (MRC special report no 111.)
37. Perry CB, Roberts JAF. Study on the variability in the incidence of rheumatic heart disease within the city of Bristol. *BMJ* 1937;2 (suppl):154–8.
38. Hutchison R. The value of pulse charts in acute carditis in childhood. *Lancet* 1922;i:1086–8.
39. Coombs CF. Rheumatic infection in childhood. *Lancet* 1927;i:579–634.
40. Wilson MG, Lim WN, Birch AM. The decline of rheumatic fever. *J Chronic Dis* 1958;7:183–97.
41. Millard D. Rheumatic fever national control programme, Jamaica. *Caribbean Cardiac Soc Bull* 1999;2:5.
42. Veasy LG, Weidmeier SE, Osmund GS, Rattenburg HD, Boucek MM, Roth SJ, et al. Resurgence of acute rheumatic fever in the intermountain area of the United States. *N Engl J Med* 1987;316:421–7.
43. Thomas GT, Besterman EMM, Hollman A. Rheumatic pericarditis. *Br Heart J* 1953;15:29–36.
44. Schwarzchild MM, Feldstein MD. A new method for the recording of heart sounds. *Am Heart J* 1934;10:453–8.
45. Besterman EMM. Use of phenylephrine to aid auscultation of early rheumatic diastolic murmurs. *BMJ* 1951;2:205–11.
46. Besterman EMM, Harrison JK. A multichannel cathode ray phonocardiograph. *Br Heart J* 1953;15:130–4.
47. Besterman EMM. Phonocardiography in acute rheumatic carditis. *Br Heart J* 1955;17:360–72.
48. Besterman EMM. The cardiac output in acute rheumatic carditis. *Br Heart J* 1954;16:8–12.
49. Portal RW. Mitral stenosis, the picture changes. astonishing decline in rheumatic fever and consequent mitral stenosis. *BMJ* 1984;1:167–8.
50. Maclagan T. The treatment of acute rheumatism by salicin. *Lancet* 1976;i:342–3.
51. Rheumatic Fever Working Party of the Medical Research council of Great Britain and the Subcommittee of Principal Investigators of the American Council on Rheumatic Fever and Congenital Heart Disease, American Heart Association. Natural history of rheumatic fever and rheumatic heart disease. Ten year report of a cooperative clinical trial of ACTH, cortisone and aspirin. *BMJ* 1965;2:607–15.
52. Besterman EMM. Closed mitral valvotomy, has it still a place? *Proceedings of 6th Asia-Pacific congress on diseases of the chest.* Bombay: 1979.
53. Virmani R, Roberts WC. Aschoff bodies in operatively excised atrial appendages and in papillary muscle. *Circulation* 1977;55:559–63.

Chapter 24

Valvular Disease, Endocarditis, and Cardiomyopathy

Celia M Oakley

In the 19th century, clinical medicine was firmly based on pathological anatomy. Indeed, in 1846 the Pathological Society of London was founded by physicians rather than pathologists. Pericarditis, valve disease, and endocarditis were described. Fatal conditions became well recognised clinically, benign ones less so. German pathologists and Irish clinicians dominated cardiology in the last century. Although aortic regurgitation was well recognised, other valve deformities were believed to be unimportant.

Valvular heart disease in Britain

Soldier's heart

The development of cardiology as a specialty in the United Kingdom stems from the study of soldiers discharged from the army during the first world war because of chest pain, dyspnoea, and palpitations. As these men were thought to have heart disease, the syndrome was dubbed "soldier's heart." In 1862 and 1864, Jacob DaCosta of Philadelphia had described similar symptoms in soldiers seen in the American Civil War. He wrote a definitive paper on "Irritable heart" in 1871, and the condition became known eponymously as DaCosta's syndrome. William Osler, who was still in Philadelphia at the time, presented a paper on "Irritable heart in civil life" in 1887.

After the retreat from Mons in 1914, many British soldiers were diagnosed with "disorderly action of the heart" or "DAH," which had become the third leading cause of discharge from the army. It was a major economic burden, as these men were incarcerated in hospital for rest and treatment lasting many months. Physicians believed that the heart condition had resulted from over exertion, hence the other designation "effort syndrome." As many of the young soldiers had systolic murmurs, the disorder was classified under valvular heart disease.

Non-cardiac origin

In 1916, after the likely aetiology of the effort syndrome had already been extensively studied by Clifford Allbutt (regius professor of medicine, Cambridge) and by W C McLean (professor of military medicine), Sir James Mackenzie came to the conclusion that the origin of soldier's heart was non-cardiac. These workers had confirmed what Osler had found – that the syndrome was not peculiar to soldiers, nor necessarily to war conditions. At a time when soldiers were executed for cowardice or for disobeying commands, it is interesting that a diagnosis of DAH, unlike one of "shell shock," carried no stigma.

The first "heart" hospital in England was set up in Hampstead; others were founded at Mount Vernon and in Colchester, where Thomas Lewis was appointed as consultant physician. Centres were also set up in France so that British troops did not have to be sent home for treatment. In 1918, Lewis wrote a monograph on *Soldier's heart and the effort syndrome*, in which the symptoms and signs were described and contrasted with those of heart disease.

Lewis' prejudice against diagnosing mitral regurgitation is shown in a discussion on the significance of apical systolic murmurs. In the context of the soldiers, he was correct, and in this he and Mackenzie were in agreement. Lewis's work on the effort syndrome during the war was recognised by his appointment as a Commander of the British Empire (CBE) and in 1921 by a knighthood. However, problems with diagnosis and lack of uniformity in assessment remained. Despite Lewis's efforts, a cardiac diagnosis was still common among the army pensioners after the war.[1][2]

Lewis on valve disease and aortic stenosis

Mackenzie and Lewis were undoubtedly the two "greats" of British cardiology in the first half of the 20th century. While Mackenzie's reputation was as a master clinician,[2a] Lewis owed his standing to electrocardiography and to his work on arrhythmias and conduction defects. Lewis wrote a textbook, *Diseases of the heart, for practitioners and students*, which was first published in 1933. The first eight chapters dealt with cardiac failure and angina pectoris. Cardiac murmurs were described, but the importance of valve disease was grossly undervalued in an era when rheumatic carditis was common. Mitral regurgitation was disregarded, and even in the third edition, in 1942, Lewis wrote the following about mitral stenosis "Although many symptoms may be complained of by patients suffering from mitral stenosis, there are none that can be ascribed properly and usefully to this deformity of the valve." Lewis wrote that aortic stenosis "is far less common than aortic regurgitation and its diagnosis should be infrequent. There are no symptoms of aortic stenosis."

In the third edition of his textbook, Lewis wrote the following on valve defects:

> The undue emphasis placed upon diseases of the cardiac valves in diagnosis was the chief reason why the prognosis of heart disease long remained so unsatisfactory. This over-emphasis resulted largely from an exaggerated notion of the extent to which valve defects burden the heart mechanically. There is no evidence to show that any valve defect imposes a burden upon the healthy heart which, even in the absence of intervening hypertrophy, will result in heart failure . . . Surgical attempts to relieve cases of mitral stenosis presenting with failure by cutting the valve have so far failed to give benefit – I think they will continue to fail not only because the interference is too drastic, but because the attempt is based upon what usually at all events is an erroneous idea that the valve is the chief source of trouble.[3]

Phonocardiogram

Up to the 1940s, the interpretation of symptoms and signs of valve disease remained rather stagnant. No major advances were made until the advent of the phonocardiogram in 1941 and the work of Aubrey Leatham at the London Hospital. Auscultation then became more precise as this technique aided detailed analysis of the sounds and murmurs.

Developments in the 1950s

At Hammersmith Hospital, John McMichael, Sheila Howarth and Peter Sharpey-Schafer started to apply the new technique of cardiac catheterisation (described by André Cournand in the United States in 1948), to the study of heart failure and of the healthy heart too. By the early 1950s, Frances Gardner at the Royal Free Hospital was making accurate diagnoses in children with congenital heart disease (previously regarded as a diagnosis in itself) and in patients with mitral valve disease before closed valvotomy. Paul Wood, who was physician at the National Heart and Brompton Hospitals, had, by this time, become the leading influence on British cardiology, his major contributions were correlation of cardiac catheterisation, haemodynamics and physical signs, and not least through his fearless demolition of ancient myths, in Britain and the United States.

Mitral valve prolapse syndrome

Wood's first significant contribution had been his definitive demonstration with Aubrey Lewis in 1941 that DaCosta's syndrome is a psychiatric disorder.[4] Interest in DaCosta's syndrome revived in the 1980s. In 1980, after Barlow's description of the billowing mitral leaflet syndrome (made following the discovery by Read that systolic clicks and late systolic murmurs were, after all, intracardiac), the mitral valve prolapse syndrome was born. The autonomic and neuroendrocrine mechanisms responsible for palpitation, shortness of breath, and syncope in patients with only mild mitral regurgitation were studied by Harisios Boudoulas and Charles Wooley in the United States and were related to DaCosta's syndrome and neurocirculatory asthenia.

Paul Wood's influence

Wood concentrated on congenital and rheumatic heart disease and their surgical treatment, and he was one of the first cardiologists to study primary pulmonary hypertension. His textbook, *Diseases of the heart and circulation*, had an enormous influence worldwide.[5] He also lectured extensively in the United States, ruffling many feathers through his dismissal of outmoded ideas, while packing the lecture theatres. His clarity of thought and incisiveness of speech were riveting, and although his acerbity could be off-putting, he also had considerable charm. His teaching further increased understanding of the haemodynamics of rheumatic and congenital heart disease, obtained through catheterisation, as correlated with physical signs, inspection, palpation, and meticulously accurate auscultation checked by phonocardiography. Cardiac pharmacology was still strictly limited and cardiac surgery still in its infancy, but the foundation of accurate diagnosis had been laid.

Infective endocarditis

Excrescences on the heart valves have been described by pathologists over the past three or four centuries. Some of these patients would have had infective endocarditis, but the different forms of endocarditis were not differentiated until late in the 19th century when it was recognised that bacteria caused disease. Thus, Sir William Osler in his *Principles and practice of medicine* published in 1892, described acute endocarditis, characterised by the presence of vegetations with loss of continuity or of substance in the valve tissues, and chronic endocarditis, which resulted in thickening, puckering, and deformity. Osler detailed a simple or benign endocarditis, which was often associated with acute articular rheumatism, and a malignant or ulcerative endocarditis, which was frequently seen with pneumonia, complicating septicaemia, or puerperal fever but was extremely rare in chorea. Osler had studied over 200 cases of malignant endocarditis in Montreal, and this was the subject of his Goulstonian Lectures delivered at the Royal College of Physicians in 1885. It was not until 1909 that he described 10 patients whose illness lasted up to 13 months before ending fatally.[6][6a]

In the United Kingdom, Thomas (later Lord) Horder popularised the diagnostic procedure of taking blood samples for culture.[7] These frequently grew a small streptococcus (now known as a viridans streptococcus). This bacterium, found in many cases of endocarditis lenta, was said by Libman to be found in no other diseases. In 1924, Libman and Sacks in the United States, differentiated atypical verrucose endocarditis, which was later known to be a feature of systemic lupus erythematosus.[8]

As infective endocarditis came to be recognised in both its acute and subacute forms, it seemed to increase in prevalence. Thomas Cotton in Colchester studied the disorder in members of the armed forces, and described finger clubbing in these patients. The disease remained fatal despite the advent of the sulphonamides in 1935, and only the availability of penicillin in 1944 brought the real possibility of cure.[9] At first, penicillin was in short supply. By 1948, when it had become more freely available, its efficacy had been proved in large numbers of patients. The advent of streptomycin, and the discovery of antibacterial synergy when it was combined with penicillin, enabled *Enterococcus faecalis* and viridans streptoccocal infections to be treated successfully. The number of deaths from infective endocarditis reported each year fell from 1200 to about 300.

Importance of dental hygiene

Infective endocarditis had been induced experimentally in animals, and it had been suggested that bacteraemia after dental extraction might be a cause. With the availability of penicillin, prophylaxis became a possibility. In the 1950 (first) edition of his book, Wood wrote that "dental hygiene is particularly important . . . tooth extraction, tonsillectomy and other ENT operations should be covered by 100 000 units of penicillin 6 hourly for 48 hours." Even more sapiently, Wood also advised that "patients should be treated early as soon as the diagnosis is clinically probable without waiting for positive results of blood cultures."[5] If Wood's advice were better heeded, the high mortality from infective endocarditis would not have continued to this day. Important and efficacious though prophylaxis is, studies have shown that most cases do not follow "unprotected" dentistry in people who are at risk, but result from bacteraemias in patients with poor oral hygiene and genetic susceptibility.[10][11]

Cardiomyopathy

Even after diseases of the myocardium were classified by Corvisart and Laennec, physicians were slow to recognise that myocardial disease could exist independently of raised blood pressure, congenital, or acquired lesions affecting the valves or basic structure of the heart. This is surprising, as Sir William Osler included a section on "Infections of the myocardium" in his famous textbook *The principles and practice of medicine* published in 1892. Here he clearly described lesions caused by disease of the coronary arteries, including sudden death from myocardial infarction due to blocking of a coronary artery, well before Herrick's 1912 paper in the *Journal of the American Medical Association.* Osler described "acute interstitial myocarditis," occurring in fevers, and also "amyloid degeneration." He noted that amyloid occurred in the intermuscular connective tissue and blood vessels and not in the myocardial fibres. Osler also recognised "dilatation and hypertrophy due to over-exertion and alcohol." He credited Bollinger with calling attention to this in beer drinkers in the German breweries who drank 20 or more litres each day, and Strumpell and Erlangen, who had told him that the condition was very common in draymen. Osler noted that at post mortem examination the valves might be healthy and the aorta smooth with no extensive arteriosclerosis or renal disease.

With this background already in place, it is perhaps surprising that clinical recognition of cardiomyopathy did not receive earlier general recognition. However, Sir James Mackenzie and Sir Thomas Lewis emphasised physiology and function rather than their clinicopathological correlations, which had been the hallmark of the previous century.[12] High blood pressure and Bright's disease of the kidneys were known causes of left ventricular hypertrophy, while diphtheria and other fevers were associated with toxic dilatation. Over exertion was blamed for hypertrophy and dilatation. In 1937, however, Lewis wrote "There are many cases of hypertrophy and of great hypertrophy of the heart in which during life and after death no source of increased work can be discovered. . . . It is clear that there must be hidden sources of increased energy expenditure or the idea that increased energy expenditure is the only cause of hypertrophy is wrong."

Dilated cardiomyopathy

The cardiomyopathies, a term first used by Wallace Brigden of the London Hospital, usually presented with heart failure associated with dilated and poorly contracting ventricles.[13] Also at the London, William Evans recognised the contribution of excessive alcohol consumption in many of these cases.[14] After the development of a morphological and functional classification of cardiomyopathies by Goodwin et al. at Hammersmith Hospital, these were called "congestive."[15] The term congestive was later changed to dilated to distinguish it from the hypertrophic type, which first became clinically recognised in 1958.

A French Pathologist, Hallopeau, is credited with the first description of the gross anatomic features of hypertrophic cardiomyopathy in 1869. The condition was also recognised by other pathologists such as Schmincke in 1907, by Bernheim, and by clinicians such as Osler, who had recognised an idiopathic hypertrophic condition of the heart in children. Nevertheless, this fascinating clinicopathological entity was largely ignored until the late 1950s.

Families with unexplained cardiomyopathies were described by LG Davies from Cardiff[16] and by William Evans from the London Hospital, but it was the paper by the forensic pathologist, Donald Teare at Guy's, entitled "Asymmetrical hypertrophy of the heart in young adults" which brought a surge of worldwide interest.[17] Teare described nine young adults who had died suddenly, which had brought their hearts to his attention. He noticed that there were two siblings, a brother and sister, which made him speculate on genetic inheritance. Interestingly, the surviving three siblings of the two young adults who had died and been described by Teare did not have murmurs or left ventricular outflow tract gradients. It was as pseudo aortic stenosis that hypertrophic cardiomyopathy first captivated attention on both sides of the Atlantic.[18]

Hypertrophic cardiomyopaphy

The year before Teare's description in the *British Heart Journal*, Russell Brock (later Sir Russell, then Lord Brock), described "Functional obstruction of the left ventricle" in the *Guy's Hospital Report*, but the patient probably did not have hypertrophic cardiomyopathy.[19] She was a late middle aged Welsh woman with severe hypertension. On admission to the Brompton Hospital for blood pressure reduction, she had no murmur. However, a loud murmur developed after an over zealous house officer (me) reduced the blood pressure too abruptly. Brock passed a percutaneous catheter into the apex of the left ventricle and threaded it into the aorta, measuring a considerable gradient. The disorder became known as idiopathic hypertrophic subaortic stenosis in the United States (where it was extensively investigated by Braunwald's group), and as hypertrophic obstructive cardiomyopathy in this country (after Goodwin's group at Hammersmith Hospital). Other names were given to these disorders, but it was the British term hypertrophic cardiomyopathy that became generally accepted. The adjective "obstructive" was removed after it was realised that outflow tract gradients are more often absent than present, as in the family recognised by Teare. Many of the published reports on the disorder over the next few years were devoted to physical and pharmacological means of altering the left ventricular outflow tract gradient.

The first case of hypertrophic (obstructive) cardiomyopathy to be diagnosed at Hammersmith Hospital had caused puzzlement because of lack of aortic valve calcification. It occurred in a middle aged man with apparent aortic stenosis but with bounding pulses despite the absence of aortic regurgitation. I took the patient to see Paul Wood at the Brompton Hospital. He, in a letter to John Goodwin, succinctly described the salient features of the condition, which are so well known today – the rapidly rising pulses, the atrial beat, the delayed ejection systolic murmur inside the apex, and the well heard aortic closure sound. Wood speculated that the patient had dynamic muscular left ventricular outflow tract obstruction that might be improved by drug treatment. This was the first patient in the world to be treated by surgical septal myectomy . . . and to survive. The man underwent operation because the surgeon, Bill Cleland, would not accept that he did not have valvular aortic stenosis and, since he had severe angina as well as multiple syncopal attacks, insisted on surgery. Upon finding a normal aortic valve but a protruding septum below it which felt "like a scirrhous carcinoma," Cleland attempted resection while protecting the myocardium in ice slush. The patient did well, his murmur and gradient cleared completely, and he proclaimed himself free from syncope or chest pain. He also developed left bundle branch block, which was at first thought to be a key element in the loss of left ventricular outflow tract obstruction. This is interesting in the light of much more recent enthusiasm for dual chamber right ventricular pacing to produce a functional left bundle branch block. Premature depolarisation of the right ventricular outflow tract septum causes paradoxical systolic motion that widens the left ventricular outflow tract during ejection. Subsequently, surgical skills improved and it was shown that the loss of gradient was not dependent upon creation of left bundle branch block.

Enthusiasm for the operation waned because of the rather high early mortality from myectomy, the increased number of patients who developed left ventricular failure in subsequent years, and the lack of evidence of any reduction in sudden death or long term benefit. However, it continued in a few specialist centres where patients with recalcitrant symptoms, gross hypertrophy, and high outflow tract gradients were referred.

Following some experimental papers on per catheter laser resection of the ventricular septum in animals, Kuhn in Germany first described transient reduction of the outflow tract obstruction after balloon occlusion of the first large septal branch of the left anterior descending coronary artery. This approach was inspired by learning of a Hammersmith Hospital patient who had lost her outflow tract obstruction after spontaneous infarction of the septum. Sigwart and his group at the Brompton Hospital in London subsequently showed that injection of alcohol into this artery to cause septal infarction brings about long lasting reduction in the outflow tract gradient.[20] Data on reduction of long term mortality and morbidity are still awaited, and there is concern that the myocardial scar may increase the risk of fatal arrhythmia.

Hypertrophic cardiomyopathy was described before the development of clinical echocardiography, which has become the ideal way of establishing the diagnosis. Systolic anterior movement of the anterior leaflet of the mitral valve was the first feature of the condition to be recognised by early primitive M-mode echo. It was described by Pridie in this country and by Shah and Gramiack in the United States. However, it is the abnormal diastolic properties of the left ventricle that are recognised to play a more important part. This is the abnormality which no treatment has successfully alleviated.[21]

Although an autosomal dominant transmission with variable penetrance was early recognised in family studies, the first genetic mutation (in the myosin heavy chain gene on chromosome 14) was found in a large French Canadian family in 1989, and at least seven different chromosomal loci, each with many different mutations, have now been discovered. All affect sarcomeric proteins. Much of this work has been carried out through cooperation between McKenna's group at St George's Hospital, London and Zideman's group at Harvard.

Restrictive cardiomyopathy

The third type of cardiomyopathy – restrictive cardiomyopathy – is the least common. It resembles hypertrophic cardiomyopathy in having a diastolic fault, but except for amyloid infiltration, the ventricular thickness is normal. The condition often simulates constrictive pericarditis clinically. At

Hammersmith Hospital, anticipation of myocardial amyloid deposition and its progression from a disorder of relaxation to one of restriction has been shown by serial echocardiography. The possibility of reducing the amyloid load by restricting the production of precursor proteins has become a reality through the work of Mark Pepys and Philip Hawkins, also at the Hammersmith.[22][23][24]

Another important infiltrative type of cardiomyopathy, sarcoidosis, was studied by Hugh Fleming at Addenbrooke's in Cambridge. He showed, in a large necropsy series, that this condition is not as rare as previously thought, and should be suspected in cases of unexplained arrythmia or heart block.[25]

The classification of the cardiomyopathies developed by Goodwin at Hammersmith Hospital persists to this day. His "congestive" group is now called "dilated" and much overlap exists between the three types. Nevertheless, the original purpose of ensuring that clinician and pathologist recognise the same condition in the same terms was successful and helped research to move on.

References

1. Fleming P. *A short history of cardiology.* Amsterdam-Atlanta: Editions Rodopi, 1997.
2. Hollman A. *Sir Thomas Lewis, pioneer cardiologist and clinical scientist.* London: Springer-Verlag, 1992.

2a. Mair A. *Sir James Mackenzie MD.* Edinburgh: Churchill-Livingstone, 1973.

3. Lewis T. *Diseases of the heart.* 3rd ed. London: Macmillan, 1944.
4. Wood P. DaCosta's syndrome or effort syndrome? *BMJ* 1941;1:767–72, 805–11, 845–51.
5. Wood P. *Diseases of the heart and circulation.* London: Eyre and Spottiswoode, 1950.
6. Osler W. Chronic infectious (sic) endocarditis. *Q J Med* 1909;2:219–30.

6a. Levy DM. Centenary of William Osler's 1885 Gulstonian lectures and their place in the history of bacterial endocarditis. *J R Soc Med* 1985;78:1039–46.

7. Horder TJ. Observations upon the importance of blood culture with an account of the technique recommended. *Practitioner* 1905;75:611–22.
8. Libman E, Sacks B. A hitherto undescribed form of valvular and mural endocarditis. *Arch Intern Med* 1924;33:701–37.
9. Christie RV. Penicillin in subacute bacterial endocarditis. Report to the MRC. *BMJ* 1948;i:1–5.
10. Bayliss R, Clarke C, Oakley C, Somerville W, Whitfield AGW. The teeth and infective endocarditis. *Br Heart J* 1983;50:506–1.
11. Working Party of the British society for Antimicrobial Chemotherapy. The antibiotic prophylaxis of infective endocarditis. *Lancet* 1982;ii:1323–6.
12. Mackenzie J. *Diseases of the heart.* London: Frowde, 1908.
13. Brigden W. Uncommon myocardial diseases in the non-coronary cardiomyopathies. *Lancet* 1957;ii:1179–84.
14. Evans W. Alcoholic cardiomyopathy. *Am Heart J* 1961;61:556–7.
15. Goodwin JF, Gordon H, Hollman A, Bishop MB. Clinical aspects of cardiomyopathy. *BMJ* 1961;1:69–79.
16. Davies LG. A familial heart disease. *Br Heart J* 1952;14:206.
17. Teare RD. Asymmetrical hypertrophy of the heart in young adults. *Br Heart J* 1958;20:1–8.
18. Goodwin JF, Hollman A, Cleland WP, et al. Obstructive cardiomyopathy simulating aortic stenosis. *Br Heart J* 1960;22:1403.
19. Brock RC. Functional obstruction of the left ventricle. *Guy's Hosp Rep* 1957;106:221.
20. Sigwart U. Non-surgical myocardial reduction for hypertrophic obstructive cardiomyopathy. *Lancet* 1995;346:211–4.
21. Goodwin JF, Oakley CM. The cardiomyopathies. *Br Heart J* 1972;34:545–52.
22. Pepys MB, Dyck RF, de Beer FC, Skinner M, Cohen AS Binding of serum amylase P component (SAP) by amylase fibrils. *Clin Exp. Immunol.* 1979;38:284–93

23. Hawkins PN. The diagnosis, natural history and treatment of amyloidosis. *J R Coll Physicians London* 1997;31:55–8.
24. Oakley CM. Amyloid heart disease and cardiomyopathies is difficult to classify. In Goodwin J, Olsen E eds. *Cardiomyopathies*. London: Springer Verlag, 1993:193–214.
25. Ghosh P, Fleming HA, Gresham GA. PG1. *Br Heart J* 1972;34:769–71.

Chapter 25

Hypertension

William A Littler

In his book, *Classic papers in hypertension*, John Swales, professor of medicine at Leicester and an international authority in the field of hypertension, collected his personal choice of publications "reporting ideas and work which has an impact on our knowledge of high blood pressure." From the 20th century he chose only three British contributors, Pickering, Platt, and Peart.[1]

Work of Pickering

No account of the history of hypertension could omit Sir George Pickering; he dominated the subject at home and abroad for nigh on 50 years.[2] In my opinion the best and most succinct account of Pickering's contribution was written by one of his former pupils, JIS Robertson, in a dedication to a book entitled *Frontiers in hypertension research.*[3]

Renin

One of Pickering's earliest contributions to the study of high blood pressure was concerned with the renin angiotensin system. In 1898, Tigerstedt and Bergman of the Karolinska Institute, Stockholm had shown that a definite and long lasting increase in arterial blood pressure could be achieved by injecting an extract of renal cortex from a freshly excised rabbit kidney into a normal rabbit. They named this substance renin. Others found their experiments difficult to repeat, and renin fell into obscurity. In 1936, Pickering and Myron Prinzmetal (a visiting American working in Sir Thomas Lewis's laboratory) were among those responsible for rediscovering renin. Later, Pickering and Cook located renin in the vascular pole of the kidney.[4]

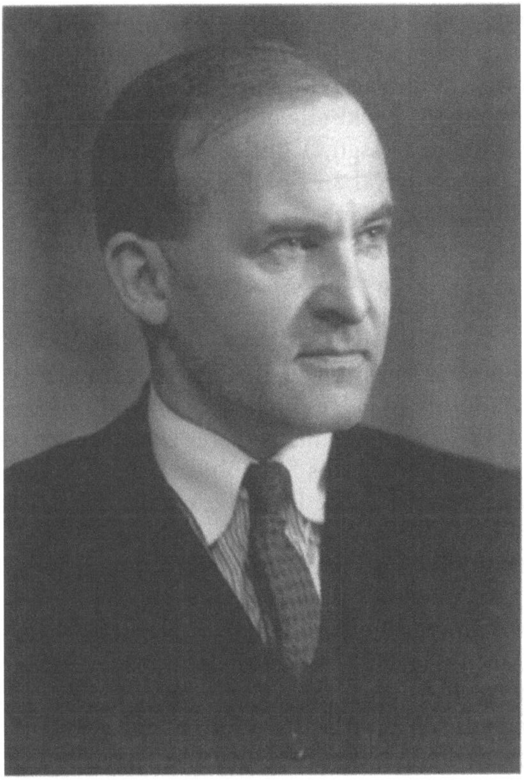

Figure 1 Sir George Pickering.

Angiotensin

In 1939, Braun-Menendes and colleagues in Buenos Aires and Irvin Page's group at the Cleveland Clinic published separately the results of independent work emanating from the observation that venous blood from ischaemic kidneys had both pressor and vasoconstrictor properties. Both groups concluded that renin acted on its plasma substrate to produce an active pressor substance. This substance was called "hypertensin" by the Argentinians and "angiotonin" by the Americans. Subsequently, the name "angiotensin" was coined. This recognised the equal contribution of the two groups to our understanding of the renin angiotensin system as a major regulator of arterial resistance and the principal hormonal system contributing to hypertension in renovascular disease.

Pickering encouraged and supported Stanley Peart in work at St Mary's Hospital Medical School which led to the isolation and subsequent amino acid sequencing of hypertensin. In two papers published in *Nature* in 1956, Peart and Elliott - working with ox plasma, ox serum, and rabbit renin - showed that hypertensin was a decapeptide with the sequence Asp.Arg.Val.Tyr.Val.His.Pro.Phe.His.Leu.[5] We now know this substance as angiotensin I. Peart and Pickering's groups combined to study the action of angiotensin in man, and showed it to be the most powerful vasoconstrictor. Brown, Lever, and Robertson, from Peart's laboratory (who subsequently became the backbone of the Medical Research Council (MRC) Blood Pressure Unit in Glasgow) undertook extensive studies on plasma renin in several physiological and pathological states. They also developed a standardised renin assay.

Battle of the knights

However, it was on the question of the "nature of essential hypertension" that Pickering made his most important contribution and sparked one of the most celebrated scientific debates of the 20th century. Pickering's principal opponent in this debate was Sir Robert (later Lord) Platt, professor of medicine at Manchester.[6] The Platt–Pickering debate was described by Swales as "fierce but good natured," and his book *Platt versus Pickering* is a comprehensive account of the whole episode and required reading for anyone claiming an interest in hypertension and clinical science.[7]

The two combatants entered the fray as equals, heavyweights of the British medical scene, unconcerned for the consequences. The debate was carried out principally through the columns of the *Lancet*, which was appropriate, given that journal's radical tradition and is often referred to with relish as "The battle of the knights." The annual meeting of the American College of Physicians also provided both combatants with a platform from which to expound their views before a wider and influential audience.

Heredity in hypertension

The origin of the dispute was Platt's paper "Heredity in hypertension" published in 1947 in the *Quarterly Journal of Medicine*.[8] "It is not a new observation that a family history suggestive of high blood pressure is commonly enlisted with patients with essential hypertension," began Platt. He then went on to detail the evidence supporting his hypothesis that essential hypertension is a specific clinical entity, conveyed by a single Mendelian dominant gene with a rate of expression of more than 90%. His observations had been made on patients who had been referred to him because they had high blood pressure.

In 1952, Pickering published his first comments on the hereditary factor in hypertension, and seemed to support Platt's views. However, within two years all had changed. This change of mind resulted largely from the analysis of blood pressure readings that Pickering and his colleagues had taken at St Mary's Hospital. The readings were from around 2000 men and women representing a sample of the general population, together with first degree relatives of people with and without hypertension. The principal conclusion was clear and unambiguous: "there is no evidence of two populations so far as blood pressure is concerned and any division between

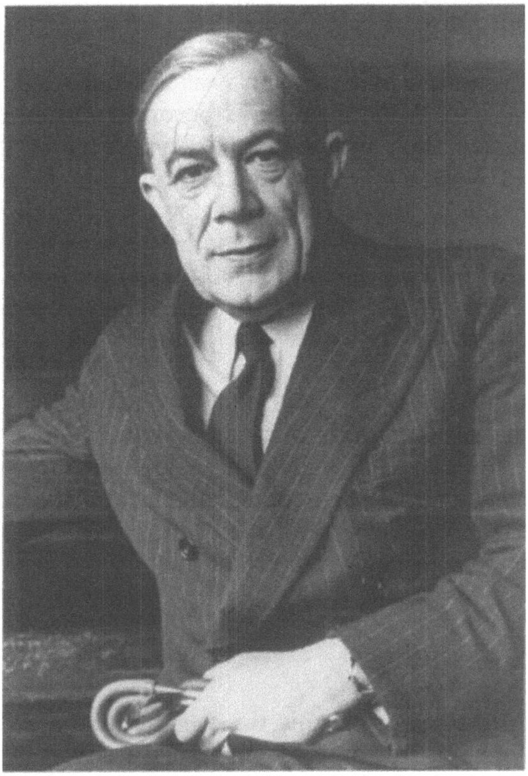

Figure 2 Lord Platt.

normal and abnormal is purely arbitrary."[9] Pickering argued that any genetic factor in hypertension was probably polygenic, and its contribution relatively modest.[10] Finally, Pickering proposed the "revolutionary" (his word) idea that essential hypertension was not a specific disease entity – the difference between normal pressure and hypertension was a quantitative, not qualitative, deviation from the norm.

Battle was joined! Platt's rebuttal was published in the *Lancet*. He defended essential hypertension as a separate entity and re-analysed the data of Pickering and his collaborators, such that the blood pressure curves showed a bimodal distribution with a "natural dividing line between normotension and hypertension."[11]

Back came Pickering. He pointed out technical reasons explaining why blood pressure distribution curves may not be smooth ("unconscious digit preference") and highlighted the pitfalls of using relatively small numbers of subjects when making predictions about whole populations. And so it went on. . . .

Achieving compromise

The "nature of essential hypertension" was a debate that lasted for nearly a decade. In the end, the audience was becoming bored and the combatants had exhausted their arguments. Pickering's views gradually gained ascendancy and became the accepted wisdom, but he lost his fight for abandoning the term hypertension in favour of high blood pressure; hypertension was more convenient. In the best British tradition, some compromise was involved. Platt acknowledged the multifactorial nature of blood pressure, while Pickering accepted that there might be a discrete subgroup of people with hypertension concealed within the blood pressure distribution curves.

With hindsight, we could be forgiven for wondering what all the fuss was about, but we should remember that our vantage point is achieved only by standing on the shoulders of these two great men. As a result of their debate, essential hypertension had been defined, the technical problems associated with blood pressure measurement had been recognised, and the need for large population studies had been established.

Epidemiological studies

Epidemiological studies of chronic diseases became a serious business in the 1950s. The impetus for the epidemiological study of hypertension came from Pickering. He was convinced that knowledge of the distribution of blood pressure in relation to age and gender, together with its determinance in the general population was needed. The landmark studies in hypertension were carried out by Miall and Oldham in the 1950s, in two south Wales communities – the miners of the Rhondda Fach and the agricultural workers in the Vale of Glamorgan.[11] These studies set the standard for all subsequent epidemiological work in this area. Miall and Oldham investigated a true random sample of the two populations, and a single observer (Miall) measured the blood pressures. They produced blood pressure frequency distribution curves that were unimodal and showed a close similarity in the pressures of first degree relatives, regardless of whether their propositi were chosen because they presented as patients with essential hypertension or came from the population at large. This was strong evidence for the inheritance being quantitative and the same for the whole range of blood pressure.

Problems of measurement

Epidemiological studies of blood pressure were impeded by inherent defects of conventional sphygmomanometer measurement – in particular, terminal digit preference and observer bias. During the 1960s, Geoffrey Rose and his colleagues at the London School of Hygiene and Tropical Medicine undertook painstaking work on measurement error and eventually produced a special sphygmomanometer for use by epidemiologists.[13] This sphygmomanometer largely excluded observer prejudice and terminal digit preference. What Rose's work told us, above all else, was that great care needed to be taken in measuring blood pressure in order to obtain useful data.

Oxford studies

Epidemiological studies have repeatedly and consistently identified high blood pressure as an independent risk factor for a number of cardiovascular disorders, particularly stroke and coronary heart disease. This has been clarified recently by Sir Richard Peto and his colleagues in Oxford. They pooled information from 418 343 adults aged 25–70 years who participated in nine prospective observational trials and who were followed for an average of 10 years. The risk of coronary heart disease was five times higher and the risk of stroke 10 times higher for people whose diastolic pressure was in the highest stratum (105 mmHg) compared with those in the lowest stratum (76 mmHg).[14]

The fetal origins hypothesis

During the last decade, David Barker and his colleagues in Southampton championed the hypothesis that retardation of growth during fetal life and infancy leads to high blood pressure and other cardiovascular risks in adult life. In a number of cohort studies, Barker has shown an inverse relation between birth weight or weight at 1 year and the blood pressure in adult life, and also an independent positive correlation between placental weight and adult blood pressure. Thus, improving the nutritional status and general well being of the mother has enormous potential for preventing the development of hypertension in the general population.[15]

Benign and malignant hypertension

Volhard and Fahr, in 1914, were the first to point out that essential hypertension might behave in one of two ways. In most patients, the course was long with little change until death came from heart failure, stroke, or an intercurrent illness. This they named "benign hypertension." However, in a few patients (usually younger ones), the disease followed a rapidly fatal course. It was heralded by the appearance of "albuminuric retinitis," and followed by progressive renal failure and uraemia. The distinctive feature of this condition was arteriolar-fibrinoid necrosis, and they named the condition "malignant hypertension."

The concept of a malignant form of essential hypertension was slow to gain acceptance. It was observed that there was practically no type of hypertension that could not become complicated by the malignant phase.

Attempts were made to incriminate infections, toxins, mental stress, or unknown factors as the mechanism by which the benign form of essential hypertension suddenly and dramatically transformed itself into the malignant phase. Pickering suggested that benign and malignant courses of hypertension merely expressed the severity of the hypertensive process irrespective of the lesion that ultimately determined it. In other words, whatever the underlying cause of hypertension, its course would become malignant if the blood pressure were sufficiently high.

"Goldblatt hypertension"

Wilson and Pickering had shown that Goldblatt hypertension could produce arteriolar-fibrinoid necrosis in animals in the same organs as in man, with the exception of the kidney whose artery had been clamped and thereby "protected" from the high arterial pressure. At the London Hospital, FB Byrom with Clifford Wilson, and later LF Dobson, carried out sophisticated experiments showing that acute fibrinoid necrosis occurred when the arterial luminal pressure increased beyond a certain point.[16] When they produced severe hypertension in rats by constricting one renal artery (the other kidney being intact), Byrom et al. showed fibrinoid lesions in the kidney with the intact artery, but not in the kidney whose artery had been clamped. The renal abnormality in the rat's unclamped kidney was identical to that of renal lesions of malignant hypertension in man.

Surgical reversal of malignant hypertension

Pickering therefore argued that if arterial pressure could be reduced sufficiently, and for long enough, the pathological changes associated with the malignant phase of hypertension could be reversed. And so it proved. With AD Wright and RA Heptinstall at St Mary's Hospital, he showed that in three histologically proved cases of malignant hypertension due to pyelonephritis, nephrectomy or subtotal adrenalectomy reduced aterial pressure and restored normal renal function.[17] In addition, the retinal changes were reversed and the patients were restored to wellbeing. With the introduction of effective hypotensive drugs these observations were to be confirmed impressively. Incidentally, Platt did not like the terms benign and malignant, when applied to hypertension. He preferred simple and compound hypertension. However, Platt agreed with Pickering that these were variants of the one disease and observed personally a transition from the benign to the malignant phase in some of his patients.

Early drug treatments

Writing about 70 years ago, John Hay, professor of medicine at Liverpool and a founder member of the Cardiac Club in 1922, expressed the opinion of many of his colleagues on the treatment of hypertension when he said, "the greatest damage to a man with high blood pressure lies in its discovery, because then some fool is certain to try to reduce it." This attitude arose against a background of treatment that included "mercury as a blue pill or a dose of calomel followed next morning by a small concentrated dose of saline."[18]

Blocking ganglionic neurotransmission

While Pickering and Platt were arguing about the nature of hypertension, important developments were taking place in its treatment and its pathological consequences. WDM Paton, working initially at the National Institute for Medical Research, Mill Hill and subsequently at University College Hospital, investigated the pharmacological properties of compounds capable of blocking ganglionic neurotransmission. He drew attention to the clinical potential of one of these compounds, hexamethonium, in hypertension.[19] The clinical effects of this drug were examined by several British workers, including P Arnold and ML Rosenheim at University College Hospital and researchers under the direction of John McMichael at the Postgraduate Medical School at Hammersmith Hospital. It was evident from their studies that hexamethonium could produce a noticeable and protracted reduction in systolic and diastolic blood pressures.

At first, ganglion blocking drugs were used only in patients with malignant hypertension or with symptomatic complicated essential hypertension. McMichael's group was among the first to confirm that the pharmacological reduction of blood pressure in malignant hypertension (hitherto a condition that was uniformly fatal) would prolong survival especially if treatment was begun before the onset of renal failure.[20] It was also shown that the pathological consequences of hypertension - such as retinitis, cardiac strain, and heart failure - could be reversed by reducing blood pressure.

Hypertension clinic

The Hammersmith group had begun to use hexamethonium in 1951, and had developed a specialist hypertension clinic with dedicated staff, a facility which now exists in many hospitals throughout the world. In the early 1950s, McMichael had the wisdom to involve his patients more actively in their own treatment by issuing them with printed instructions on their drug therapy. These instructions included an explanation of the nature of hypertension and the likely side effects of the drug treatment - a practice well ahead of its time.

Trial ethics

The introduction of an effective drug treatment for hypertension in the 1950s resulted in a considerable improvement in mortality and morbidity for patients, particularly those with malignant hypertension and hypertensive heart failure. Yet, up to 1964, no properly controlled clinical trial in the treatment of hypertension had been published. Indeed many doctors at the time considered it unethical to carry out such a trial given the apparent benefits of antihypertensive drugs. In 1963, the *British Medical Journal* published an editorial entitled, "Ethics in human experimentation." It attacked those doctors in general, and Sir Austin Bradford-Hill in particular, who thought advocates of the controlled trial resisted any kind of code of conduct or the voluntary consent of the human subjects involved.[21]

The basis for primary prevention

Against this background, Michael Hamilton and his colleagues in Chelmsford published a landmark paper in the *Lancet* in 1964 - an article that is often under appreciated, particularly in the United States.[22] Hamilton's trial aimed to determine whether blood pressure reduction would affect the incidence of strokes caused by high blood pressure in patients aged less than 60 years with symptomless, uncomplicated, benign essential hypertension. The patients had to have a diastolic blood pressure of at least 110 mmHg, sustained over three months of outpatient observation entailing at least three visits. These entry criteria would later become the standard for subsequent trials. The study was conducted over a period of six years in men and women, and involved hard clinical end points, including death and cardiovascular complications. Although the study was under powered by today's standards, it produced very important results that have been substantiated many times subsequently. These were that blood pressure reduction should be recommended for patient's with sustained diastolic blood pressure of greater than 110 mmHg, even though they were free of symptoms or complications of hypertension, in order to prevent strokes and other complications. This important paper established the basis for primary preventative treatment of hypertension.

Research at the Hammersmith in the 1950s and 1960s

The 1950s and 1960s were exciting times. The development of antihypertensive drugs and a specialist clinic in hypertension provided the focus for clinical investigations of these agents. At the Postgraduate Medical School the MRC Clinical Pharmacology Research Group was established. It was centred on the hypertension clinic, which helped to popularise clinical pharmacology as an academic discipline within the United Kingdom. Not surprisingly, since many of those subsequently appointed to chairs in this discipline had worked at the Hammersmith, clinical pharmacologists have had a long and strong reputation in hypertension research.

Prognosis of treated hypertension

The name of Colin Dollery became synonymous with hypertension research. He and Alistair Breckenridge, together with their colleagues from the MRC unit, produced an important audit of the Hammersmith hypertension clinic in 1969 which addressed the question of the prognosis of treated hypertension.[23] Reviewing the 16 year experience from 1952, they compared treatment in the eight years when ganglion blocking drugs were used with a similar period in which adrenergic blocking drugs and diuretics were prescribed. Most of their findings were unsurprising; during the second period the survival was better, presumably because of better treatment and the accumulated knowledge of patient management. They made two important observations that were to point the way to future research which would confirm their validity. The first was that survival was determined by the blood pressure achieved by treatment, rather than the pretreatment levels. The second was the noticeable increase in the number of deaths from myocardial infarction in patients with non-malignant hypertension as the treatment of hypertension improved. During their second period of study, Dollery and Breckenridge found that myocardial infarction was the major cause of death.

Treating patients with mild hypertension

The important findings of Hamilton and his colleagues were subsequently confirmed by the large Veterans Administration cooperative trial carried out in the United States: this trial was placebo controlled, double blinded, and involved men with diastolic blood pressures ranging from 90–112 mmHg. The study showed that lowering blood pressure was beneficial in patients whose diastolic blood pressure exceeded 104 mmHg and reduced the incidence of cerebrovascular accidents, heart failure, and malignant hypertension. The trial confirmed the Hammersmith observations that myocardial infarction was a common complication of mild to moderate hypertension and did not seem to be significantly affected by antihypertensive drugs. But the trial produced no clear mandate for treating patients with mild hypertension (diastolic blood pressure 90 mmHg to 104 mmHg). These results set the questions to be answered in the next series of trials – namely, should mild hypertension be treated and does treatment of mild hypertension reduce the severity of coronary artery disease?

β blockers

JW (later Sir James) Black made an outstanding contribution to cardiovascular therapy with his invention and development of the β adrenoceptor blocking drugs, widely used in angina, arrhythmias, hypertension, and recently in heart failure. While at Glasgow University in the 1950s, Black initiated the concept that in treating coronary heart disease, a reduction in cardiac oxygen consumption would be better than an increase in coronary flow. His idea that sympathetic over activity might have a deleterious effect on patients with angina or cardiac arrhythmias led him to pursue the then novel idea of developing drugs to inhibit the effect of the sympathetic nervous system on the heart via the noradrenaline receptor sites on heart muscle cells. Black began his work in 1958, at the laboratories of Imperial Chemical Industries, and the fruits of his search for drugs to block β adrenergic receptors first appeared in a landmark article in the *Lancet* in 1962.[24] Bradycardia was the main clinical feature, and interestingly the paper attracted no editorial review or correspondence. Nethalide, known better as pronethalol, was the world's first β blocker. It was succeeded by the widely used propranolol and later by several other compounds. For this imaginative concept and for his other inventive work in clinical pharmacology, Sir James was jointly awarded the Nobel Prize for physiology or medicine in 1988.

The credit for the discovery of the antihypertensive effect of β blocking drugs in man belongs to Brian Prichard of University College Hospital. In 1964, he published the results of a double blinded trial of pronethalol in patients with angina.[25] Prichard observed that the supine blood pressure was, on average, 8.3–5.7 mmHg lower in patients taking pronethalol than in those given placebo, a statistically significant difference. In the 11 patients in his study, who were also hypertensive, he observed a considerably greater fall in blood pressure in the absence of any postural hypotension. Pronethalol did not survive either, but its successor propranolol did, and became perhaps the most important cardiac drug of the decade. In 1964, Prichard and Gillam showed that propranolol exerted a considerable antihypertensive effect and used it to treat high blood pressure.[26] β blockers remain the first line drugs for the treatment of hypertension and are recommended by all authoritative bodies from WHO to the national hypertension societies of most countries.

MRC trial of drug treatment in mild hypertension

The landmark MRC trial of drug treatment for mild hypertension was carried out in the United Kingdom and began in 1973.[27] The working party running the trial was chaired by Sir Stanley Peart and included some of the leading figures in hypertension research such as Colin Dollery, Bill Miall, Geoffrey Rose, and Tony Lever. The trial was set up to establish whether drug treatment of mild hypertension (phase V diastolic blood pressure 90–109 mmHg) would be associated with a 40% reduction in mortality from stroke and in the number of non-fatal strokes. The effects of treatment on fatal and non-fatal coronary events were also assessed. There were two subsidiary objectives – to compare the course of blood pressure in the groups taking bendrofluazide and propranolol and to compare the incidence of adverse reactions to these two drugs. The population screened was drawn from 176 general practices across the United Kingdom. A total of

695 000 invitations to attend for screening were sent out and 515 000 (74%) were accepted. Altogether 17 354 patients, men and women aged 35–64 years, were randomly allocated at entry to take bendrofluazide (10 mg), propranolol (up to 240 mg), or placebo tablets. The primary results showed that antihypertensive treatment made no difference to mortality from all causes. However, while the incidence of all cardiovascular events fell in the groups taking active treatment - significantly so with regard to stroke - treatment made no difference to the overall incidence of coronary events.

Role of meta-analysis

Although there has been remarkable agreement among published trials on the effect of treatment on stroke, this has been less impressive for ischaemic heart disease. Peto and his colleagues in Oxford made an important contribution to the way that we interpret clinical trial data, especially in the use of the statistical technique of meta-analysis. Meta-analysis allows an overview of all available data, including smaller studies that do not have enough power to give statistically significant results and those in which trends are non-significant. Meta-analysis is able to pool disparate studies, and where findings are reasonably consistent it provides robust overall conclusions. Meta-analysis of observational studies has shown a linear relation between the level of diastolic blood pressure throughout the whole pressure range and the risk of stroke or ischaemic heart disease, with a fourfold greater risk of stroke and a twofold greater risk of ischaemic heart disease at a diastolic blood pressure of 105 mmHg compared with one of 90 mmHg. Reversal of risk produced by lowering blood pressure has been shown for drug treatment. A meta-analysis of the intervention trials in hypertension indicates that with an average reduction of blood pressure of 5 mmHg to 6 mmHg, the odds for stroke fall by 35%–40% and those for ischaemic heart disease by 20%–25% within five years of treatment.[28]

In conclusion

With the increasing specialisation in medicine, it is not surprising that hypertension has become a speciality in its own right over the past 30 years. National and international societies have been formed to bring together all those with an interest in the subject; the British Hypertension Society is now the main forum in Great Britain. However, with an estimated prevalence of 15%–20%, hypertension continues to be a common problem for all doctors.

References and notes

1. Swales JD. *Classic papers in hypertension, blood pressure and renin.* London: Science Press Ltd, 1987.
2. Sir George White Pickering (1904–80) decided as a young doctor that he wanted an academic career, not one in private medical practice, and he became an assistant in Sir Thomas Lewis's department of clinical research at University College Hospital in 1929. Lewis's mission was to apply scientific methods to clinical medicine, and Pickering eagerly embraced the discipline of clinical science. Pickering then developed his interests in the control of the circulation and on high blood pressure, and he became a close friend and devoted disciple of Lewis from whom he took over the editorship of *Clinical Science.* Pickering became professor of medicine at St Mary's Hospital in 1939, where he created a department in which an atmosphere of critical enquiry spread to everyone. His last appointment was in 1956, when he became the regius professor of medicine in Oxford and his scientific distinction was recognised by his election in 1960 as a fellow of the Royal Society.
3. Robertson JIS. Foreword. In: Laragh JH, Buhler FR, Seldin DW eds. *Frontiers of hypertension research.* New York: Springer-Verlag, 1981.
4. Pickering GW. *High blood pressure.* 2nd ed. London: J and A Churchill, 1987.
5. Elliott DF, Peart WS. Amino acid sequence in hypertension. *Nature* 1956;177:527–8.
6. Sir Robert (later Lord) Platt (1900–78) was appointed to the staff of the Royal Infirmary Sheffield at the age of 31. His hospital work and large private practice enabled him to develop a special interest in hypertension, which he continued when he was appointed professor of medicine in Manchester in 1946. His department became internationally known for its study of renal disease. Platt was president of the Royal College of Physicians of London from 1957–62. He made a great contribution to British medical life by organising the building of the college's new home in Regent's Park and by his leadership in the college's campaign against smoking.
7. Swales JD. *Platt versus Pickering, an episode in recent medical history.* London: The Keynes Press, 1985
8. Platt R. Heredity in hypertension. *Q J Med* 1947;16:111–21.
9. Hamilton M, Pickering DW, Roberts JAF, Sowry GSC. The aetiology of essential hypertension. The arterial pressure in the general population. *Clin Sci* 1954;13:11–35.
10. Pickering GW. The genetic factor in essential hypertension. *Ann Intern Med* 1955;43:57–62.
11. Platt R. The nature of essential hypertension. *Lancet* 1959;i:159–64.
12. Miall WE, Oldham PD. Factors influencing arterial blood pressure in the general population. *Clin Sci* 1958;17:409–44.
13. Rose GA, Holland WW, Crowley JA. Sphygmomanometer for epidemiologists. *Lancet* 1964;i: 296–300.
14. McMahon S, Peto R, Cutler J, Collins R, Sorlie P, Neaton J, et al. Blood pressure, stroke and coronary heart disease. Part One. Prolonged differences in blood pressure prospective observational studies corrected for the regression dilution bias. *Lancet* 1990;335:765–74.
15. Barker DJP, Bull AR, Osmond G, Simmons SJ. Fetal and placental size and risk of hypertension in adult life. *BMJ* 1990;301:259–62.
16. Wilson Clifford, Byrom FB. Renal changes in malignant hypertension. *Lancet* 1939;i:136–9.
17. Pickering GW, Wright AD, Hepintinstall RH. The reversibility of malignant hypertension. *Lancet* 1952;ii:952–6.
18. Hay J. The significance of a raised blood pressure. *BMJ* 1931;2:43–7.
19. Paton WDM, Zaimis EJ. The pharmacological actions polymethylene bistrinethylammonium salts. *Br J Pharmacol* 1949;4:381–400.
20. McMichael J, Murphy EH. Methonium. Treatment of severe and malignant hypertension. *J Chron Dis* 1955;1:527–35.
21. Anonymous. Ethics in human hypertension. [Editorial] *BMJ* 1963;2:122.
22. Hamilton N, Thompson EN, Wisniewski TKM. The role of blood pressure control in preventing complications of hypertension. *Lancet* 1964;i: 235–8.
23. Breckenridge A, Dollery CT, Parry EHO. Diagnosis of treated hypertension. *Q J Med* 1969;39:411–29.
24. Black JW, Stevenson JS. Pharmacology of a new adrenergic beta receptor blocking compound (Nethalide). *Lancet* 1962;ii:311–14.
25. Prichard BNC. Hypotensive effect of pronetholol. *BMJ* 1964;1:1227–8.
26. Prichard BNC, Gillam PMS. Use of propranolol (Inderal) in the treatment of hypertension. *BMJ* 1964;2:725–7.
27. Medical Research Council Working Party. MRC trial of treatment of mild hypertension: principal results. *BMJ* 1985;291:97–104.
28. Collins R, Peto R, Goodwin J, McMahon S. Blood pressure and coronary heart disease. *Lancet* 1990;336:370–1.

Chapter 26

Atherosclerosis Research after the Second World War

Michael F Oliver

This chapter focuses on the research into the causes of atherosclerosis that was conducted in the United Kingdom during the first 25–30 years after the second world war. Brief comments will also be made about the later development of ideas initiated during these early years, but no attempt will be made to provide a comprehensive review of UK research activities during the last 25–30 years of the century. This is partly because of the extent of the advances made and partly because it is often difficult to see these in perspective.

Early post war history

In the United Kingdom after the war, heart disease was a clinical subject dominated by the mitral valve and by congenital heart disease. Academic studies into the pathogenesis of vascular diseases or their clinical consequences were not encouraged and received little funding or attention. Osler, who saw only 40 patients with angina during all his years of clinical experience, and none during his 10 years in Montreal, had written in 1898 "it is too narrow a view to suppose the aetiology identical with that of arteriosclerosis. The one is so common and the other comparatively rare."[1] Coronary disease was regarded as an inevitable consequence of ageing, and the possibility of investigations or treatment did not arise before the 1950s. For example, Moschowitz states in a monograph in 1942, "it is hardly likely that any method of therapy will ever be discovered which will restore diseased vessels to their normal texture. Nor can arteriosclerosis be prevented, no more than grey hair or wrinkles."[2]

There was another attitude that retarded interest in the coronary arteries and atherosclerosis. Paul Dudley White, the most influential American cardiologist, stated in the third edition (1947) of his textbook that "coronary disease is not heart disease," thus reiterating a popular misunderstanding by cardiologists of the day.[3] In order to overcome the semantic rigidity,

White proposed the term "coronary heart disease." However, this did not establish it as a specific entity since he stated that coronary sclerosis as a cause of heart disease varied in different parts of the world "according to the frequency of such other causes as rheumatic heart disease, hypertension and syphilitic aortitis." At that time, the cause of coronary atheroma was variously ascribed to faulty cholesterol metabolism, local arterial strain or overwork, hypertension, infection, allergy, endocrinopathy, and heredity . . . "but none has been proved or even consistently found."[3]

Increasing incidence of coronary heart disease

There was some awareness before the second world war, in the United Kingdom and in the United States, that the clinical manifestations of coronary artery disease, angina, and myocardial infarction were increasing in incidence, but supporting data were few. One reason for the underdiagnosis of clinically manifest coronary heart disease was the commonly held belief that if a patient recovered from a coronary or survived for more than a few years, the original diagnosis must have been wrong.

In 1949, in a careful clinical and epidemiological survey, Ryle and Russell in Oxford, concluded that the increase in the incidence of ischaemic or coronary heart disease was real and not solely a consequence of changing habits in diagnosis or death certification.[4] Ryle and Russell:

- Documented a 15 fold increase in coronary deaths since 1921
- Identified for the first time a gender difference, with a 5:1 male:female ratio at the age of 45–54 years
- Recorded an excess of deaths in socioeconomic group I (ascribed possibly to the stress such people have to undergo together with inheritance of an ambitious and conscientious personality)
- Described a geographic difference within the United Kingdom, with deaths from coronary heart disease being more common in the north.

Later, the Registrar General's statistical tables of 1920–55 showed that there had been a much larger increase (70 fold) in coronary deaths during this period, and that their prevalence in the north was more than twice that in the south.

In 1950, Paul Wood – one of the foremost UK cardiologists at that time – wrote in the first edition of his textbook "the cause of human atheroma is unknown."[5] He did, however, quote an hypothesis that had been published two years earlier by Gordon (from the Public Health Department in Ilford, Essex).[6] This was that lipid-laden macrophages in the blood may penetrate the arterial intima and lead to irreversible lesions. Gordon pointed out that flow in the coronary arteries is intermittent and that the pressure changes there would favour the deposition of "lipophages" more in these arteries than in those farther from the heart where flow is more sustained. He also believed that hypertension facilitated this process.

In 1951, Morris analysed the autopsy records of one pathologist in the London Hospital between 1908 and 1949. He concluded that in spite of an increase in coronary deaths since 1930, there was no increase in either the incidence or the severity of coronary atheroma.[7] Morris later cautioned that to group coronary heart disease and cerebrovascular disease together as "atherosclerosis" was not justified clinically or epidemiologically from the pathology in the relevant arteries.[8] For example, although coronary heart disease was uncommon last century, cerebrovascular disease was common, and, furthermore, the high incidence of coronary heart disease seen in middle aged men is not evident for cerebrovascular disease.

Thus, around 1950, interest in atherosclerosis and coronary heart disease was low and sporadic. It was based mostly on studies of pathology and epidemiology. Laboratory research into lipid metabolism, fibrin/platelet pathophysiology, or arterial endothelial function had not begun.

Risk factors

The risk factor concept was not defined in the 1950s – or even in the 1960s – and no formal epidemiological or demographic studies were published in the United Kingdom at that time. But interest was developing.

Cigarette smoking

In 1954, Doll and Hill in London were the first to suggest that cigarette smoking might be associated with coronary heart disease.[9] This proposition came from their prospective studies of a link with lung cancer. They showed that male doctors in the United Kingdom who smoked more than 25 cigarettes daily had 25% more coronary heart disease than non-smokers. The relevance of cigarette smoking to coronary heart disease was contested for many years, and even into the 1970s. For example, the first report of an expert committee of the World Health Organization (WHO), writing on preventive aspects of ischaemic heart disease in 1958, states "recent evidence on the relation of smoking to coronary heart disease is contradictory."[10] While the US Framingham study firmly placed cigarette smoking as a major and exponential risk factor for coronary heart disease, the relevant survey was not published until 1967.[11]

Hypertension

There are sporadic references to the relation between raised blood pressure and coronary heart disease between 1940 and 1960, but it was recognised more as a risk factor for stroke. For example, White does not mention the relation between hypertension and coronary disease in his 1947 textbook.[3] At that time, there was more focus on blood pressure itself, and much of the writing was on the pathophysiology of the circulation.

Hypertensive heart disease, retinopathy, and encephalopathy were recognised complications requiring treatment, but coronary heart disease was rarely attributed.

The arterial lesion was called hyaline thickening of the intima, and Wood stated in the second edition of his textbook (1956) that vascular changes found in association with hypertension "have been proved to play no part in its production. Atherosclerosis is innocent in this respect."[12] Nor, it seems, did he consider that atherosclerosis might be worsened by increased arterial pressure. While conceding that angina may occur more frequently in the hypertensive patient, Wood took the view that coronary blood flow is greatly increased in hypertension and that, by inference, this protects the myocardium. The WHO study group of 1957 was equally cautious about any causal relation and confined its attention to screening, clinical features, and drug therapy without considering atherosclerosis as related in anyway.[13]

There was a polemical debate between Pickering of Oxford[14] and Platt of Manchester[15] concerning the nature and origin of hypertension. The former took the view that it was the manifestation of a skewed unimodal distribution curve and the latter contested this by stating that the distribution was bimodal and that hypertension was an inherited trait. Neither considered that there was any relation between hypertension and atherosclerosis.

Lipids

Research into the relation between blood lipids and coronary heart disease really began in 1949, when Gofman in the United States described the separation by the ultracentrifuge of lipids into lipoprotein classes according to their densities and flotation rates.[16][17] In 1950, he identified the Sf 12–20 lipoprotein flotation band (or low density lipoprotein (LDL) as we now know it) as "atherosclerogenic." At that time there was also interest in the plasma concentrations of phospholipids. It was believed that visible lipaemia was inversely related to the plasma lecithin concentration,[18] and a high cholesterol/phospholipid (C/P) ratio was thought to favour cholesterol deposition in the arterial wall.

In Edinburgh in 1953, Oliver and Boyd [19] established the extent of raised plasma cholesterol and phospholipid concentrations in 200 patients who had had a myocardial infarct compared with age matched controls. By using paper electrophoresis to measure the α (now recognised as high density or HDL lipoproteins) and β (now recognised as low density or LDL lipoproteins) lipoproteins, they translated Gofman's studies into clinical cardiology,[20] and proposed a low α/β ratio as an atherogenic index. The tardy recognition in the United Kingdom of any relation between plasma cholesterol or cholesterol-rich lipoproteins and coronary heart disease reflects the paucity at that time of biochemical training among UK physicians. Physiology, with a dominance of flow and pressure, was the preferred background for cardiologists.

By 1956, Wood conceded that abnormalities in blood lipids are a major influence in the pathogenesis of vascular diseases. He gave four pages of his textbook over to this subject.[12] This was a major advance for current cardiological opinion, particularly since two years earlier, at a meeting of the British Cardiac Society, Wood had dismissed Oliver's presentation of the above data "as irrelevant."

In 1957, Besterman, working at St Mary's, London reported that a pre-β band on lipid electrophoresis was also commonly seen in patients admitted to hospital with coronary heart disease.[21] This was probably the first identification of the role of triglycerides (later, very low density lipoproteins; VLDL) in coronary heart disease.

It took another 20 years for cardiologists in Britain to recognise the importance of lipoprotein abnormalities in the genesis of coronary heart disease, but even now, most patients in the United Kingdom with coronary heart disease and stroke do not have their plasma lipids measured.[22]

Nutrition

In the United States in 1950, Keys proposed that the concentration of plasma cholesterol is proportional to the intake of dietary saturated fat.[23] He based this proposition on studies of the effects of changing dietary calorie and fat intake in man, and subsequently on comparative studies between the populations in Naples, Madrid, and Minnesota. The suggestion was consolidated in 1970 by his Seven Countries study.[24] Keys was a physiologist and pioneer nutritionist who recognised for the first time that risk could be population based and not just individually based.

In 1955, Keys' theory received support from Bronte-Stewart (later to become director of the Medical Research Council Atheroma Research Unit in Glasgow). He showed a parallelism between the intake of dietary saturated fats and serum cholesterol concentrations when contrasting the incidence of coronary heart disease in Bantus (very low), Cape coloureds (intermediate), and whites (high) in South Africa.[25] In 1956, Bronte-Stewart showed for the first time that saturated fats raise and unsaturated vegetable and fish oils lower serum cholesterol concentrations.[26] He stated that " a possible common difference between animal fats and hydrogenated vegetable fat, on the one hand, and natural vegetable oils and marine oils, on the other, is not the cholesterol ... content ... but the proportion of highly unsaturated and saturated fatty acids in the diet." In 1960, Gresham and Howard (Cambridge) showed that feeding rats 5% cholesterol and butter led to thrombosis, while substituting butter with unsaturated arachis oil led to atherosclerosis.[27] Gresham and Howard were probably the first UK group to study spontaneous atherosclerosis in the aortas of non-human primates and to report (with fatty acid analyses) its induction in baboons by months of cholesterol feeding.[28]

Meanwhile, in 1956, Sinclair (Oxford) published in the *Lancet* (in perhaps the longest letter ever) his hypothesis that atherosclerosis and resultant vascular diseases might be the result of a deficiency of essential fatty acids in the diet rather than an excess of dietary saturated fats.[29] Sinclair focussed on arachidonic acid, which, by definition, cannot be synthesised in the body. He also argued that there might be a dietary deficiency of natural antioxidants. In both respects, he was later proved to be right. However, for many years he had to contend with the American obsession (with the exception of the notable studies of Ahrens [30]) that an excess of saturated fats is the sole dietary explanation for these conditions.

Physical inactivity

Between 1953 and 1958, the possibility of an inverse relationship between physical activity and coronary heart disease was proposed for the first time by Morris [31]. His studies of London Transport drivers and conductors [32] suggested that men in physically active jobs have less coronary heart disease, less coronary atheroma, and that their disease occurs later and is less frequently fatal. While the basis for these conclusions was not rigorous, subsequent surveys have supported the concept.

The arterial wall

In 1946, before Morris's London Hospital study,[7] Duguid, a respected pathologist in Newcastle, had proposed that thrombosis in the coronary arteries was the key feature of the increasing incidence of atherosclerosis.[33][34] He put forward the "encrustation hypothesis," stating that thrombosis is an important factor in the growth of the plaque and not just a terminal event leading to occlusion of the lumen. Like Rokitansky 100 years earlier, Duguid recommended that we should be studying factors that "govern fibrin formation in the circulating blood," and considered that thrombi are initiated on the arterial intima by platelet clumping or local failure of fibrinolysis. In 1951, Crawford and Levene (London) showed that fibrin could be incorporated into aortic intima.[35] Duguid also stated that the thrombosis hypothesis left unresolved the problem of the importance of the fatty changes in atherosclerotic lesions.

As early as 1951, Geiringer, working in Edinburgh, became interested in the nutrition of the arterial wall.[36] He was soon followed by Crawford at St Georges Hospital, London and by Adams in Cambridge. Crawford defined the sources of blood supply to the arterial wall and showed that new capillaries derived from the vasa vasorum cannot grow into the inner third of the media or the intima because of the high intraluminal pressure.[37] Adams used enzyme histochemistry to distinguish smooth muscle cells from other cells such as macrophages in the arterial wall and showed that the media is a site of low enzyme activity.[38]

Atherosclerosis was not given a separate chapter in Florey's first edition (1954) of lectures on pathology. But by the time the second edition was published in 1956, French in Oxford was able to report studies of the function of the vascular endothelium at a time when the interest of morbid anatomists was mostly confined to gross pathology.[39] He showed that in cebus monkeys the severity of the induced lesions was related more to the proportions of β (or LDL) lipoproteins in the plasma than to the total cholesterol concentrations. The same interest was taken up by Elspeth Smith in Cambridge, who showed the similarity between extracellular intimal lipid and serum LDL in human aortas.[40] At that time, Walton in Birmingham used antilipoprotein sera labelled with fluorescein to show unequivocally by immune histology that LDL (then called LpB) was present in atheromatous lesions.[41] Later, using immunofluorescence, he also showed the presence of LDL in xanthomata and corneal arcus. Smith then reported that cholesterol/LDL concentrations in serum taken from patients a week before death were correlated strongly with LDL concentrations in aortic intima.[42]

In Edinburgh, Fulton, using magnified stereo-arteriography post mortem, confirmed Duguid's views about the role of early mural thrombus in the genesis of atheromatous lesions.[43] He also identified the importance of the coronary collateral circulation, showing that patients with advanced coronary heart disease (long histories of relentless angina) had very extensive intercoronary anastomoses. This was not only due to dilatation but to increased growth of small arteries. He suggested chronic local myocardial ischaemia as the cause, and considered that this might be a result of endothelial dysfunction, predicting the intense investigation in the 1990s of endothelial vasodilator and vasoconstrictor substances.[44]

Thrombosis research

In Oxford during the war, Macfarlane had been studying the mechanisms of haemostasis and the classic theory of fibrin formation. He took the view that coagulation is physiologically offset by natural inhibitory processes. In the immediate post war years, Macfarlane focussed on the causes of thrombosis, regarding it as an uncommon abnormality that was particularly related to local endothelial damage.[45] He considered that thrombosis was the resultant of several factors that all happened to operate in the same direction at the same time, and he did not think that identification of a "prethrombotic state" in the blood of certain patients would be likely. A prescient comment that applies today. Macfarlane's observations presaged the work of Moncada and Vane in the early 1970s on endothelial release of prostaglandins (see next section), and of Moncada in the late 1980s on the vasodilatory function of nitric oxide.[46]

In 1955, Poole and Robinson, also working in Oxford, showed that the removal of fat from human plasma lengthened the coagulation time and that this could be corrected by adding fat and chyle. They proposed that chylomicra had an active coagulatory component and that the ethanolamine phosphatide content was probably responsible.[47] These studies seem to be the first relating the blood lipid composition to blood coagulation. Later,

Woolf, working with Crawford, demonstrated the presence of lipoproteins in thrombi.[48]

French summarised thrombosis research in the United Kingdom in 1956 by stating: "Whether the formation of a thrombus is determined by some particular feature of the lesions or by a change in the blood as a whole is unknown. If this tendency to thrombosis could be controlled, there is no real evidence that atherosclerosis would continue to have a serious effect on the normal life-span."[40]

Platelet morphology

Studies of thrombosis were advanced in the late 1950s and thereafter by Born's development of light scattering for optical assessment of the morphology of platelets. Using an early development of this technique, he showed that platelets contain high concentrations of adenosine triphosphate, which is released when plasma is clotting, and that they aggregate in response to adenosine diphosphate as well as to catecholamines.[49] Born proposed that thrombotic platelet aggregation might occur in vivo through the formation of adenosine diphosphate from adenosine triphosphate released from platelets.[50][51] Born also identified that aspirin has an anti-platelet aggregatory effect. This was followed by the seminal observations of Vane, for which he was awarded a Nobel prize, that the effects of aspirin, as well as its anti-inflammatory action, are due to inhibition of the synthesis of prostaglandins, later shown to be due to cyclo-oxygenase inhibition.[52]

Moncada and Vane showed that indomethacin and aspirin prevented the release of prostaglandin from the spleen. They proposed that the generation of prostaglandin X by the endothelium might be the mechanism underlying their unique ability to resist platelet aggregation.[53]

An obstacle to progress in thrombosis research was the debate in the 1960s over whether thrombosis followed myocardial infarction or preceded it. This was not really resolved until Fulton showed through pre-mortem injections of radiolabelled fibrinogen that thrombosis often preceded myocardial infarction.[54] Much later, Davies and Thomas[55] demonstrated very convincingly the role of thrombosis in sudden cardiac death, and subsequent angiographic studies showed that thrombolysis can reduce the incidence of myocardial infarction.

Fibrinogen

Meanwhile, on the basis that there may not have been much, if any, increase in atheroma over the years when coronary heart disease mortality had been increasing,[7] Meade and Chakrabarti initiated in 1972 a series of studies of the components of the blood, particularly fibrinogen and factor VII.[56] Later, in the seminal Northwick Park study they were able to show for the first time that raised fibrinogen is an independent predictor of coronary heart disease.[57] In 1981, Smith (now in Aberdeen) suggested that fibrinogen might be converted to fibrin within atherosclerotic plaques, leading to sequestration of LDL.[58] Raised fibrinogen is now recognised as a predictor of arterial disease in the brain and legs and also of disease progression and recurrence.

Lipid and lipoprotein research

Interest in lipids and lipoproteins was growing (see lipids in section on risk factors above), and was focusing on absorption studies. In 1953, the Edinburgh group showed that the plasma of patients with coronary heart disease became more intensely lipaemic than that of controls after a standard fat meal, and that heparin-induced clearing of postprandial turbidity was slower in these subjects.[59] In Oxford, Robinson demonstrated that a comparable chylomicra clearing system exists physiologically,[60] and Mitchell showed that platelet rich plasma clears less rapidly and completely than platelet poor plasma, and suggested that there is an inhibitory factor in platelets (see section on thrombosis).[61] These studies identified lipoprotein lipase as a key enzyme.

Gender differences

While studying possible interpretations of the gender difference in coronary heart disease, the Edinburgh group discovered that plasma lipids undergo regular changes during the menstrual cycle, with cholesterol lowest at ovulation when oestrogen levels are highest.[62] They studied extensively the effects of pregnancy and sex, thyroid, adrenal, and pituitary hormones on plasma lipoproteins. These studies also showed that normal ovarian function was crucial for normal lipid metabolism, particularly plasma HDL concentrations. The loss of ovarian function, either spontaneously or through bilateral ovariectomy, leads to an increase in the β/α (LDL/HDL) ratio and the premature development of coronary heart disease.[63]

Fibrate development

The first fibrate was developed as a result of the laboratory-based Edinburgh studies – it ultimately became clofibrate. In 1953, it was noted that an insecticide used in France led to a profound reduction of plasma cholesterol, and ICI (the manufacturers) asked Boyd and Oliver to study the mechanism of action. After 5 years of study (mostly in animals) the effectiveness of a reformulated, related compound as a cholesterol lowering agent was confirmed in hypercholesterolaemic men as Atromid and Atromid-S.[64] This led to the establishment of the first and largest (15 000 men) clinical trial of the value of lowering raised cholesterol concentration – the WHO clofibrate trial – in Edinburgh, Prague, and Budapest (see clinical trials).[65]

Beneficial role of HDL

In 1976, Miller and Miller (brothers) proposed that increased plasma concentrations of HDL (or Sf 0–20 or α lipoproteins) might be protective against coronary heart disease and atheroma.[66] Norman Miller was working in Edinburgh at that time. The idea that any cholesterol carrying lipoprotein might have a beneficial role was revolutionary, but soon received confirmation from the Tromso heart study.[67] Two years later, Shepherd (of Glasgow) showed that a diet high in polyunsaturated fats, already being recommended by many bodies, lowers HDL, possibly reducing the benefit.[68] The HDL hypothesis has stood the test of time - even to the extent that many guidelines on the prevention of coronary heart disease now recommend the use of the HDL/LDL ratio as a measure for introducing treatment.

Organisational developments

The Atherosclerosis Discussion Group, 1958

The Atherosclerosis Discussion Group (now the British Atherosclerosis Society) was founded in 1958 and provided the first UK forum for exchanging knowledge on basic atherosclerosis research and its clinical application. It was the first atherosclerosis society in Europe. Sir Howard (later Lord) Florey was the first chairman, and stated the "the principal aim of this Group is to obtain an exchange of facts and of views concerning the aetiology, pathogenesis and treatment of atherosclerosis between individuals whose interests and experiences differ widely." Subsequent chairman included Pickering (Oxford), Macfarlane (Oxford), Crawford (London), and Oliver (Edinburgh).

Journal of Atherosclerosis Research, 1961

An important development in 1961 was the initiation of this international journal. It had a British, European, and American editor, and soon became the principal organ in the United Kingdom for publishing basic atherosclerosis research. At that time, the *British Heart Journal* was primarily a clinical journal and did not seem favourably disposed to publishing basic or clinical science. The first British editors in series were Oliver (Edinburgh) and Adams (Cambridge). Later, this journal became *Atherosclerosis*.

The Medical Research Council's Atheroma Research Unit, 1962–5

This was established in the Western Infirmary in Glasgow in 1962 under the directorship of Bronte-Stewart, who had established an impressive reputation as a clinical scientist and epidemiologist working on atherosclerosis and coronary heart disease in Cape Town. The main focus of the research of this MRC unit was the physiology and pathophysiology of absorption and excretion of cholesterol in man, and the relation of lipids to blood coagulation. Bronte-Stewart confirmed that plasma cholesterol and LDL concentrations are partly related to the degree of saturation or unsaturation of dietary fatty acids, but he died within 3 years, at the early age of 44, before the work of the atheroma unit could really be established.

In 1966 the MRC transformed the unit into one on hypertension and kidney research. No other government-sponsored atheroma research unit has been established since. In 1969, however, an MRC Lipid Metabolism Unit was initiated at Hammersmith under Myant. The brief was "investigation and treatment of patients with disorders of lipid metabolism, particularly those leading to premature ischaemic heart disease." With Lewis, Myant established the first lipid clinic in the United Kingdom. This was taken over by Thompson, who investigated the potential of the cell separator as a means of lowering cholesterol in patients with the familial hypercholesterolaemia homozygote (see below).

Cardiovascular survey methods

During the 1960s, as epidemiological surveys increased, it became apparent that there was a need to standardise methods. Under the auspices of the WHO, Rose from the London School of Hygiene and Blackburn from Minneapolis led the way. They produced a manual of principles, protocols, survey questionnaires, and standards to be applied to physical examination of people and patients.[69]. This has acted as a *vade mecum* for generations of researchers developing field studies of cardiovascular diseases.

Major research developments after 1970

Lipid metabolism

The key development in this area took place in the United States in 1973. Goldstein and Brown reported a defect in the regulation of 3-hydroxy-3-methylglutaryl coenzyme A reductase (HMG CoA) activity in patients with familial hypercholesterolaemia. This led them to identify the crucial role of LDL receptors in the regulation of plasma cholesterol concentrations[70] and to receive the award of a Nobel prize. Shepherd et al. in Glasgow followed in 1979 with evidence supporting the Brown-Goldstein hypothesis that LDL receptors play a key role in governing LDL metabolism.[71] Myant in London then delineated the physical characteristics of LDL, the LDL receptor, and apolipoprotein B.[72] These developments led to the statin drugs, which through their inhibition of mevalonate synthesis up-regulate LDL receptors and reduce plasma LDL concentrations (see clinical trials).

Family and genetic studies

Interest in familial clusters of coronary heart disease occurred fairly late, although, in 1953, Gertler and White (Paul Dudley) in the United States had reported the characteristics of 100 young men with coronary heart disease and recorded that a family history was common when coronary heart disease occurred prematurely.[73] Rose in London took this a stage further by describing family patterns of coronary heart disease,[74] and Joan Slack's studies (London) in the late 1960s of first degree relatives of patients with coronary heart disease were innovatory.[75][76] Slack found that more than half of the male relatives of patients with familial hypercholesterolaemia had already developed coronary heart disease before the age of 50 years. Myant focussed particularly on the genetic polymorphism of LDL receptors and of the human apoB gene, proposing routes that may eventually lead to successful gene therapy for homozygous familial hypercholesterolaemia.[77]

These observations were followed by many studies of the relation between homozygous and heterozygous familial hypercholesterolaemia with premature coronary heart disease, particularly by Thompson (London), who pioneered plasma aphoresis for these patients.[78] Studies of mutant lipoproteins followed,[79] and in 1985 Humphries (also in London) elaborated on the polymorphisms in the LDL receptor gene and their use in the possible diagnosis of familial hypercholesterolaemia in children.[80]

From the time of the publication of the Northwick Park study on fibrinogen,[56] the interest in Europe in the relation of fibrin/fibrinogen to the arterial wall grew rapidly. Humphries soon reported genetic variations at the fibrinogen gene locus and assessed the contribution of these polymorphisms to coronary heart disease.[81]

Epidemiology

There was no relatively simple method of measuring plasma triglycerides before 1969, although it had been known since Gofman's publications that the Sf 100–400 fraction in the ultracentrifuge was particularly rich in triglycerides and relatively poor in cholesterol.[16] The Scandinavians' interest in the relation between triglycerides and coronary heart disease [82] was a key part of the cross sectional Edinburgh–Stockholm survey.[83] In this study, many characteristics were contrasted in 100 men aged 40 in each of the two cities in order to find out why the coronary heart disease rate in Edinburgh was three times that for young men in Stockholm. The survey showed that Edinburgh men were shorter, had significantly higher plasma triglyceride concentrations, and a greater insulin response to a standard glucose load, but that there was no difference in LDL or HDL concentrations. This was the first identification of insulin resistance as a risk factor for coronary heart disease and of the metabolic syndrome X.[84]

Through the 15 year Whitehall study of civil servants, Reid et al. (including Rose) identified in 1976 that the age adjusted coronary heart disease mortality was 10 times greater in the top decile of risk (based on smoking, blood pressure, and cholesterol) relative to the lowest.[85] These finding reinforced the Framingham study results.

While there was increasing enthusiasm in the United States for strategies to prevent coronary heart disease, the focus on prevention did not really occur in the United Kingdom until Rose proposed that a relatively small shift to the left of the distribution curve of any risk factor would probably make a major impact on the incidence of the disease in the whole population.[86] This was a new concept 20 years ago.

Rose and colleagues identified in 1978 that the relation of coronary heart disease to social class structure in the United Kingdom had changed over the previous 20 years from a predominance in socioeconomic classes 1 and 2 to an increasing mortality in classes 4 and 5.[87] They ascribed this partly to a relative reduction of cigarette smoking in the more educated social classes and to "a higher consumption of sugar and wholemeal bread" in those less well off. More recently, Marmot has shown through extensive analyses of the records of Whitehall civil servants that one of the chief causes of the excess of coronary heart disease mortality in the lower social classes is impoverishment of life, inability to better themselves, and frustration.[88] In the 1980s, in contrast to the United states, little improvement in morbidity or mortality from coronary heart disease was seen in the least privileged in the United Kingdom. Scotland, together with East Karelia in Finland, had the highest rates in the world. This has continued into the 1990s and has been ascribed by Marmot to "a trailing behind with respect to changes in life style."

In the late 1970s, Shaper initiated the British regional heart study of 7735 men aged 40–59, which focused on the marked excess of coronary heart disease in the north compared with the south.[89] This study, which now has a 20 year follow up, showed many of the same associations between risk and coronary heart disease that had been identified in the United States by the Framingham survey, but particularly strong associations between coronary heart disease mortality in various UK towns were shown with blood pressure, cigarette smoking, and heavy drinking. It also seems that the environment of the town to which people migrate is more important than the environment of their birth place.[90]

Barker (Southampton) took the view that variations in adult diet, cigarette smoking, and drinking habits did not explain adequately why the highest coronary heart disease rates are in the industrial areas in the north of the United Kingdom and some less affluent areas in the west.[91][92] He proposed that retardation of growth during critical periods of fetal life and infancy increases the risk of coronary heart disease in adult life, and that these result from unbalanced nutrition during pregnancy.

Confirming Sinclair's 1956 hypothesis that an essential fatty acid deficiency might contribute to coronary heart disease,[28] the Edinburgh group provided evidence 30 years later that a relative deficiency of adipose linoleic acid exists in patients with angina compared with controls.[93] This is consistent with the fact that diets with a high ratio of polyunsaturated/saturated fats are more effective in preventing coronary heart disease than low fat diets. They also found that there are significantly more patients with angina in the lowest population distribution of the antioxidant vitamins E and C.[94] The relevance of this latter observation has increased subsequently with the recognition that LDL needs to be oxidised to be incorporated into the arterial intima.

The problem of measuring a thrombotic tendency has troubled atherosclerosis research for years. It may be so labile and evanescent that its identification is impossible. But an important contribution came from Meade et al. working at Northwick Park Hospital, London These authors published the first of a series of seminal reports indicating that raised plasma fibrinogen and factor VIIc are major risk factors for subsequent coronary heart disease.[95] Furthermore, raised fibrinogen is an independent factor and at least as strong for coronary heart disease mortality as raised blood cholesterol.[57]

Arterial wall

Consideration of how symptoms arise from coronary atherosclerosis must focus on the atheromatous plaque, and knowledge of the pathology in the arterial wall underlying acute myocardial infarction began to be resolved in the 1980s. This was as a result of relating coronary angiograms taken during life with detailed pathological studies. Foremost in Britain were the seminal studies of Davies.[96][97] (See chapter 20 by Davies). He demonstrated that fissuring of atheromatous plaques, progressing to the formation of intraluminal thrombosis, is the dynamic progress that leads to these acute manifestations of coronary heart disease and also to ischaemic death. It became clear that plaque composition is a major determinant of the risk of an ischaemic event, and now ultrasound and thermal imaging enable lipid rich vulnerable plaques to be identified. Furthermore, there is now evidence from clinical regression trials (see below) that lowering of LDL cholesterol leads to improved plaque stability, possible by replacing the lipid core with collagen.

Clinical trials on the reduction or prevention of atheromatous coronary heart disease

The concept of placebo-controlled randomised clinical trials did not emerge until the middle 1960s. Even although these were first developed in the United Kingdom,[98] statistical calculations of power were not properly recognised until the 1970s,[99][100] and the crucial importance of numbers was not delineated until even later when a group in Oxford (led by Peto) was established to coordinate many clinical trials.[101]

An early clinical trial conducted in Edinburgh in 1956, which preceded the definition of a discipline for the conduct and design of clinical trials, was a small controlled five year pilot trial of oestrogen. This was undertaken on the somewhat naive basis that oestrogens might be protective in men since women with normal ovarian function have less coronary heart disease. The trial was conducted in 100 men with coronary disease in order to determine whether plasma cholesterol concentrations and coronary events would be reduced by oestrogen.[102] Plasma lipids were reduced, but there was no benefit in terms of coronary events. Too large a dose of oestrogen was used, gynaecomastia developed, and there was a significant increase in the incidence of venous thromboembolism in the men treated with oestrogen. This went unnoticed until the introduction of the oral contraceptive some years later. In 1968, Inman and Vessey (London) reported an increased incidence in coronary heart disease, cerebrovascular accident, and pulmonary infarction in women taking oral contraceptives,[103] and it has become clear subsequently that these adverse effects were related to the high concentration of oestrogen used.

There have been two UK clinical trials of the effects of changing dietary fats on the incidence of coronary heart disease. The first in 1970 (the MRC trial using a soya bean oil based diet), was too underpowered statistically and badly designed to make it possible to reach any conclusion, although there was not even a hint that such a diet might be beneficial.[104] The second, larger, and better designed trial was conducted in the 1980s by Burr (Cardiff).[105] It suggested that a regular consumption of fish is protective against further coronary events in coronary heart disease patients. This beneficial effect of omega-3 fatty acids has been reinforced recently by the Lyon heart trial.[106]

Six clinical trials – three of clofibrate and three of statins – were carried out in the United Kingdom between 1965 and 1995 to determine whether cholesterol lowering drugs reduce the incidence of coronary heart disease or affect the progress of atherosclerosis related diseases by reducing plasma cholesterol and LDL.

Two clofibrate trials conducted in the 1960s showed a favourable trend as a result of reducing high plasma cholesterol levels in patients with coronary heart disease, but they were too small to be definitive.[107] The WHO clofibrate trial was the first major double-blind randomised primary prevention trial and is still the largest study of lipid lowering ever to be conducted.[65] It was established in 1965 in Edinburgh, and later in centres in Budapest and Prague; the statistical monitoring was conducted in London. Altogether 10 627 men aged 30–59 who were in the upper third of the cholesterol distribution were randomised to receive clofibrate or a placebo (1 g olive oil) daily for 5.3 years. Additionally, there were 5118 men from the lowest third of the cholesterol distribution who received the placebo. Non-fatal myocardial infarction was significantly reduced by 25% and the primary endpoint of myocardial infarction and coronary heart disease death by 20%. But non-coronary heart disease mortality was increased, and the data were compatible with an adverse effect of clofibrate or of cholesterol lowering.

From 1976, when the first results of the WHO clofibrate trial were published, this increase in non-coronary heart disease mortality played an important part for nearly 20 years in raising scepticism about the value of cholesterol lowering. While a recent meta-analysis of lipid lowering trials suggests that the increase in non-coronary heart disease mortality occurred only in the clofibrate trials,[108] this doubt continued until 1994 with the publication of the landmark Scandinavian simvastatin survival study (4S).[109] This trial was carried out in 4444 coronary heart disease patients. It showed a 26% reduction in plasma cholesterol and a 36% reduction in LDL cholesterol with a 29% reduction in total mortality, due to a 41% reduction in coronary heart disease mortality and a 33% reduction in non-fatal myocardial infarction. There was no increase in non-coronary mortality.

The next important trials conducted in the United Kingdom were atheroma regression studies using angiography to quantify the extent of change in atheromatous lesions in the coronary arteries of patients with known coronary heart disease. These trials were randomised and placebo controlled. In the 2-year St Thomas's atherosclerosis regression study, cholesterol lowering by cholestyramine and diet reduced the extent of lesions.[110] In the larger, Multicentre Antiatheroma Study (MAAS), based in the United Kingdom, simvastatin reduced plasma LDL values by 30%, and over the 4 years of the study showed significant regression and non-progression of lesions with the development of fewer small lesions.[112] Along with comparable "regression" trials in the United States and Holland, it was possible to conclude in the early 1990s that marked lowering of cholesterol (and LDL) by statins slowly reduces existing arterial lesions and prevents the development of new lesions.

The first definitive primary prevention trial using a statin was the West of Scotland prevention (WOSCOPS) trial.[112] This was conducted in Glasgow in 6595 middle aged men with a moderately high blood cholesterol concentration and mostly without known vascular disease. The report in 1995 showed results very similar to the 4S secondary prevention trial and established clearly that cholesterol lowering with a safe and effective drug (pravastatin) will reduce the incidence of coronary heart disease without incurring a penalty of increased non-cardiac deaths or unacceptable side effects. This positive result has recently been confirmed by the similar US Air Force/Texas coronary atherosclerosis prevention study (AFCAPS/TexCAPS).[113] These results are now altering the attitude of cardiologists to risk reduction.

The British doctors' trial of aspirin should also be mentioned.[114] This was randomised but not blinded: 5139 male physicians received daily aspirin (500 mg) or no treatment over 6 years. Total mortality was 14% lower (NS) in the aspirin treated group, but the incidence of myocardial infarction or stroke was not reduced. In contrast, the larger, double-blind placebo controlled American physicians' health study showed a highly significant reduction (44%) in myocardial infarction, primarily in those over 50 years.[115]

In conclusion

It is not possible, nor would there be any purpose, to try to reach any conclusion or provide an abstract about atherosclerosis research in the United Kingdom since the second world war. Studies of the relations between thrombosis, lipoproteins, and the arterial wall proceeded rapidly in the 1950s. However, little or no interest was shown by cardiologists and clinicians until 20–25 years later. Before 1975, presentations were made to the Medical Research Society, to biochemical, physiology, and pathology societies and the Atherosclerosis Discussion Group but seldom to the British Cardiac Society where most papers were clinical. Likewise, publication of results of atherosclerosis research went to general journals, such as the *Lancet*, and specialised journals such as *Atherosclerosis Research*, *Clinical Science*, and *Molecular Medicine*, *Lipid Research*, and the *European Journal of Clinical Investigation.*

While many studies have been omitted, and others described superficially, it is hoped that this review will prove to be a useful background for future advances, and provide some knowledge and perspective regarding the early contributions made by investigators in the United Kingdom.

References

1. Osler W. *Angina pectoris and allied states.* New York: Appleton Press, 1897.
2. Moschowitz E. *Vascular sclerosis with special reference to arteriosclerosis.* New York: Oxford University Press, 1942.
3. White PD. *Heart disease.* 3rd ed. New York: Macmillan, 1947.
4. Ryle JA, Russell WT. The natural history of coronary disease. A clinical and epidemiological study. *Br Heart J* 1949;11:370.
5. Wood P. *Diseases of the heart and circulation.* 1st ed. London: Eyre and Spottiswoode, 1950.
6. Gordon I. Mechanism of lipophage deposition in atherosclerosis. *Arch Pathol* 1948;44:247–60.
7. Morris JN. Recent history of coronary disease. *Lancet* 1951;i:1–7, 69–73.
8. Morris JN. *Uses of epidemiology.* 1st ed. Edinburgh: E & S Livingstone, 1957.
9. Doll R, Hill AB. Lung cancer and other causes of death in relation to smoking. *BMJ* 1956;2:1071.
10. World Health Organization. *Classification of atherosclerotic lesions, Standards of methodology and of sites of lesions.* Geneva: WHO, 1958. (Technical report series no 143.)
11. Kannel WB, Castelli WB, McNamara P. Coronary profile: a 12 year follow-up in the Framingham study. *J Occup Med* 1967;9:611.
12. Wood P. *Diseases of the heart and circulation.* 2nd ed. London: Eyre and Spottiswoode, 1956.
13. World Health Organization. *Arterial hypertension and ischaemic heart disease: preventive aspects.* Geneva: WHO, 1962. (Technical report series no 231.)
14. Pickering GW. *High blood pressure.* 1st ed. London: Churchill, 1955. (2nd ed, 1966.)
15. Platt R. The nature of essential hypertension. *Lancet* 1959;ii:55–60.
16. Gofman JW, Lindgren F, Elliott H, Mantz W, Hewitt J, Stissowr B, et al. The role of lipids and lipoproteins in atherosclerosis. *Science* 1950;111:166.
17. Gofman JW, Jones HB, Lyon TP, Lindgren F, Strisower B, Coleman D, et al. Blood lipids and human atherosclerosis. *Circulation* 1952;5:119–34.
18. Ahrens EH, Kunkel HG. The stabilisation of serum lipid emulsions by serum phospholipids. *J Exper Med* 1949;90:409–24.
19. Oliver MF, Boyd GS. The plasma lipids in coronary artery disease. *Br Heart J* 1953;15:387–90.
20. Oliver MF, Boyd GS. Serum lipoprotein patterns in coronary sclerosis and associated conditions. *Br Heart J* 1955;30:410–13.
21. Besterman EMM. Lipoproteins in coronary artery disease. *Br Heart J* 1957;19:503–15.
22. ASPIRE Steering Group. Action of secondary prevention through intervention to reduce events. *Heart* 1996;75:334–42.

23. Keys A, Mickelsen O, Miller E O, Chapman CB. The relation in man between cholesterol levels in the diet and in the blood. *Science* 1950;112:79–87.
24. Keys A. *Coronary heart disease in seven countries. Circulation* 1970;41(suppl 1).
25. Bronte-Stewart B, Keys A, Brock JF. Serum cholesterol, diet and coronary heart disease. An inter-racial survey in the Cape Peninsula. *Lancet* 1955;ii:1103–8.
26. Bronte-Stewart B, Antonis A, Eales L, Brock JF. Effects of feeding different fats on serum-cholesterol level. *Lancet* 1956;i:521–6.
27. Gresham GA, Howard AN. The independent production of atherosclerosis and thrombosis in the rat. *Br J Exp Pathol* 1960;41:395–402.
28. Gresham GA, Howard AN, McQueen J, Bowyer DE. Atherosclerosis in primates. *Br J Exp Pathol* 1965;46:94–103.
29. Sinclair HM. Deficiency of essential fatty acids and atherosclerosis etcetera. *Lancet* 1956;i:381–3.
30. Ahrens EH. Nutritional factors and serum lipid levels. *Am J Med* 1957; 23:928–52.
31. Morris JN, Heady JA, Raffle PAB, Roberts CG, Parks JW. Coronary heart disease and physical activity of work. *Lancet* 1953,ii:1053, 1111.
32. Morris JN, Crawford MD. Coronary heart disease and physical activity of work. *BMJ* 1958;2:1485.
33. Duguid JB. Thrombosis as a factor in pathogenesis of coronary atherosclerosis. *J Pathol Bacteriol* 1946;58:207–12.
34. Duguid JB. Pathogenesis of atherosclerosis. *Lancet*1949;ii:925–7.
35. Crawford T, Levene CI. Incorporation of fibrin in the aortic intima. *J Pathol Bacteriol* 1952;64:523–8.
36. Geiringer E. Intimal vascularisation and atherosclerosis. *J Pathol Bacteriol* 1951;63:201–11.
37. Crawford T. Morphological aspects in the pathogenesis of atherosclerosis. *J Atheroscler Res* 1961;1:3–25.
38. Adams CWM, Bayliss OB. The relationship between diffuse intimal thickness, medial enzyme failure and intimal lipid deposits in various human arteries. *J Atherosclerosis Res* 1969;10:327–39.
39. French JE. Atherosclerosis. In: Florey H, ed. *General pathology.* 2nd ed. London: Lloyd-Luke, 1956.
40. Smith EB. The influence of age and atherosclerosis on the chemistry of aortic intima. *J Atherosclerosis Res* 1965;5:224–40.
41. Walton KW, Williamson N. Histological and immunofluorescent studies of the evolution of the human atheromatous plaque. *J Atherosclerosis Res* 1968;8:599–624.
42. Smith EB, Slater RS. Relationship between low-density lipoprotein in aortic intima and serum-lipid levels. *Lancet* 1972;i:463–69.
43. Fulton WFM. Chronic generalized myocardial ischaemia with advanced coronary artery disease. *Br Heart J* 1956;18:341–54.
44. Fulton WFM. The dynamic factor in enlargement of coronary arterial anastomoses and paradoxical changes in the subendocardial plexus. *Br Heart J* 1964;26:39–50.
45. Macfarlane RG. Reactions of blood to injury. In: Florey H, ed. *General pathology.* 2nd ed London: Lloyd-Luke, 1958.
46. Moncada S, Palmer RMJ, Higgs EA. Biosynthesis of nitric oxide from L-arginine: a pathway for the regulation of cell function and communication. *Biochem Pharmacol* 1989;38:1709–15.
47. Robinson DS, Poole JCF. The similar effect of chylomicra and ethanolamine phosphatide on the generation of thrombin during coagulation. *Q J Exp Physiol* 1956;41:36–49.
48. Woolf N, Pilkington TRE, Carstairs KC. The occurrence of lipoprotein in thrombi. *J Pathol Bacteriol* 1966;91:383–7.
49. Born GVR. Changes in the distribution of phosphorus in platelet-rich plasma during clotting. *Biochem J* 1958;68,695–704.
50. Born GVR. Aggregation of blood platelets by adenosine diphosphate and its reversal. *Nature* 1962;194:927–9.
51. Born GVR, Cross MJ. The aggregation of blood platelets. *J Physiol* 1963,168: 178–95.
52. Vane JR. Inhibition of prostaglandin synthesis as a mechanism of action for aspirin-like drugs. *Nature New Biol* 1971;231:232–5.
53. Moncada S, Gryglewski R, Bunting S, Vane JR. An enzyme isolated from arteries transforms prostaglandin endoperoxides to an unstable substance that inhibits platelet aggregation. *Nature* 1976;163: 663–5.
54. Fulton WFM. Does coronary thrombosis cause myocardial infarction or vice-versa? In: Weatherall D, ed. *Advanced medicine.* London: Pitman Medical, 1978:138–47.
55. Davies MJ, Thomas A. Thrombosis and acute coronary artery lesions in sudden cardiac ischaemic death. *N Engl J Med* 1994;310:1137–40.
56. Meade TW, Chakrabarti R. Arterial disease research: observation or intervention. *Lancet* 1972;ii:913–6.
57. Meade TW, Mellows S, Brozovic M, Miller GJ, Chakrabarti R, North WRS, et al. Haemostatic function and ischaemic heart disease: principal results of the Northwick park heart study. *Lancet* 1986;ii:533–7.

58. Smith EB, Staples EM. Haemostatic factors in human aortic intima *Lancet* 1981;i:1171–4.
59. Oliver MF, Boyd GS. The clearing by heparin of alimentary lipaemia in coronary artery disease. *Clin Sci* 1953;12:293–7.
60. Robinson DS, Harris PM, Poole JCF, Jeffries GH. The effect of a fat meal on the concentration of free fatty acids in human plasma. *Biochem J* 1955;60:xxxvii.
61. Mitchell JRA. Inhibition of heparin clearing by platelets. *Lancet* 1959;i:169–72.
62. Oliver MF, Boyd GS. Changes in the plasma lipids during the menstrual cycle. *Clin Sci* 1953;12:217–22.
63. Sznajderman M, Oliver MF. Spontaneous premature menopause, ischaemic heart disease and serum lipids. *Lancet* 1963;i:962–5.
64. Oliver MF. Further observations on the effects of Atromid and of ethylchlorophenoxyisobutyrate on serum lipid levels. *J Atherosclerosis Res* 1963;3:427–44.
65. Report from the Committee of the Principal Investigators. A cooperative trial in the primary prevention of ischaemic heart disease using clofibrate. *Br Heart J* 1978;40;1069–118.
66. Miller GJ, Miller NE. Plasma high density lipoprotein concentration and development of ischaemic heart disease. *Lancet* 1975;i:16–19.
67. Miller NE, Forde OH, Thelle DS, Mjos OD. The Tromso heart study: high density lipoprotein and coronary heart disease: a prospective case control study. *Lancet* 1977;i:1965–8.
68. Shepherd J, Packard CJ, Patsch JR, Gotto AM, Taunton OD. Effects of dietary polyunsaturated and saturated fat on the properties of high density lipoproteins and the metabolism of apolipoprotein A1. *J Clin Invest* 1978;61;1582–92.
69. Rose GA, Blackburn H. *Cardiovascular survey methods.* Geneva, World Health Organization, 1968.
70. Brown MS, Goldstein JL. A receptor mediated pathway for cholesterol homeostasis. *Science* 1986;232:34–47.
71. Shepherd J, Bicker S, Lorimer AR, Packard CJ. Receptor mediated low density lipoprotein catabolism in man. *J Lipid Res* 1979;20:999–1006.
72. Myant NB. *The biology of cholesterol and related steroids.* London: Heinemann, 1981.
73. Gertler MM, White PD. *Coronary heart disease in young adults.* Cambridge, MA: Harvard University Press, 1953.
74. Rose GA. Familial patterns in ischaemic heart disease. *J Epidemiol Community Health* 1964;18:75–80.
75. Slack J, Evans KA. The increased risk of death from ischaemic heart disease in first-degree relatives of 121 men and 96 women with ischaemic heart disease. *J Med Genet* 1966;3:239–57.
76. Slack J. Risks of ischaemic heart disease in familial hyperlipoproteinaemia. *Lancet* 1969;ii:1380–82.
77. Myant NB. *Cholesterol metabolism, LDL and the LDL receptor.* San Diego and London: Academic Press, 1990.
78. Thompson GR, Lowenthal R, Myant NB. Plasma exchange in the management of homozygous familial hypercholesterolaemia. *Lancet* 1975;i:1208–11.
79. Higgins MJ, Lecamwasam DS, Galton D. A new type of familial hypercholesterolaemia. *Lancet* 1975;ii:737–40.
80. Humphries SE, Kessling AM, Horsthemke B, Donald JA, Seed M, Jowett N, et al. A common DNA polymorphism of the low-density lipoprotein (LDL) receptor gene and its use in diagnosis. *Lancet* 1985;i:1003–5.
81. Humphries SE, Cook M, Dubowitz M, Stirling Y, Meade TW. Role of genetic variation at the fibrinogen locus in determination of plasma fibrinogen concentrations. *Lancet* 1987;i:1452–5.
82. Carlson LA, Böttiger LE. Ischaemic heart disease in relation to fasting values of plasma triglycerides and cholesterol. *Lancet* 1972;i:865–70.
83. Logan RL, Riemersma RA, Thomson M, Oliver MF, Olsson AG, Walding G. et al. Risk factors in ischaemic heart disease in normal men, aged 40. *Lancet* 1978;i:949–55.]
84. Reaven GM. Role of insulin resistance in human disease. *Diabetes* 1988;37:1595–607.
85. Reid DD, Hamilton PJS, McCartney P, Rose G, Jarrett RJ, Keen H. Smoking and other risk factors for coronary heart disease in British civil servants. *Lancet* 1976;ii:979–84.
86. Marmot MG, Adelstein AM, Robinson N, Rose AG. Changing social-class distribution of heart disease. *BMJ* 1978;2:1109–12.
87. Marmot MG. Life style and national and international trends in coronary heart disease mortality. *Postgrad Med J* 1984;60:3–8.
88. Rose GA. Strategy of prevention: lessons from cardiovascular disease. *BMJ* 1981;282:1847–50.
89. Shaper AG, Pocock SJ, Walker M, Cohen NM, Wale CJ, Thomson AG. British regional heart study: cardiovascular risk factors in middle aged men in 24 towns. *BMJ* 1981;283:179–86.
90. Elford J, Phillips AN, Thomson AG, Shaper AG. Migration and geographic variations in ischaemic heart disease in Great Britain. *Lancet* 1989;i:343–6.
91. Barker DJP, Osmond C. Infant mortality, childhood nutrition, and ischaemic heart disease in England and Wales. *Lancet* 1986;i:1077–81.

92. Barker DJP. Winter PD, Osmond C, Margetts B, Simmonds SJ. Weight in infancy and death from ischaemic heart disease. *Lancet* 1989;ii:577–80.
93. Wood DA, Butler S, Riemersma RA, Thomson M, Oliver MF. Adipose tissue and platelet fatty acids and coronary heart disease in Scottish men. *Lancet* 1984;ii:117–21.
94. Riemersma RA, Wood DA, Macintyre CAA, Elton RA, Gey KF, Oliver MF. Risk of angina pectoris and plasma concentrations of vitamins A, C, and E and carotene. *Lancet* 1991;337:1–5.
95. Meade TW, North WRS, Chakrabarti R, Stirling Y, Haines AP, Thompson SG. Haemostatic function and cardiovascular death: early results of a prospective study. *Lancet* 1980;i:1050–4.
96. Davies MJ, Thomas AC. Plasma fissuring – the cause of myocardial infarction, sudden ischaemic death, and crescendo angina. *Br Heart J* 1985;53:363–73.
97. Davies MJ. Stability and instability: two faces of coronary atherosclerosis. *Circulation* 1996;94:2013–20.
98. Hill AB. *Statistical methods in clinical and preventive medicine.* Edinburgh and London: E & S Livingstone, 1962.
99. Armitage P. *Statistical methods in medical research.* Oxford: Blackwell, 1971.
100. Armitage P. *Sequential medical trials.* New York: Wiley, 1972.
101. Yusuf S, Collins, Peto R. Why do we need some large, simple randomised trials? *Stat Med* 1984;3:409–20.
102. Oliver MF, Boyd GS. Influence of reduction of serum lipids on prognosis of coronary heart disease – a five year study using oestrogen. *Lancet* 1961;ii:499–505.
103. Inman WHW, Vessey MP. Investigation of death from pulmonary, coronary and cerebral thrombosis and embolism in women of child-bearing age. *BMJ* 1968;2:193–9.
104. Controlled trial of soya-bean oil in myocardial infarction – (MRC trial). *Lancet* 1968;ii:693–700.
105. Burr ML, Fehily AM, Gilbert JF, Rogers S, Holliday RM, Sweetman PM, et al. Effects of changes in fat, fish, and fibre intakes on death and myocardial reinfarction: diet and reinfarction trial (DART). *Lancet* 1989;ii:757–61.
106. De Lorgeril M, Salen P, Martin J-L, Monjaud I, Delaye J, Mamelle N. Mediterranean diet, traditional risk factors, and the rate of cardiovascular complications after myocardial infarction: final report of the Lyon diet heart study. *Circulation* 1999;99:779–85.
107. Dewar HA, Oliver MF. Secondary prevention trials using clofibrate: a joint commentary on the Newcastle and Scottish trials. *BMJ* 1971;4:784–6.
108. Gould LA, Rossouw JE, Santanello NC, Heyse JF, Furberg CD. Cholesterol reduction yields clinical benefit. A new look at old data. *Circulation* 1995;91:2274–82.
109. Scandinavian Simvastatin Survival Study Group. Randomised trial of cholesterol lowering in 4444 patient with coronary heart disease: the Scandinavian simvastatin survival study (4 S). *Lancet* 1994;344:1383–89.
110. Watts GF, Lewis B, Brunt JNH, Lewis ES, Coltart DJ, Smith LDR, et al. Effects on coronary artery disease of lipid-lowering diet, or diet plus cholestyramine, in the St Thomas' atherosclerosis regression study (STARS). *Lancet* 1992;339:563–9.
111. MAAS Investigators. Effect of simvastatin on coronary atheroma: the multicentre anti-atheroma study. *Lancet* 1994;344:633–38.
112. Shepherd J, Cobbe SM, Ford I, Isles CG, Lorimer AR, Macfarlane PW, et al. Prevention of coronary heart disease with pravastatin in men with hypercholesterolemia. *N Engl J Med* 1995;333:1301–7.
113. Downs JR, Clearfield M, Weis S, Whitney E, Shapiro DR, Beere PA, et al. Primary prevention of acute coronary events with lovastatin in men and women with average cholesterol levels. Results of AFCAPS/TexCAPS. *JAMA* 1998;279:1615–22.
114. Peto R, Gray R, Collins R, Wheatley V, Hennekens C, Jamrozik K, et al. Randomised trial of prophylactic aspirin in British male doctors. *BMJ* 1988;296:313–16
115. Physicians' Health Study. Final report of the aspirin component of the ongoing physicians' health study. *N Engl J Med* 1989;321:129–35.

Chapter 27

Clinical Coronary Heart Disease

Desmond Julian

Cardiologists did not regard coronary heart disease as an important part of their specialty until well after the second world war. General practitioners or general physicians cared for most patients with angina and myocardial infarction, and it was not until the advent of coronary care units and the development of techniques such as arteriography and echocardiography that it was appreciated (at least in the United Kingdom) that cardiologists had an essential role in the diagnosis and management of coronary heart disease.

Myocardial infarction – 1945–60

The diagnosis of myocardial infarction in the early years after the second world war depended largely upon the medical history, supplemented by the three lead electrocardiogram. Portable electrocardiograms were relatively rare, and because the records were photographic and needed developing, they were difficult to use in the home, where most patients were treated. Although chest leads had been developed in the 1930s, they were not used widely until the 1950s. Thus, in the textbook *Diseases of the Heart* written by the Glasgow cardiologist Fitzgerald Peel in 1947, all the tracings illustrated were of three leads.[1] However, when Paul Wood's first edition of *Diseases of the Heart and Circulation* came out in 1950,[2] there were many examples of 12 lead records. Confirmation of the diagnosis by measuring cardiac enzymes was not available until the 1960s.

Bed rest

Management was confined largely to the relief of pain by opioids and to bed rest, which was implemented strictly. In Thomas Lewis's third edition, published in 1946, a total of 200 words were devoted to the treatment of myocardial infarction.[3] These included the following:

> Rest in bed should continue for from 6 to 8 weeks to ensure firm cicatrisation of the ventricular wall; during the whole of this period the patient is to be guarded by day and night nursing and helped in every way to avoid voluntary movement or effort. Patients have lost their lives and especially those who have early recovered from their symptoms by neglect of these precautions.

All physicians advised prolonged bed rest at this time, although some were less draconian than Lewis. Peel, for example, disagreed with the 6 weeks minimum and thought that patients with milder disease might become ambulatory at 4 weeks. Nonetheless, he recommended total bed rest and no visitors for the first 2 weeks. As late as 1959, Wood was still recommending 3 to 6 weeks bed rest or longer, depending on the severity of the infarction.[4]

Anticoagulants and pressor drugs

In the 1950s, two other forms of treatment were coming to the fore – anticoagulants and pressor drugs. Wright et al. had published results of a non-randomised study initiated by a special committee of the American Heart Association in which 432 patients treated with oral anticoagulants were compared with 368 controls.[5] Mortality was 15% in the treated patients and 24% in the controls. The enthusiasm engendered in the United States by these findings soon spread to the United Kingdom, especially after Gilchrist and Tulloch reported in 1954 that oral anticoagulants halved mortality in a study of 321 patients.[6] Because of this, many physicians began to admit patients with myocardial infarction to hospital for treatment. But there were also many sceptics such as William Evans who derided the use of "rat poison."[7] In 1959, Wood recommended heparin followed by oral anticoagulants, but he believed the claims of reductions in mortality were exaggerated.[4] He pointed out that the incidence of pulmonary embolism at that time was 15%, but only about 3% of patients with myocardial infarction died of this cause, and systemic embolism was responsible for no more than 2% of deaths.

After the report of Griffiths et al. in 1954, pressor amines became standard treatment of shock.[8] Wood stated dogmatically that "Shock has been treated actively in recent years and its mortality has been reduced from 80% to 50%." This was the widespread belief at this time. Other drugs were used with caution. Nitrates were considered to be contraindicated, and there were anxieties about using digitalis. Oxygen and mercurial diuretics were given to patients with acute cardiac failure.

Mortality associated with in-hospital treatment for acute myocardial infarction was high. In 1962, Peel reported a 28 day mortality of 28%.[9] On the basis of experience in the 1950s, Peel had formulated a prognostic index. The index was in widespread use internationally until 1969 when it was replaced by a more up to date index developed by Robin Norris of Auckland.[9][10]

Myocardial infarction – 1960 onward

In the preface to his second edition of *Diseases of the Heart and Circulation*,[4] published in 1956, Wood applauded the rapid advances made by cardiology in the preceding years, especially in the field of congenital heart disease and acquired valve disease. However, he made no mention of ischaemic heart disease.

The coronary care unit

It is reasonable to ascribe the sudden explosion of interest in coronary disease to the work on closed chest cardiac resuscitation undertaken by Kouwenhoven et al. of Johns Hopkins which was published in 1960.[11] The obvious potential of this technique and the difficulties of applying it effectively in the hospital environment of the time led Julian in 1961 to put forward the idea of what came to be known as the coronary care unit.[12] The setting up of these units developed rapidly in North America and Australia, but only slowly in the United Kingdom. However, there was an increasing interest in the haemodynamic aspects of acute heart attacks – important observations were being made by Jack Shillingford's group in the Hammersmith Hospital, London[13] and Kenneth Donald's team in Edinburgh.[14]

The eminent epidemiologists Archie Cochrane and Geoffrey Rose questioned the effectiveness of coronary care units. In 1972, Cochrane wrote, "the battle for coronary care is just beginning," and he was enthusiastic about the possibility of randomised controlled studies to test their effectiveness.[15] Rose was very critical of the early units for not comparing their experiences before and after the introduction of coronary care.[16] In fact, many such comparisons were made, and reasons were given for the difficulty, if not the impossibility, of conducting valid controlled trials of coronary care units.[17] Nonetheless, randomised trials were undertaken of home versus hospital treatment in Bristol and the south west of England,[18] and in Nottingham.[19] Both studies concluded that there was little or no benefit from hospital treatment, but it is obvious, in retrospect, that they were not powered to answer the question, and patients were entered so late into the trials that it was most unlikely that a benefit could be shown. However, criticisms of the coronary care unit influenced strongly the policy of the Department of Health, which failed conspicuously to support their development in the United Kingdom.

Prevention and treatment of arrhythmias

At first, the primary concern of coronary care units was treating cardiac arrest. However, it seemed that ventricular fibrillation was frequently preceded by what were termed "warning arrhythmias," and attention was focused on the vigorous suppression of arrhythmia. This focus was epitomised by the work of Lown, who stated at the first international conference on coronary care (held in Edinburgh in 1967) that he had never seen primary ventricular fibrillation because it could be prevented by the use of lidocaine (lignocaine) for warning arrhythmias. Intense efforts to detect and treat arrhythmias resulted, and nurses were taught that detection was a prime responsibility. However, it was subsequently claimed that detection was of little value.[20][21] Many units began to use intravenous lignocaine routinely until it was found that this practice might increase rather than reduce mortality in myocardial infarction.

Pre-hospital coronary care

Frank Pantridge of Belfast pioneered the concept and practice of pre-hospital coronary care in 1966.[22] Mobile coronary care was achieved at the Royal Victoria Hospital, Belfast by sending out an appropriately equipped ambulance manned by a doctor. Pantridge was soon able to report successful resuscitations outside hospital, but his initiative was not followed widely in the United Kingdom because its cost effectiveness was doubted. However, several centres, notably Brighton, soon started schemes utilising specially trained and equipped ambulance personnel. The Department of Health was sceptical about this approach, as were many ambulance staff, and mobile care was resisted until the mid 1980s. In 1986, the British Heart Foundation mounted a major charitable campaign to provide ambulances with defibrillators (provided there were reassurances that ambulance staff had been trained suitably). A few years later, the Department changed its viewpoint. It actively encouraged the training of ambulance personnel in resuscitation techniques and supplied the remaining ambulance services with defibrillators. As a consequence, by the 1990s, virtually all ambulance services provided good quality resuscitation carried out by well trained paramedics.

Pump failure

It soon became apparent that coronary care units were reducing the mortality due to arrhythmias and conduction disorders, but little, if any, advance was being made in the prevention and management of the serious complications of acute heart failure and cardiogenic shock. The Myocardial Infarction Research Unit (MIRU) programme in the United States contributed, inter alia, to two important developments – the introduction of invasive monitoring (mainly through the use of the Swan–Ganz catheter) and the concept of limiting the size of the infarct. In the United Kingdom, unlike the United States, invasive monitoring was not taken up very widely except in specialised units. Heart failure and shock in the acute phase of infarction were managed largely on traditional lines until the benefits of the early use of angiotensin converting enzyme inhibitors were shown by the Oxford based ISIS-4 study of infarct survival and the Italian GISSI-3 studies in the early 1990s.[23][24]

Limiting infarct size

Because of the poor outcome of treating pump failure and cardiogenic shock, there was great optimism that strategies that reduced infarct size in animal experiments would do the same in humans. Numerous trials were undertaken with drugs such as calcium antagonists and hyaluronidase, but only the trials with β blockers showed a beneficial effect.[25] In fact, the benefit achieved in the largest trial (ISIS-1)[25] seemed to be due mainly to the prevention of cardiac rupture rather than limitation of infarct size. Although many British coronary care units participated in this trial, few British cardiologists incorporated routine intravenous β blockade into their practice. In a recent survey, only 0.5% of patients with acute myocardial infarction in British hospitals received intravenous β blockade.[26]

Fibrinolytic and antithrombotic therapy

Undoubtedly, reperfusion with thrombolytic agents was second only to the introduction of the coronary care unit itself in improving the management of myocardial infarction. Although first introduced in the 1950s, and strongly advocated by Chazov of Moscow at the Edinburgh conference in 1967, it took the Oxford based ISIS-2[27] and the Italian GISSI[28] studies of streptokinase in the mid 1980s to influence cardiological practice generally. By the time these studies were published, it was evident that genetically engineered tissue plasminogen activator produced more effective thrombolysis – although at the risk of an increase in cerebral haemorrhage. ISIS-3 [29] and GISSI-2 [30] were set up to compare these agents, and it was concluded that there was little to choose between them. The relatively cheap drug, streptokinase, therefore became the agent of choice in the United Kingdom. It remains so, despite evidence from GUSTO[31] and other studies that tissue plasminogen activator and similar drugs are better, at least in high risk patients.

As in other countries, there was concern in Britain that too few eligible patients were receiving thrombolytic therapy, and that those given this treatment were prescribed it too long after the onset of symptoms. The British Heart Foundation hosted a conference that produced guidelines on the use of thrombolysis and recommended that the time from first medical care to starting thrombolytic therapy should not exceed 90 minutes.[32] Rawles and the GREAT study investigators in Scotland had shown that general practitioners could administer thrombolytic treatment faster and more effectively than was possible if the drug was given only in hospital.[33]

In a survey of 39 British hospitals undertaken between 1992 and 1995, the Myocardial Infarction Audit Group[34] reported that 71.6% of patients with proved myocardial infarction received thrombolytic therapy.[34] This was a high figure by international standards, but the groups selected to participate may have had a better than average performance in delivering thrombolysis.

The finding of ISIS-2[27] that aspirin also reduced mortality was very important and passed swiftly into practice in the United Kingdom. A recent survey in three cities (Brighton, York, and Cardiff) showed that aspirin was administered to 88% of patients during the acute phase.[35]

Percutaneous transluminal coronary angioplasty

Studies in the United States and continental Europe have shown that angioplasty is at least as effective as thrombolysis. However, relatively few coronary care units in the United Kingdom have been suitably staffed and equipped to undertake emergency percutaneous coronary angioplasty, and so, to date, this treatment has been confined largely to tertiary centres.

Secondary prevention after myocardial infarction

In the 1950s and 1960s, attention was focused on the use of anticoagulants in the long term prevention of recurrent infarction and death. Paul Wood recommend their use in 1956, but felt that they were still under trial.[4] In the Medical Research Council's subsequent long term trial of anticoagulants, published in 1964, 21.3% of the control group compared with 14.9% of the intervention group died at a mean follow up of 25 months ($p = 0.03$).[36] Some took this as convincing evidence of efficacy. For example, Gilchrist of Edinburgh, who had experienced a myocardial infarction that year, continued to take warfarin until his death 30 years later! Others were sceptical. Mitchell of Nottingham pointed out that the trial was stopped prematurely when it seemed that a "positive" result was likely, and

Abbreviations for studies and study groups

AIRE:	Acute Infarction Ramipril Efficacy
BHAT:	β Blocker Heart Attack Study
GISSI-1:	Gruppo Italiano per lo Studio Della Streptokinase Nell'Infarto Miocardico
GISSI-3:	Gruppo Italiano per lo Studio Supravvivenza nell'infarto Miocardico
GREAT:	Grampian Region Early Anistreplase Trial
GUSTO:	Global Utilization of Streptokinase and Tissue plasminogen activator for Occluded coronary arteries
HINT:	Holland Interuniversity Nifedipine/metoprolol Trial
ISIS:	International Study of Infarct Survival
RITA-3:	Randomised Intervention Treatment of Angina
SAVE:	Survival And Ventricular Enlargement
TRACE:	Trandolapril Cardiac Evaluation

the participants thought it unethical to continue the trial.[37] Cardiologists were divided in their views on this topic, but when it seemed that aspirin was also effective, few physicians continued to prescribe anticoagulants routinely.

β blockade for secondary prevention was first studied in the early 1970s. Two small Swedish studies suggested benefit, but the multicentre international study on practolol,[38] based in the United Kingdom, ended unfortunately and prematurely. The study had intended to recruit 4000 patients, but after 3053 subjects had been randomised, it was found that the drug produced an oculo-cutaneous syndrome and plastic peritonitis. The study was promising in that there was a nearly significant reduction in mortality (8.2% in the placebo group, 6.3% in the practolol group; $p = 0.051$). Physicians were then wary of β blockers, and the subsequent negative propranolol study of only 729 patients was probably too small to show any benefit.[39] However, when the Norwegian timolol study [40] and the American BHAT study[41] showed that β blockers were effective in preventing reinfarction and reducing mortality, prescribing these drugs after infarction became standard practice. British physicians have remained cautious, probably because of fears of inducing or aggravating heart failure, and the recent European secondary prevention study[42] has shown that only 34% of British patients who had had an infarct were discharged home on β blocker treatment compared with 54% across Europe and 77% in Sweden.

Antiarrhythmic drugs were never used as enthusiastically in British hospitals as they were elsewhere, perhaps because Holter monitoring after infarction was infrequent. The only major British study of an antiarrhythmic drug in this context was similar to other studies in that it showed a non-significant increase in mortality in patients taking mexiletine compared with those on placebo.[42]

The suggestion that angiotensin converting enzyme inhibitors given a few days after the onset of myocardial infarction might prevent infarct expansion and the development of heart failure in patients was proved convincingly by the AIRE study based in Leeds.[43] This study, whose conclusions were similar to those of the SAVE[44] and TRACE[45] studies, led to the routine use of angiotensin converting enzyme inhibitors during the acute period in patients who had experienced heart failure or in those with seriously impaired left ventricular function.

Unstable angina

Heberden recognised that there was a high risk of death if angina was becoming rapidly more severe.[46] In the succeeding two centuries this has been commented on frequently, both in medical and lay publications. Herrick had pointed out that myocardial infarction was often preceded by attacks of angina.[47] This phenomenon was well documented by Stowers and Short from Aberdeen.[48] They noted in 1970 that 55% of patients with proved myocardial infarction had experienced the onset or intensification of attacks of chest pain in the preceding two months.

The topic was bedevilled by problems of nomenclature. Many terms were used to describe the syndrome, including "impending acute coronary occlusion," "intermediate coronary syndrome," "coronary failure," "pre-infarction angina," and "the prodromal syndrome." Wood used "impending infarction" and "acute and sub-acute coronary insufficiency."[49] Objections were raised to several of these descriptions because they implied foreknowledge of the outcome, whereas most patients did not proceed to either myocardial infarction or death, even in the absence of treatment. The term "unstable angina" was adopted widely in the early 1970s onward and has remained popular.

Anticoagulants and aspirin

The natural history of unstable angina was much debated. In 1961, Wood reported a 30% mortality and 22% myocardial infarction rate at 2 months in 50 patients who had not received anticoagulants.[49] He claimed to have reduced the mortality to 6% by using heparin. Others had also reported a very high complication rate, but in 1972, Krauss et al. from Boston reported a 1% mortality and a 7% myocardial infarction rate in hospital in 100 patients with acute coronary insufficiency.[50]

In a community survey in Edinburgh in the early 1970s, patients with new or worsening angina were seen promptly in a special chest pain clinic.[51] Of 251 patients taking no treatment other than nitrates who were followed for 6 months, 31 (13%) developed myocardial infarction and nine (4%) died. Because of the relatively low incidence of adverse events in this and other studies at that time, the initial enthusiasm for anticoagulants waned. Fulton and Julian wrote in 1977, "Although there are still those who use either heparin or oral anticoagulants for this syndrome, most physicians have now abandoned this form of treatment."[52] In the mid 1980s, both the United States Veterans Administration study [53] and the study of Cairns et al.[54] from Canada showed the effectiveness of aspirin in unstable angina. Aspirin therapy then became standard practice and the debate continued about the concomitant use of heparin and other anticoagulants.

Nitrates had been used traditionally to treat this condition, and β blockers became popular in the 1970s. About the same time, the role of spasm in rest angina had been shown by coronary angiography, and it was thought that this might play an important part in the unstable angina syndrome. Since it had been observed that calcium antagonists (notably nifedipine) could reverse coronary spasm while β blockers might aggravate it, β blockers with nitrates were replaced by calcium antagonists as first line treatment in many units. This trend was reversed after publication of the HINT trial, which showed that in this context nifedipine alone was worse than placebo, but could be usefully added to a β blocker when the latter was not fully effective on its own.[55]

Role of coronary angiography

Practice regarding the role of coronary angiography in the management of unstable angina differed appreciably. In the 1970s, some units started to undertake routine early angiography in the belief that coronary artery bypass surgery was urgently indicated in this condition. This enthusiasm was dampened when studies from the United States suggested no benefit from urgent surgery.

A recurrence of enthusiam for angiography occurred when it was shown that coronary angioplasty could dramatically relieve symptoms in patients who did not respond to drug treatment, and subsequently in most centres angiography and angioplasty were largely restricted to this group. The precise indications for these procedures remain uncertain but are being studied in the RITA-III trial. Practices in the United States and the United Kingdom were compared by the Antithrombotic Therapy in Acute Coronary Syndromes Research Group in 1998.[56] The study found that coronary angiography was performed in 61% of cases in the United States but in only 22% in the United Kingdom. Revascularisation in the absence of recurrent angina was performed in 19% and 4% respectively.

Variant angina

In 1959, Prinzmetal described what is now the eponymous or variant angina syndrome.[57] Few cases were described in the United Kingdom until Attilio Maseri, then of Pisa, reported an impressive series in which the condition had resulted from coronary artery spasm in the presence of vessels that seemed otherwise normal.[58] Interest in variant angina intensified when Maseri became professor of cardiology at the Royal Postgraduate Medical School in 1979. It then became common practice to infuse ergometrine during cardiac catheterisation, especially in patients with unstable angina. It soon became apparent that pure spasm was responsible in only a few cases, but that tonic changes could be a material factor in both stable and unstable angina.

Stable angina

Diagnosis

Since the time of Heberden, the diagnosis of stable angina has depended fundamentally on the history, and it remains so. However, with increasing knowledge of the possible causes of the syndrome, and with effective and specific means of preventing and treating it, the aetiology and the severity of the underlying lesion must be determined in each patient. The physical examination is important in establishing the underlying diagnosis, and was particularly so formerly when disorders such as syphilitic aortitis and mitral stenosis could be responsible. In recent years, the only relatively common non-coronary causes in the United Kingdom have been aortic stenosis and cardiomyopathy. Consequently, most cases are due to coronary artery disease and the main issue is to confirm the diagnosis and to assess the extent of disease and its impact on the myocardium.

Master had introduced the two-step exercise test in 1935, and his method was widely practised in the United Kingdom.[59] In 1956, Wood wrote, "the only reliable test . . . is to obtain an electrocardiogram immediately after effort when characteristic depression of the RS-T segment, with or without inversion of the U wave, clinches the diagnosis."[60] Another technique that was popular in some centres at this time was to take electrocardiograms while the patient breathed 10% oxygen for 20 minutes. Wood did not regard this test highly because of its poor sensitivity and specificity.

In the 1960s, it was recognised that the Master test was inadequate, and Swedish and American investigators developed new methods – a bicycle ergometer and a treadmill respectively. Different centres in the United Kingdom followed one or other method, but eventually most cardiology units adopted the treadmill because cycling is unfamiliar to many British patients. Sowton and Balcon developed atrial pacing as an alternative method of inducing stress in patients with suspected angina.[60]

Nuclear imaging, as a technique for measuring blood flow and myocardial function, is described in Chapter 12. Although highly developed in some places, its use in assessing angina has been limited largely to tertiary centres in the United Kingdom.

Coronary angiography arrived in the United Kingdom not long after Mason Sones of Cleveland described it in 1962,[61] but it was not commonly used for diagnosis until coronary artery bypass surgery had become established. Practice has varied widely between centres. In some, almost all patients with suspected angina are catheterised routinely, while in others the procedure is confined to patients in whom intervention seems likely. (See also Chapter 11.)

Treatment

Until the introduction of β blockers in the 1960s, management of stable angina pectoris had not changed very much since the beginning of the century. Emphasis was always placed on the general management of the patient, with particular caution with regard to exercise and the avoidance of physical and mental stress. Wood (himself a heavy smoker) recommended that cigarette smoking should be limited to 10–15 a day.[4]

Sublingual glyceryl trinitrate was the standard agent for preventing and treating angina, but long acting nitrates were not considered effective, except by a few enthusiasts. Several treatments were used, including theophylline preparations, perhexilene, prenylamine, and khellin. Khellin, an extract of *Ammi visnaga*, an eastern Mediterranean plant, was said to be effective, but it was poorly tolerated and was largely abandoned. It has, however, re-emerged in the synthetic preparation of amiodarone.

β blockade for angina was introduced in the late 1960s and rapidly became widely used. In general, it was prescribed for patients for whom sublingual nitrate treatment was insufficient.

Verapamil was the first calcium antagonist drug to be used (although its precise pharmacology was not initially understood). It was mainly reserved for patients who did not respond to β blockers, and the danger of combining verapamil with β blockade was soon appreciated. Nifedipine followed in the 1970s and was taken up with enthusiasm, particularly for patients in whom coronary artery spasm was thought to be a factor. Combined treatment with nifedipine and a β blocker became popular, and remains so.

Coronary artery surgery for angina developed relatively slowly in the United Kingdom (see Chapter 16). The Vineberg operation was practised on a limited scale, but the success of saphenous vein bypass grafts in relieving angina was soon apparent, and a number of major centres adopted the technique. Questions about the effectiveness of coronary bypass surgery in reducing mortality led to participation in the European coronary surgery study. [62]

Percutaneous transluminal coronary angioplasty was introduced shortly after Grüntzig's original description of the technique in the *Lancet* in 1977.[63] The development of this therapeutic method is discussed in detail in Chapter 11.

Guidelines for managing stable angina

Because of the number of treatments available for managing angina pectoris, and their varying cost, several guidelines have been issued. A Working Party of the Joint Audit Committee of the British Cardiac Society and the Royal College of Physicians of London published recommendations on the investigation and management of stable angina pectoris in 1993.[64] An important objective was to lay down standards by which the quality of care provided by health professionals and health authorities could be judged. An updated version of this report was published in 1999.[65] Concern about the escalating expense of treating angina led to the publication in 1998 of *Resource allocation for chronic stable angina: a systematic review of effectiveness, costs, and cost-effectiveness of alternative interventions* – a report by the Health Economics Research Group.[66]

In conclusion

At the end of the century, despite the enormous fall in mortality, coronary heart disease remains the greatest single cause of death and morbidity in the United Kingdom. Indeed, with the ageing population and better survival among those who would previously have died from the disorder, the prevalence of coronary heart disease in the community is set to rise. Only when primary prevention is successful will the burden of coronary heart disease diminish.

References and notes

1. Peel AAF. *Diseases of the heart*. London: Oxford University Press,1947:292.
2. Wood P. *Diseases of the heart and circulation*. London: Eyre and Spottiswoode, 1950.
3. Lewis T. *Disease of the heart*. 3rd ed. London: Macmillan, 1946:60.
4. Wood P. *Diseases of the heart and circulation*. 2nd ed. London: Eyre and Spottiswoode, 1956 (reprinted 1959).
5. Wright IS, Marple CD, Beck DF. Report of the committee for the evaluation of anticoagulants in the treatment of coronary thrombosis with myocardial infarction. *Am Heart J* 1948;36:801–15.
6. Gilchrist AR, Tulloch JA. Anticoagulants in coronary disease. *BMJ* 1954;2:720.
7. William Evans. (1895–1988) Cardiologist on the staff of the National Heart and London Hospitals. Proud to be a Welshman, he was both a lay preacher and a Druid. He enjoyed controversy. He held strong views on the dangers of anticoagulants and stated that he could recognise incompetence when he saw it but not mitral incompetence. He made important contributions to electrocardiography and was perhaps the first (with Clifford Allbutt) in 1929 to undertake a controlled trial in angina.
8. Griffiths.GC. The treatment of shock associated with myocardial infarction. *Circulation* 1954;9:527–32.
9. Peel AAF, Semple T, Wang I, Lancaster WM, Dall JLC. A coronary prognostic index for grading the severity of myocardial infarction. *Br Heart J* 1962;24:745–60.
10. Norris RM, Brandt PWT, Caughey DE, Lee AJ, Scott PJ. A new coronary prognostic index. *Lancet* 1969;i:278–81.
11. Kouwenhoven WB, Jude JR, Knickerbocker GG. Closed-chest cardiac massage. *JAMA* 1960;173:1064–7.
12. Julian DG. Treatment of cardiac arrest in acute myocardial ischaemia and infarction. *Lancet* 1961;ii:840–4.
13. Thomas M, Malmcrona R, Shillingford JP. Hemodynamic changes in patients with acute myocardial infarction. *Circulation* 1965;31:811–8.
14. Mackenzie GJ, Taylor SH, Flenley DC, McDonald AH, Staunton HP, Donald KW. Circulatory and respiratory studies in myocardial infarction and cardiogenic shock. Lancet 1964;ii:825–8.
15. Cochrane AL. *Effectiveness and efficiency*. London: Nuffield Hospital Trust, 1972.
16. Rose G. The contribution of intensive coronary care. *Br J Prev Soc Med* 1965;29:147–50.
17. Oliver MF, Julian DG, Donald KW. Problems in evaluating coronary care units. *Am J Cardiol* 1967;20: 465–74.
18. Mather HG, Morgan DC, Pearson NG, et al. Myocardial infarction: a comparison between home and hospital care for patients. *BMJ* 1976;1:925–9.
19. Hill JD, Hampton JR, Mitchell JRA. A randomised trial of home versus hospital management for patients with suspected myocardial infarction. *Lancet* 1978;i:837–41.
20. Lie KI, Wellens HJJ, Downar E, Durrer D. Observations on patients with primary ventricular fibrillation complicating myocardial infarction. *Circulation* 1975;52:75–9.
21. Campbell RWF, Murray A, Julian DG. Ventricular arrhythmias in first 12 hours of acute myocardial infarction. *Br Heart J* 1981;46:351–7.
22. Pantridge JF, Geddes JS. A mobile coronary care unit in the management of myocardial infarction. *Lancet* 1967;ii:271–3.
23. ISIS-4 Collaborative Group. Fourth international study of infarct survival. A randomised factorial trial assessing early oral captopril, oral mononitrate, and intravenous magnesium sulphate in 58 050 patients with suspected acute myocardial infarction. *Lancet* 1995;435:669–85.
24. Gruppo Italiano per lo Studio Supravvivenza nell'infarto Miocardico. GISSI-3. Effect of lisinopril and transdermal glyceryl trinitrate singly and together on 6 week mortality and ventricular function after acute myocardial infarction. *Lancet* 1994;343:1115–22.
25. ISIS-1 Collaborative Group. Randomised trial of intravenous atenolol among 16 027 cases of suspected acute myocardial infarction: ISIS-1. *Lancet* 1986;ii:57–66.
26. Woods KL, Ketley D, Lowy A, et al. β-blockers and antithrombotic treatment for secondary prevention after acute myocardial infarction. *Eur Heart J* 1998;19:74–9.
27. ISIS-2 Collaborative Group. Randomised trial of intravenous streptokinase, oral aspirin, both or neither among 17 187 cases of suspected acute myocardial infarction. ISIS-2. *Lancet* 1988;i:349–60.
28. Gruppo Italiano per lo Studio Della Streptokinase Nell'Infarto Miocardico.(GISSI). Effectiveness of intravenous thrombolytic treatment in acute myocardial infarction. *Lancet* 1986;i:397–402.
29. ISIS-3 (Third International Study of Infarct Survival) Collaborative Group. ISIS-3: a randomised comparison of streptokinase vs tissue plasminogen activator vs anistreplase and of aspirin plus heparin vs aspirin alone among 41 299 cases of suspected acute myocardial infarction. *Lancet* 1992;339:753–70.

30. The International Study Group. In-hospital mortality and clinical course of 20 891 patients with suspected acute myocardial infarction randomised between alteplase and streptokinase with or without heparin. *Lancet* 1990;336:71–5.
31. The GUSTO Investigators. An international randomized trial comprising four thrombolytic strategies for acute myocardial infarction. *N Engl J Med* 1993;329:673–82.
32. Weston CF, Penny WJ, Julian DG. Guidelines for the early management of patients with myocardial infarction. British Heart Foundation Working Group. *BMJ* 1994;308:767–71.
33. GREAT Group. Feasibility, safety, and efficacy of domiciliary thrombolysis by general practitioners. Grampian region early anistreplase trial. *BMJ* 1992;305:548–53.
34. Birkhead JS. Thrombolytic treatment for myocardial infarction; an examination of practice in 39 United Kingdom hospitals. Myocardial Infarction Audit Group. *Heart* 1997;78:28–33.
35. Norris RM. *Sudden cardiac death and acute myocardial infarction in three British health districts, The UK heart attack survey*. London: British Heart Foundation, 1999.
36. Medical Research Council. Second report of the working party on anticoagulant therapy in coronary thrombosis. *BMJ* 1964;2:837–43.
37. Mitchell JRA. Anticoagulants in coronary disease-retrospect and prospect. *Lancet* 1981;i:257–62.
38. Multicentre International Study. Improvement in prognosis of myocardial infarction by long-term β-adrenoceptor blockade using practolol. *BMJ* 1975;3:735–40.
39. Baber NS, Wainwright Evans D, Howitt G, et al. A multicentre propranolol post-infarction trial in 49 hospitals in the United Kingdom, Italy and Yugoslavia. *Br Heart J* 1980;44:419–21.
40. Norwegian Multicenter Study Group. Timolol-induced reduction in mortality and reinfarction in patients surviving myocardial infarction. *N Engl J Med* 1981;304:801–7.
41. Beta-blocker Heart Attack Study Group (BHAT). A beta-blocker heart attack trial. *JAMA* 1981;246:2073–74.
42. Chamberlain DA, Jewitt DE, Julian DG, et al. Oral mexiletine in high-risk patients after myocardial infarction. *Lancet* 1980;ii:1324–7.
43. The Acute Infarction Ramipril Efficacy (AIRE) Study Investigators. Effect of ramipril on mortality and morbidity of survivors of acute myocardial infarction with clinical evidence of heart failure. *Lancet* 1993;342:821–8.
44. Pfeffer MA, Braunwald E, Moyé LA, et al. Effect of captopril on mortality and morbidity in patients with left ventricular dysfunction after myocardial infarction. *N Engl J Med* 1992;327:669–77.
45. Kober L, Torp-Pedersen,C, Carlsen JE, et al. for the Trandolapril Cardiac Evaluation Study Group. A clinical trial of the angiotensin-converting-enzyme inhibitor trandolapril with left ventricular dysfunction after myocardial infarction. *N Engl J Med* 1995;333:1670–4.
46. Heberden W. Some account of a disorder of the breast. *Med Trans R Coll Physicians Lond* 1772;2: 59.
47. Herrick JB. Clinical features of sudden obstruction of the coronary arteries. *JAMA* 1912;59:2015–20.
48. Stowers M, Short D. Warning symptoms before major myocardial infarction. *Br Heart J* 1970;32:833–8.
49. Wood P. Acute and subacute coronary insufficiency. *BMJ* 1961;1:1779–82.
50. Krauss KR, Hutter AM Jr, De Sanctis RW. Acute coronary insufficiency: course and follow-up. *Circulation* 1972;45(suppl I):66–71.
51. Fulton M, Duncan B, Lutz W, et al. Natural history of unstable angina. *Lancet* 1972;i:860–4.
52. Fulton M, Julian DG. Unstable angina. In: Julian DG ed. *Angina pectoris*. Edinburgh: Churchill Livingstone, 1977.
53. Lewis HD Jr, Davis JW, Archibald DG, et al. Protective effects of aspirin against acute myocardial infarction and death in men with unstable angina. *N Engl J Med* 1983;309:396–403.
54. Cairns JA, Gent M, Singer J, et al. Aspirin, sulfinpyrazone or both in unstable angina. *N Engl J Med* 1985;313:1369–75.
55. The Holland Interuniversity Nifedipine/Metoprolol Trial (HINT) Research Group. Early treatment of unstable angina in the coronary unit. *Br Heart J* 1986;56:400–13.
56. Adams PC, Skinner JS, Cohen M, McBride R, Fuster V. Acute coronary syndromes in the United States and the United Kingdom: a comparison of approaches. The Antithrombotic Therapy in Acute Coronary Syndromes Research Group. *Clin Cardiol* 1998;21:348–52.
57. Prinzmetal M, Kennamar R, Merliss R, Wada T, Bor N. A variant form of angina pectoris. *Am J Med* 1959;27:375–88.
58. Maseri A, Severi S, Nes MD, et al. Variant angina: one aspect of a continuous spectrum of vasospastic myocardial ischemia. Pathogenetic mechanisms, estimated incidence and clinical and coronary arteriographic findings in 138 patients. *Am J Cardiol* 1978;42:1019–35.
59. Master AM, Rosenfeld I. Two-step exercise test: current status after 25 years. *Modern Concepts Cardiovasc Dis* 1967;36:19–24.
60. Balcon R, Maloy WE, Sowton E. Clinical use of atrial pacing test in angina pectoris. *BMJ* 1968;610:91–2.

61. Sones FM Jr, Shirey EK. Cine coronary arteriography. *Modern Concepts Cardiovasc Dis* 1962;31:735–38.
62. European Coronary Surgery Study Group. Coronary artery bypass surgery in stable angina pectoris: survival at two years *Lancet* 1979;ii:889–93
63. Grüntzig AR. Transluminal dilatation of coronary artery stenosis. *Lancet* 1978;i:263.
64. Working Party of the Joint Audit Committee of the British Cardiac Society and the Royal College of Physicians of London. The investigation and management of stable angina pectoris. *J R Coll Physicians* 1993;27:267–73.
65. De Bono D for the Joint Working Party of the British Cardiac Society and the Royal College of Physicians of London. Investigation and management of stable angina: revised guidelines 1998. *Heart* 1999;81:546–55.
66. Sculpher MJ, Pettigrew M, Kelland JL, Elliott RA, Holdright DR, Buxton MJ. Resource allocation for chronic stable angina: a systematic review of effectiveness, costs, and cost-effectiveness of alternative interventions. *Health Technol Assess* 1998;2:10.

Chapter 28

Leaders of British Cardiology

Arthur Hollman, Gaston E Bauer and Mark Silverman

Russell Claude Brock, Lord Brock of Wimbledon, 1903–1980

Arthur Hollman

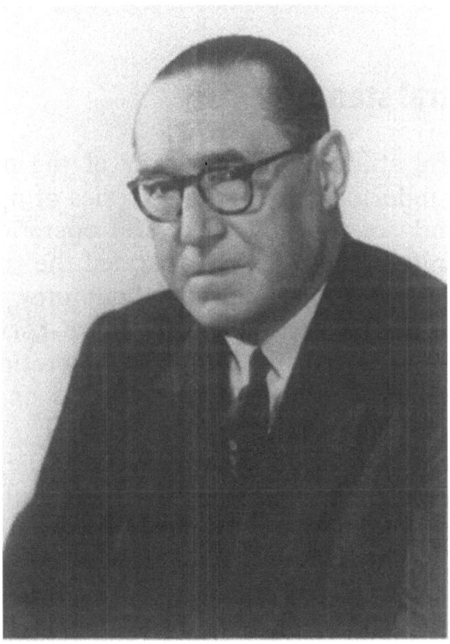

Figure 1 Lord Brock of Wimbledon (with permission of the Royal College of Surgeons of England).

Russell Brock was a notable pioneer of cardiac surgery, known worldwide for his achievements. He was born in London, educated at Christ's Hospital School, and entered Guy's Hospital Medical School at the age of 17. As a medical student, he showed the brilliance and force of character which were to mark his whole career, winning prizes and two gold medals. At the age of 25 he became a Hunterian professor, and a Rockefeller scholarship in 1929 enabled him to work under Evarts Graham in St Louis, which gave him his interest in thoracic surgery. Graham in 1922 had been the first surgeon to operate on mitral stenosis, though without success.

Brock continued to work at Guy's and was appointed to the staff both there and at the Brompton Hospital in 1936. His work in thoracic surgery led to two monographs, *The anatomy of the bronchial tree* and *Lung abscess*. In 1947, he created a thoracic surgical unit at Guy's and turned his attention to the possibilities of operating on mitral and pulmonary stenosis. He argued that a stenotic heart valve was a simple obstruction that could be relieved by surgery. Also in 1947, Alfred Blalock of Johns Hopkins was a visiting surgeon at Guy's and demonstrated the Blalock–Taussig operation for Fallot's tetralogy. Brock treated a series of patients with this operation, but considered that a direct attack on the pulmonary valve would be a better approach. He invented a valvulotome and published three successes in June 1948, later writing a monograph *The anatomy of congenital pulmonary stenosis*. In the meantime, Thomas Holmes Sellors had achieved the world's first pulmonary valvotomy at Harefield Hospital England in December 1947.

Operation for mitral stenosis

Brock made a careful study of the anatomy of the mitral valve, and in September 1948 he undertook the first of a series of operations for mitral stenosis, independently of the first successful operations which had just been done in the United States. Brock separated the commisures with his finger, and named the procedure a mitral valvulotomy. The name was later changed, on advice, to the etymologically more correct valvotomy. Six successful cases were reported in 1950, in collaboration with the cardiologist Maurice Campbell whom he praised for his unstinted cooperation and medical and moral support.[1]

The appointment of Paul Wood as cardiologist at the Brompton Hospital enabled Brock to begin cardiac surgery there too, and to establish a very productive partnership with Wood. He devised percutaneous left ventricular puncture to assess aortic valve stenosis, but aortic valvotomy proved a more difficult problem. Brock started open heart surgery at Guy's with his senior registrar, Donald N Ross, using veno-venous cooling for repair of atrial septal defect.

A perfectionist

Brock was not an easy man to know. He was a perfectionist who allowed neither himself nor those with whom he worked any margin for inaccuracy. Anything slipshod was anathema to him and he would not tolerate lack of clinical detail or intelligent analysis. Brock would never offer a patient less than his best – and did not see why anyone else should do so either. He would do anything to help a young surgeon's career if he felt that he lived up to his own standards, and beneath a layer of shyness there lay a rich vein of generosity. Away from work he had a good sense of humour and had quotations – mostly biblical – for any occasion, but he was not easy to talk to socially. Brock felt deeply about the personal aspects of illness in his patients and about the needs and aspirations of his pupils.[2] His surgical colleagues said that while he was a great thinker, he was not a natural surgeon and technically not brilliant. In the operating theatre he was on edge and often difficult and demanding.

From 1949 onwards and despite his heavy clinical and teaching commitments, Brock concerned himself increasingly in the work of the Royal College of Surgeons of England. He was president from 1963–6 and gave a fine Hunterian Oration in 1960. Brock maintained that private practice was complementary to the NHS and he promoted the Private Patients Plan, of which he became president.

Brock had considerable literary distinction. He edited *Guy's Hospital Reports* for 25 years and showed his interest in history with a book on the famous Guy's surgeon, Sir Astley Cooper. Outside work, he had an extensive knowledge of antique furniture and prints, and he had an especial interest in the history of London Bridge and its environs. He did much to restore the operating theatre at old St Thomas's Hospital.[3] At his death, he was described as one of the great figures in medicine of the last half century.

References

1. Brock RC. Pulmonary valvulotomy for the relief of congenital pulmonary stenosis. *BMJ* 1948;i:1121–6.
2. Obituary. Lord Brock, MS, FRCS, FRCP. *BMJ* 1980;ii:814.
3. Anonymous. Russell Claude Brock. *Lives of the fellows of the Royal College of Surgeons, 1974–82.* London: Royal College of Surgeons, 1982.

Sir Thomas Lewis, 1881–1945

Arthur Hollman

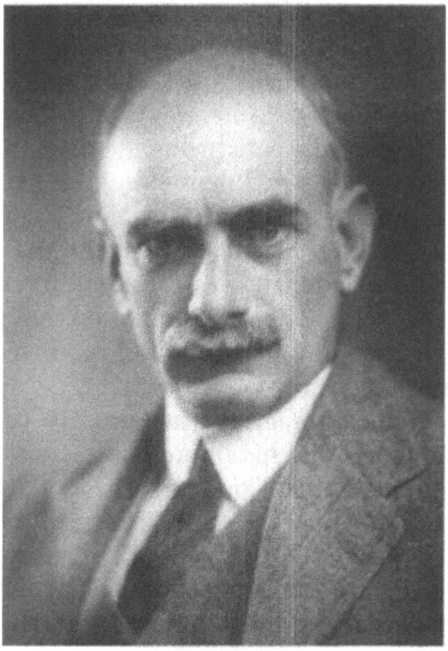

Figure 2 Sir Thomas Lewis.

Thomas Lewis is best known for his pioneer research in electrocardiography and electrophysiology, and for his studies in heart disease. However, cardiology was only one of his interests. It needs to be emphasised that his chief mission in life was that of applying the scientific method to the study of clinical problems, a discipline that he called clinical science.

Lewis was born in Cardiff and came from an old Welsh family. He was educated at home by his mother and a tutor, and after attending college in Cardiff he went to London. He qualified from University College Hospital in 1905 and stayed there for the rest of his professional life.[1]

From the start, Lewis was attracted to the cardiovascular system, and while still a house physician he wrote five papers on the pulse and blood pressure. He also did physiological research in the laboratory of EH Starling at University College on the relation between pericardial and arterial pressures. However, it was the influence of James Mackenzie in 1908 that catalysed Lewis's decision to study cardiac irregularities, and he mastered the then new and difficult technique of electrocardiography with the Einthoven string galvanometer. Lewis visited Einthoven in Leiden and became a firm friend and admirer. Their collaboration enhanced the progress of electrocardiography.

Lewis's monograph *The mechanism of the heart beat* was written in 1911 after only three years' research. It became the standard work in English on the subject – "the bible of electrocardiography" as it was called in the United States. Lewis summarised this work in two small books for the general physician. These were *Clinical electrocardiography* and *Clinical disorders of the heart beat*, still in print 25 years later. He elucidated the nature of nearly all cardiac arrhythmias and later proposed that atrial fibrillation and flutter were due to a circus movement in the atria (Chapter 10).

The newly designed Cambridge Instrument Company galvanometer could record two electrocardiograms simultaneously. This enabled Lewis in 1914 to precisely record the spread of the excitation wave in the dog heart, which laid a foundation for cardiac electrophysiology. Physicians from the world over came to learn from the master, and he was invited to give four lectures in Canada and the United States. Lewis was still only 33 years of age.

Soldier's heart and cardiac studies

The world war then stopped Lewis's research and he took charge of the Military Heart Hospital in England. There he made a scientific study of so called soldier's heart, a non-cardiac disorder, which he termed the effort syndrome. He devised a successful method of treatment using graded physical exercises. After the war he studied endocarditis, identified the pathology of the congenital bicuspid aortic valve, and was the first to demonstrate the *x* ray appearance of the aortic arch in coarctation. Lewis emphasised the importance of diagnosing heart failure by inspecting the jugular veins, and he would not accept that digitalis was beneficial in heart failure with normal rhythm (Chapter 1). He made a serious error in saying the symptoms and heart failure in mitral stenosis were not caused by the contracted valve orifice but by myocardial disease, and he opposed surgery for this condition. However, Lewis was not against cardiac surgery in general, and one of his patients was among the first in Britain to have a patent ductus ligated by Mr OS Tubbs about 1943.

End of cardiac research

Lewis signalled the end of his cardiac research in 1925 by publishing the very fine third edition of his book, now entitled *The mechanism and graphic registration of the heart beat.* It is one the classics of cardiology in the 20th century. He was now able to devote himself entirely to the promotion and acceptance of clinical science, saying, "it is requisite that medicine should renew its strength to wield its chief weapon, the experimental method."[2] For the next 20 years he and his assistants in his department of clinical research, men and women like Pickering, Wayne, Grant, and Janet Vaughan, successfully unravelled the mechanisms of disease. He investigated intermittent claudication and showed that the pain of muscular ischemia was due to a chemical substance, factor P, a study that was extended to the pain of angina pectoris. The triple response of the skin to injury was shown to be due to liberation of a histamine like substance. The mechanism of Raynaud's disease was elucidated and he wrote an excellent book on *Vascular disorders of the limbs*. Lewis undertook a long and very perceptive study of the difficult subject of pain, identifying the double pain response of the skin and mapping out segmental areas of referred pain. Intellectually, this was among his best work and he summarised it in a monograph, *Pain*.

Lewis was a hard taskmaster, and his assistants found it difficult to keep up with his intense activity and insistence on very high standards. However, they all came to have high personal regard for him and for his quietly done acts of kindness. Lewis had a burning desire to establish clinical research as a permanent and full time career. To this end he founded the Medical Research Society in 1930, at a time when very few opportunities were available for such a career. With James Mackenzie he had founded the journal *Heart* in 1909, which he changed in 1933 to *Clinical Science*. He edited these journals for 35 years - the longest editorship in British science this century.

An inspiring clinical teacher and clinician

Lewis was an inspiring clinical teacher who stressed the importance of thinking logically and taking nothing for granted without evidence. He taught his students the need for accurate observation and although some found him intimidating, they appreciated the clarity of his teaching which made cardiology an exciting topic for them. In 1933, he distilled his teaching into a book *Diseases of the heart*. This was written in compelling, clear English and soon became the preferred text for students and practitioners. It sold thousands of copies in the United States. It had a unusual chapter on "Conversing with the patient and his friends."

Lewis's scientific distinction was recognised when the Royal Society awarded him their highest honour, the Copley Medal. But Lewis was no backroom scientist. He gave careful and personal attention to his patients, in the ward and in the outpatient clinic, both of which he attended conscientiously.[3] He was interested in the philosophy and history of medicine, and the first four of his courses of undergraduate lectures dealt with the way diseases were named and classified, with the nature of disease and with the discovery of new remedies. Those lectures must have been unique in any medical school.

Away from work Lewis pursued his hobbies of fishing, bird watching and photography during his two-month annual holiday and did so with the same energy that he applied to his research, making copious notes of his findings. He loved to share these hobbies with his wife and three children, and he made a fine collection of bird photographs some of which he published in *British birds*.

Thomas Lewis had myocardial infarcts at the ages of 45 and 53. He never had angina of effort and died in cardiac failure at the age of 63.

References

1. Drury AN, Grant RT. Thomas Lewis, 1881-1945. *Obit Notices Fell Roy Soc Lond* 1945;5:179–202.
2. Lewis T. *Clinical science, illustrated by personal experiences.* London, Shaw and sons, 1934.
3. Hollman A. *Sir Thomas Lewis, pioneer cardiologist and clinical scientist.* London, Springer-Verlag, 1997.

Sir James Mackenzie, 1853–1925

Arthur Hollman

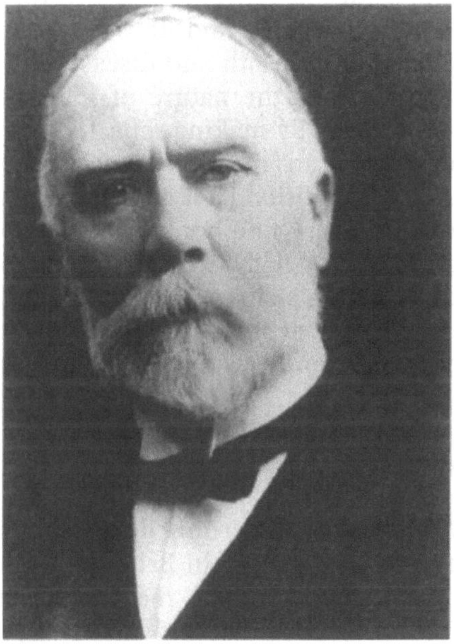

Figure 3 Sir James Mackenzie.

James Mackenzie was the inspiration for the new generation of cardiologists at the beginning of the century. His research on arrhythmias and his wide vision of medicine in general commanded the attention of discerning young workers such as John Hay of Liverpool and Thomas Lewis in London. What is surprising is the fact that Mackenzie's career up to the age of 54 had been entirely in general practice. He came from a poor Scottish family, and having been a pharmacist for four years, he entered medical school at Edinburgh and graduated in 1878. He was then offered a good academic post, but he could not afford to take it up and instead he went into general practice in the manufacturing town of Burnley in Lancashire.[1]

For Mackenzie, with his quite original and enquiring mind, his 28 years as a practitioner gave him special opportunities to study disease. In particular, he was able to follow patients for many years. He soon came to realise that he could not understand or explain many features of a patient's illness and he set himself the task of understanding the mechanism of symptoms and physical signs and their prognostic significance. He did original work on referred pain and he was the first to describe hyperaesthetic skin in association with visceral disease.

Mackenzie's work on the heart

In 1892, at the age of 39, Mackenzie started his outstanding work on the heart. He modified the Dudgeon sphygmograph so that it could record the venous as well as the arterial pulse, and he was the first to systematically investigate venous pulsation in health and disease. His greatness lay in his recognition that by this means the nature of many cardiac irregularites could be analysed and proved. By making repeated recordings over several years, Mackenzie showed that atrial activity ceased when the heart became completely irregular – the condition later shown to be atrial fibrillation. He presented all his work in a very fine book *The study of the pulse, arterial venous and hepatic* in 1902. It had 335 illustrations of pulse recordings, all done with the polygraph on strips of smoked paper measuring 14 cm × 2 cm. A few years later Mackenzie invented an ink writing polygraph which made recording much easier and was widely adopted.

The move to London

Mackenzie's book was hailed by discerning doctors in Europe and America, but his work was less well recognised in Britain and this led him to move to London in 1907 in order to promote recognition of his research. This was a bold move at the age of 54, and it took him two years to get a hospital appointment at the Mount Vernon Hospital for Chest Disease in Hampstead. However, Sir Wiiliam Osler recognised his genius and he was elected to the prestigious Association of Physicians, which Osler had just founded.

In London, he had the spare time to write a textbook on *Diseases of the heart* and, ironically, it was this rather than his research that brought him wide acclaim. He insisted that it was the functional capacity of the heart which mattered, and not just the presence of murmurs or extrasystoles – "A heart is what a heart can do." This was the beginning of functional classification and a very important change in thinking at that time. But Mackenzie was cautious about the benefit of measuring the blood pressure, and said of the electrocardiograph, "its limitations in clinical medicine are great." Mackenzie was not keen on the use of instruments in diagnosis.

He was appointed lecturer in cardiac research at the London Hospital in 1910, but the staff denied him beds until 1913 when he founded the cardiac department, the first of its kind in Britain.[2]

Mackenzie, Lewis, and *Heart*

Mackenzie was always keen to learn from cardiac physiologists and it was probably from a visit to Starling's laboratory at University College London that he came to meet Thomas Lewis in 1908. He urged Lewis to study cardiac arrhythmias and this catalysed Lewis's pioneer work with the electrocardiogram. Together they decided that a new journal was required for the study of the circulation, and Mackenzie asked Lewis to be the first editor of *Heart* in 1909.

The war

Mackenzie appointed John Parkinson as his chief assistant at the London in 1913 but the world war intervened. Mackenzie soon recognised that thousands of soldiers were being wrongly diagnosed as having heart disease and at his urgent appeal the Military Heart Hospital was founded at Hampstead. There a thorough study was made of "soldier's heart." His scientific distinction was amply recognised by his election in 1915 as a fellow of the Royal Society, and in the same year he received the honour of knighthood.

Return to Scotland

After 11 years in London, Mackenzie realised that his work there was impeding his former great interest in investigating the early stages of disease. He had already written a book, now in its third edition, on *Symptoms and their interpretation*. Thus, at the age of 65, he returned to Scotland and founded an Institute for Clinical Research in the university town of St Andrews in order to create a long-term study of the investigation and prevention of common diseases. It was his vision that it was essential to document patients' symptoms for a long time in order to understand their significance and prognosis. The town was small with a stable population and his idea, started in Burnley, of following patients for many years was a forerunner of the Framingham project in America. Indeed, Paul D White visited Mackenzie there.

While in Scotland, Mackenzie returned to his former interest in pain, with the publication of a monograph on angina pectoris. He summarised five years' work at the institute in his book, *The basis of vital activity*, and he explained his philosophy of practice in another, *The future of medicine*. Mackenzie laid great emphasis on the importance of assessing the severity of heart disease by the response of the heart to effort – the patient's exercise tolerance – rather than basing it on heart murmurs and irregularities. His views on heart failure are analysed in Chapter 1.

Mackenzie, aged 47, had an episode of atrial fibrillation after running, and at age 54 he had a two hour episode of cardiac pain – not then labelled cardiac infarction or coronary thrombosis, terms that in fact he never used. Increasingly severe angina of effort forced him to return to the warmer climate of London where he died after another infarct in 1925.[3]

Described by contemporaries

Mackenzie's great contribution to the development of cardiology and the affection which he inspired in his colleagues were fully recognised when he was made the only honorary member of the newly created Cardiac Club in 1922. His work and personality were described by his colleagues. John Hay of Liverpool said that he was, "Tall, 6ft 2 inches, a massive head and rough-hewn features, and – at most times – a kindly humourous twinkle in his shrewd blue-grey eyes, but withal a dour man and one who did not suffer fools gladly."[4] Sir John Parkinson described him as, "a tall and massively built Scot with a noble head set with searching yet sympathetic eyes and bearing a sober expression often relieved by a smile. He was agreeable and courteous to strangers, genial and happy with his friends, and most perfectly happy in his home."[5] Sir Thomas Lewis wrote:

> The patient was the lodestone of all his work. He was intolerant of authoritative statement and of traditional utterance. He was the first authority in clinical medicine on whose lips I frequently heard the words, 'I don't know.' A warm hearted man, oft touched by emotion, more often stirred by enthusiasm, a hard and tireless worker whose converse with his fellows was enlivened by a bright and blunt humour.[6]

References

1. Mair A. *Sir James Mackenzie, MD 1853–1925, general practitioner.* Edinburgh and London, Churchill Livingstone, 1953.
2. Obituary. Sir James Mackenzie. *BMJ* 1925;i:242–44.
3. Hollman A. How John Parkinson did the post mortem on Sir James Mackenzie. *Br Heart J* 1993;70:587–8.
4. Hay J. Sir James Mackenzie. *Liverpool Med-Chir J* 1930;70:161–76.
5. Parkinson J. Sir James Mackenzie. The centenary of his birth. *Br Heart J* 1954;15:125–7.
6. Lewis T. Sir James Mackenzie. *Heart* 1925;12:i–vii.

Sir John McMichael, 1904–93

Arthur Hollman

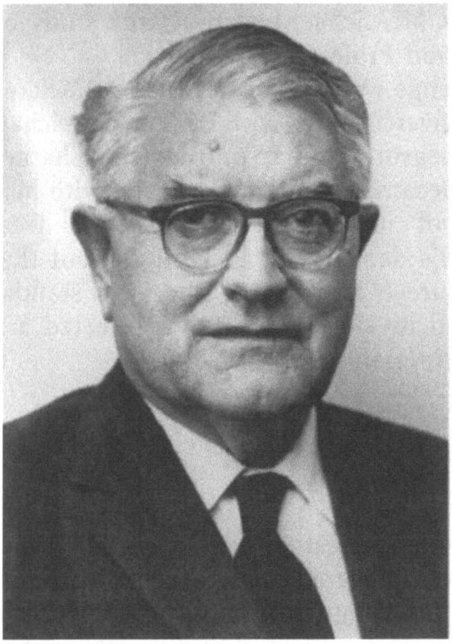

Figure 4 Sir John McMichael (with permission of the Royal College of Physicians of London).

John McMichael came from a poor Scottish family, but with scholarships he was able to qualify in medicine from Edinburgh in 1927. Early on, he decided to pursue a career in academic and experimental medicine, and with the support of a Beit memorial fellowship, he made an animal study in Aberdeen of pressure and flow in the portal circulation. This led to a study of splenic disease under Dr JW McNee at University College Hospital, London in 1932. In London, he met men active in clinical research such as Sir Thomas Lewis, GW Pickering, EJ Wayne, FT Smirk, and HP Himsworth. To study the systemic venous circulation McMichael mastered the acetylene technique for measuring cardiac output. Between 1934 and 1938, he made an important and original investigation of heart failure in Edinburgh, where he was a lecturer in human physiology and had a clinical appointment at the Royal Infirmary.

Hammersmith Hospital

In 1938, Francis Fraser appointed McMichael to a readership at Hammersmith Hospital, latterly named the British Postgraduate Medical School. This was a momentous move for him. Soon afterwards, with the outbreak of war, Fraser had to leave and at the age of 35, McMichael was in charge of the department. Wartime problems gave him the stimulus for two seminal investigations. Hepatitis was prevalent in the army, and in 1941, using percutaneous liver biopsy, McMichael began a large study of liver disease with Dr Sheila Sherlock and Professor JH Dible.[1]

The second challenge was that of traumatic shock, and this initiated an acclaimed series of investigations with EP Sharpey-Schafer using right heart catheterisation to measure cardiac output (see Chapters 1, 7, and 11).[2] Hypertension then became a main interest, and with his associates he made important studies of its clinical features and treatment. McMichael supported Platt in his debate with Pickering about the mode of distribution of blood pressure (Chapter 25). The high standard of his scientific work was recognised in 1957 when he was elected a fellow of the Royal Society – a rare distinction for a clinician.

Contentious positions

McMichael had a wide interest in cardiovascular disease and he attacked two positions that he considered were based on unsound evidence. The first was the use of oral anticoagulant therapy for myocardial infarction. This treatment was then so well endorsed that it was almost heresy to question it, but he was able to identify the flaws in the trials. The second was McMichael's contention that there was not enough evidence from clinical trials to support the recommendation that the whole population should have a lower fat diet.

For 21 years McMichael was the head of the department of medicine, and his achievements in this post rank as high as his clinical and research work. He created a fine department of clinical and academic research. Charles Newman, the dean, wrote, "He was a perfect 'Director' of research, quite happy to let his team carry out their own ideas . . . while gently seeing to it that no-one stretched freedom into licence."[3]

A fine teacher

The Hammersmith became synonymous with high class investigative medicine and doctors from all over the world vied to get a junior appointment. At the weekly staff rounds, McMichael encouraged anyone, however junior, to speak, providing they gave fact and not opinion. McMichael wrote, "Although many of our staff are brilliant to the point of being prima donnas . . . the school is remarkably united and free from the disrupting influences of personal rivalry." This was his doing. He was a fine teacher and explained that "This School does not instruct for any examination drill but rather attempts to educate by training reasoning power."[4]

McMichael's interest in postgraduate education led to his appointment as Director of the British Postgraduate Medical Federation from 1966–71. He was very concerned that so little money was available for research and he became deeply involved in establishing the British Heart Foundation, serving as chairman of its council. The foundation responded by endowing a chair in cardiovascular medicine in his name at Hammersmith. As a trustee of the Wellcome Trust from 1960–77, he gave valuable advice on clinical science and it was entirely his idea to establish their senior clinical fellowship scheme. McMichael had no major hobbies, but while at the trust he developed a deep interest in the history of medicine. This led him to speak on the development of cardiology in Britain in the 20th century when he had the honour of being the Harveian Orator of the Royal College of Physicians in 1975.[5] His formal association with cardiology reached its peak with his election as president of the British Cardiac Society from 1968–72, and with his presidency of the successful World Congress of Cardiology in London in 1970. In 1965 his eminence in British medicine was recognised by a knighthood.

After the death of his second wife, he married Dr Sheila Howarth his former colleague at Hammermsith Hospital and widow of Peter Sharpey-Schafer. At the age of 78 he had a severe stroke, and until his death nearly 11 years later he was cared for with admirable devotion by his wife. McMichael was a world figure in medicine and he became an honorary member of several foreign medical associations and received many honorary degrees.

References

1. Dollery CT. Sir John McMichael. *Biographical memoirs of the Royal Society* 1995;41:283–96.
2. McMichael J. Foreword. In: Verel D, Grainger H, eds. *Cardiac catheterisation*. Edinburgh: Churchill Livingstone, 1969.
3. Newman CE. John McMichael. *Postgrad Med J* 1966;42:738–40.
4. Mc Michael J. The postgraduate medical school: the present situation. *Postgrad Med J* 1966;42:740–43.
5. McMichael J. *A transition in cardiology: the Mackenzie Lewis era. The Harveian oration of 1975.* London: Royal College of Physicians, 1976.

Sir John Parkinson, 1885–1976

Gaston E Bauer

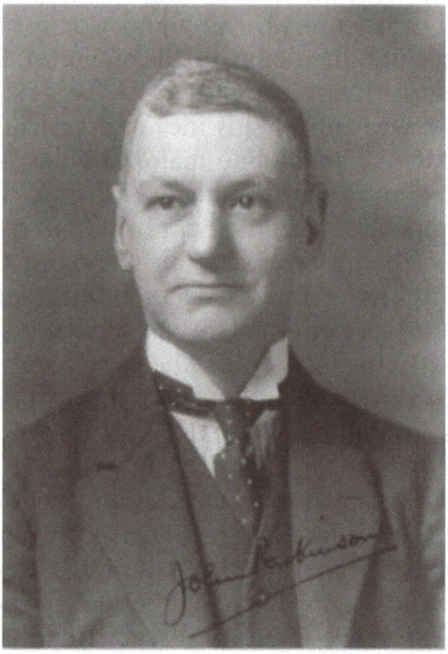

Figure 5 Sir John Parkinson.

John Parkinson was the best known and most influential British cardiologist of the second quarter of the 20th century. He excelled as a practising physician, as a teacher and as a clinical investigator, making important contributions in several fields of heart disease. He supported the creation of British and international societies for cardiology and was honoured in many countries. He accomplished all these achievements with humility and modesty. The 1950, first edition of Paul Wood's influential British textbook on heart disease was dedicated to Parkinson.

Early days

John Parkinson was born in Lancashire and graduated from the London Hospital in 1907. After being on the resident staff, he studied in Germany for one year and then returned to the London Hospital where in 1913 he became the chief assistant to Sir James Mackenzie.[1] His first significant paper reported the lack of benefit of strychnine in heart failure.[2] It was not the only or the last time that Parkinson exposed the ineffectiveness of an established treatment or procedure.[2]

In the same year – 1913 – a young colleague from Boston, Paul Dudley

White, visited Mackenzie's clinic and was welcomed by Parkinson. This visit led to a close professional and personal friendship lasting for 60 years.

During the first world war, Parkinson was in the Royal Army Medical Corps and worked at the Military Heart Hospital at Hampstead. He published four papers on soldier's heart before taking charge of a military heart centre at Rouen from 1917–19.

Head of the London Hospital cardiac department

In 1920, at the age of 35 years, Parkinson became the physician in charge of the cardiac department of the London Hospital. He succeeded Mackenzie, who had retired to his native Scotland in 1918. He was also appointed to the staff of the National Heart Hospital, and in 1922 he became a founder member of the Cardiac Club, the forerunner of the British Cardiac Society.

He studied atrial flutter and fibrillation with D Evan Bedford and Maurice Campbell, and heart block with Stokes–Adams seizures and repetitive paroxysmal tachycardia with William Evans and Cornelio Papp. With Campbell in 1929, he showed the value of quinidine in reverting atrial fibrillation and in maintaining sinus rhythm.[3]

Parkinson's interest in the diagnosis of cardiac infarction led to a landmark paper with D Evan Bedford in 1928.[4] A further report describing the serial electrocardiographic changes was published in *Heart* in the same year.[5] He then developed an interest in the use of radiology in the diagnosis of heart disease, particularly with regard to cardiac enlargment and failure, valvular heart disease, and abnormalities of the thoracic aorta. It was in cardiac radiology that some of his greatest contributions to the better understanding of heart disease were accomplished.

The Wolff–Parkinson–White syndrome

With Louis Wolff, a Boston colleague, Paul Dudley White had collected a series of electrocardiograms showing a short PR interval and bundle branch block in apparently healthy individuals with attacks of paroxysmal tachycardia and fibrillation. He took the tracings to John Parkinson who retrieved similar electrocardiograms from the collection at the London Hospital. Their combined experience of 11 cases was published in the *American Heart Journal* in 1930. Louis Wolff later wrote a full account of the discovery of the Wolff–Parkinson–White syndrome.[6]

Lectures and teaching

Parkinson was in great demand as a teacher and lecturer and he participated regularly in highly regarded graduate courses. Visitors from all over the world attended his outpatient clinics. As a teacher, Parkinson's contributions were significant not only in what they added to existing knowledge but in his ability to criticise outdated ideas. A good example is found in his 1936 Lumleian Lectures on "Enlargement of the heart," in which he showed the superiority of radiology over physical examination in determining heart size. He wrote "Nothing has been added to medical knowledge through cardiac percussion since the beginning of this century and in the light of x-rays it will shrink into obsolescence."[7] The Harveian Oration of 1945 was delivered by Parkinson at the Royal College of Physicians with the president Lord Moran in the chair. He said, "Under your presidency there has been freedom in that those who pursue a particular branch of medicine have felt they were no less physicians than those who choose the traditional and excellent field of general medicine."

Parkinson's oration included a brief historical overview: "In the 17th century rheumatism was disengaged from gout, in the 18th century rheumatism became engaged to the heart and in the 19th century wedded to it." He proposed that a rheumatic fever committee should be created to coordinate research and that more country hospitals should engage in treatment and research, with supervisory clinics being established in the cities. Parkinson expressed the hope that the college would "take a lead in this great and Christian endeavour."[8] It was his vision that helped to establish the special unit for juvenile rheumatism at the Canadian Red Cross Memorial Hospital at Taplow, Buckinghamshire. In 1947, he was awarded the Fothergillian Gold Medal of the Medical Society of London, and in 1948 a very well deserved knighthood was bestowed on him for his services to cardiology.

Sir John gave another important address in 1949, when he delivered the Carey Coombs Memorial Lecture at the University of Bristol. The title, "The radiology of rheumatic heart disease," combined two of his favourite interests.[9]

The 1950s

In 1950, Sir John Parkinson was 65 and he retired from his consultant posts at the London Hospital and the National Heart Hospital. He was a prominent figure at the First World Congress of Cardiology in Paris in 1950 and assisted in the creation of the International Society of Cardiology of which he was elected the first honorary member. After attending the Second World Congress in the United States in 1954, he went to Boston and for the first time he met Louis Wolff and was photographed with him and Paul White. He was elected as the first president of the British Cardiac Society in 1952 and was made an honorary fellow of the American College of Physicians and an honorary member of many national cardiac societies.

Retirement

After the war, Sir John and Lady Parkinson moved from Devonshire Place to an elegant house in Hampstead where their charming garden had fine rose beds. Parkinson had always been a very good friend to the younger members of the profession and he used to invite all the members of the Junior Cardiac Club to a reception in Hampstead each year. He retired from consulting practice at the age of 74 and died at the very good age of 91.

In 1951 the *British Heart Journal* dedicated an issue to him with a foreword by Paul Dudley White who wrote:

> Not only do I represent the vast number of his friends all over the world, but I voice a widespread opinion in the simple statement that this man has exerted with the utmost modesty one of the most important influences for the good of medicine in his time. Of all the physicians that I have met none has so well exemplified the highest type of three fold service-practice, teaching and research.[10]

References

1. Wolstenholme GEW, ed. Sir John Parkinson. *Lives of the fellows of the Royal College of Physicians of London, continued to 1983.* London: Royal College of Physicians,1984:443–6.
2. Parkinson J, Rowlands R A. Strychnine in heart failure. *Q J Med* 1913;7:42.
3. Parkinson J, Campbell M. The quinidine treatment of auricular fibrillation. *Q J Med* 1929;22:281.
4. Parkinson J, Bedford D E. Cardiac infarction and coronary thrombosis. *Lancet* 1928;i:4.
5. Parkinson J, Bedford DE. Successive changes in the electrocardiogram after cardiac infarction (coronary thrombosis). *Heart* 1928;14:195.
6. Wolff L. The Wolff–Parkinson–White syndrome. *Am J Cardiol* 1965;15:553.
7. Parkinson J. Enlargement of the heart. *Lancet* 1936;i:1337, 1391.
8. Parkinson J. Rheumatic fever and heart disease. The Harveian oration. *Lancet* 1945;ii:657.
9. Parkinson J. The radiology of rheumatic heart disease. *Lancet* 1949;i:895.
10. White PD. Sir John Parkinson,M.D. *Br Heart J* 1951;33: 421–2.

Paul Hamilton Wood, 1907–1962

Mark E Silverman

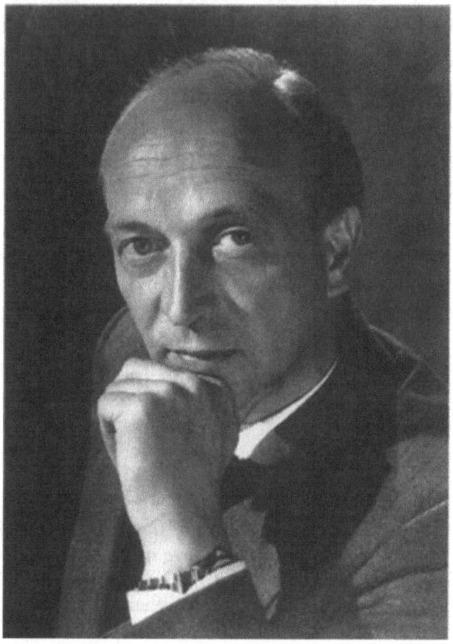

Figure 6 Dr Paul Wood. (Reprinted from American Journal of Cardiology 1972;30:ii with permission of Excerpta Medica Inc.)

Paul Wood, the charismatic leader of British and European cardiology during the middle of the 20th century, was internationally admired for his bedside teaching, clinical investigation of heart disease, and an important textbook of cardiology.[1–4] Born in 1907 in India, where his father was an English district commissioner in the Indian Civil Service, Wood was educated in England and Australia, graduating from the University of Melbourne in 1931.[1] After two years as a house physician at Christchurch General Hospital in New Zealand, where he met Betty Guthrie his future wife, Wood travelled to London in 1933 to take the membership examination of the Royal College of Physicians and complete his medical training.[2] Initially, he leaned towards a career in neurology; however, as resident medical officer at the National Heart Hospital from 1934–5, Wood soon realised that cardiology was the specialty path to future success.

Hammersmith Hospital

Francis Fraser, the first professor of medicine at the newly formed Royal Postgraduate Medical School at the Hammersmith Hospital, recognised Wood's promise and, in 1934, chose him to be his first assistant in charge of cardiology.[5] At the Hammersmith, Wood, still only 27, was assigned 30 medical beds, an outpatient clinic, and full consulting responsibilities as a full time clinician-investigator. Three years later Wood also became physician to outpatients at the National Heart Hospital, where he joined Evan Bedford, Maurice Campbell, William Evans, and John Parkinson on the consulting staff.[2] During this period, Wood began to develop his unique quantitative approach to the grading of clinical data, which he minutely recorded on voluminous data cards, taking full advantage of his remarkable talent for observation and bedside examination.[2] From John McMichael, Peter Sharpey-Schafer, and others at the Hammersmith, he learned the new technique of cardiac catheterisation and a critical approach to research. Soon he was correlating clinical data with cardiac physiology and beginning to publish his landmark studies.

The Second World War

With the advent of the second world war, Wood was assigned to the effort syndrome unit at Mill Hill where he studied 200 patients and, in 1941, published a lengthy report on this disorder.[6] This was also the subject for his Goulstonian Lecture to the Royal College of Physicians, which he gave in the same year. Wood's military career, which earned him an OBE, lasted from 1942 to 1947, and was spent in North Africa and Italy. It provided him with an opportunity to complete a textbook on cardiology, but the manuscript was stolen and the book had to be rewritten after the war.[2]

Textbook

Diseases of the heart and circulation was published in 1950 and gained Wood worldwide recognition as the European authority on heart disease.[2,7] The book, characterised by Wood's lucid and personal style of writing and replete with his broad experience and a fresh physiological approach to cardiology, was widely appreciated and compared favourably with the leading American textbooks of cardiology. The second edition, published in 1956, contained Wood's vast experience of 900 patients with congenital heart disease, and is considered his masterpiece. An unfinished third edition was completed by others after Wood's death.

Institute of Cardiology

In 1947, Wood left Hammersmith Hospital to become dean of the newly formed Institute of Cardiology at the National Heart Hospital on Westmoreland Street as well as director of the cardiology department at the Brompton Hospital.[1,2,8] At the National Heart Hospital, he created a renowned teaching and research environment that attracted postgraduate students from Britain and around the world to learn by his example. The Brompton Hospital appointment provided an opportunity for Wood to develop his own catheter laboratory and to work closely with Russell Brock, one of the pioneers of cardiac surgery. In addition, from 1948–54, Wood consulted regularly on the rheumatic fever ward at Taplow, a Canadian Red Cross Hospital outside London, where he studied the natural history of rheumatic fever, the auscultatory signs, and the effect of treatment.[2]

Wood's research work

Phonocardiography, developed by Aubrey Leatham and others, became a major research tool in Wood's analysis of heart sounds and jugular venous recordings. His analysis of the jugular venous pulse was filmed in 1957 and has become the classic teaching on the subject (now available on video through the Wellcome Institute for the History of Medicine, London). Wood's many publications, compiled from his detailed notes on each patient, wedded the bedside examination, electrocardiogram, and chest *x* ray to the underlying cardiac physiology, bringing a scientific understanding to the clinical data.[1–4] This has become the foundation for much of our current understanding about atrial septal defect, mitral stenosis, aortic stenosis, tricuspid stenosis, Eisenmenger's syndrome, and constrictive pericarditis.[2] Wood introduced accuracy into the preoperative assessment of patients with cardiac disease. In addition, he contributed importantly to electrocardiography, was an early advocate of anticoagulation for unstable coronary disease, observed that polyuria was associated with atrial arrhythmias, and was one of the first to describe the physical findings and postulate about the mechanism of muscular subvalvar aortic stenosis (now known as hypertrophic cardiomyopathy).[1,9]

Lectures

Wood's fame as a writer, teacher, and diagnostician led to many invitations to speak to a British and international audience. He delivered the Goulstonian Lecture to the Royal College of Physicians (1941), the St Cyres Lecture (1950), The Strickland Goodall Lecture (1954), the Croonian Lecture (1958), the Fahr Lecture (1958), and the Nathanson Lecture (1959), and was appointed the Arthur Sims Commonwealth travelling professor (1961). Between 1949 and 1962, his teaching took him to South Africa, Australia,

New Zealand, Prague, Beirut, the United States (on four occasions), and to Canada.[2]

Intimidation with charm

Wood was a slightly built, pale looking man with penetrating steel-blue eyes, a sharp nose, and a balding forehead. His distinctive personality – dominating, sarcastic, and combative mixed with a lacerating humour and considerable charm – impacted forcefully upon others.[1,2] He enjoyed speaking frankly and critically, never coating his remarks with tact to soften their blow, a style that appealed to some while intimidating and offending others. Privately, however, to those few who were close friends, he could display a charming, more relaxed, and entertaining side. He was an avid gardener and planned his extensive flowerbeds with the same intensity and meticulous care with which he would approach a research project.[2]

At the bedside, in front of an admiring crowd of postgraduate students, registrars, and staff, he was renowned for his showmanship and dazzling ability to sleuth out the diagnosis using a Sherlock Holmes style of deduction. His agile mind worked rapidly, sifting and comparing, quantifying and analysing, accepting and discarding one set of logic then another until he was satisfied that he had reached the correct diagnosis. Always in search of the best solution, he was open to challenge and willing to change his mind for those brave few whose arguments were sufficiently powerful.[2,9]

A great legacy

The incessant demands that seeing patients, teaching, and lecturing made on his time; the burden of writing the third edition of his textbook; and his heavy smoking eventually took their toll.[2,10] In early July 1962, Wood had a heart attack and was admitted to the Middlesex Hospital under the care of Walter Somerville.[9] Characteristically, he made it clear that he would not allow resuscitation in the event that his heart should arrest, fearing that he might survive without his full mental powers. Several hours later, he arrested and his last wish was granted. On 13 July 1962, at the age of only 54, Paul Wood, the leading force of British cardiology and the inspiration and role model for many postgraduate students, died leaving a legacy of great accomplishments as an important transition figure between the old and the new era of cardiology.

In 1972, a tribute issue of the *American Journal of Cardiology* was dedicated to Paul Wood. E Grey Dimond, Wood's friend and the guest editor of the supplement, commented:

> His textbook of 1950, his lectures, articles, and bedside teaching were sufficient signals that an exceptional man was at the National Heart Hospital in London England, and has happened throughout medical history, all paths led there. In those

exciting years when the clinician was harvesting the rich vineyard offered by cardiac catheterization, angiocardiography, electrocardiography and cardiac surgery, Wood proved himself a master, and as happens with masters, to him came students, and from him went disciples.[1]

References

1. Dimond EG. Paul Wood revisited. *Amer J Card* 1972;30 (Suppl):121–196.
2. Silverman ME. "To die in one's prime:" the story of Paul Wood. *Amer J Card* 2000;85:75–88.
3. Campbell M. Paul Wood. *Brit Heart J* 1962;24:661–665.
4. Unsigned obituary. Paul Hamilton Wood. *The Lancet* 1962;2:205–206.
5. Fraser F. *The British Postgraduate Medical Federation, The First Fifteen Years.* London: The Athlone Press, 1967.
6. Wood P. DaCosta's syndrome (or effort syndrome). *Brit Med J* 1941;1:767–772;805–811.
7. Wood P. *Diseases of the Heart and Circulation.* London: Eyre and Spottiswoode, 1956.
8. Fraser F. The training of specialists. *Brit Med J* 1948;1:135–139.
9. Somerville J. Paul Wood. *Heart* 1998;80:612–619.
10. Dimond EG. *Take Wing!* Kansas City: The Lowell Press, 1991.

Index

A

Ablation 140
Action on Smoking and Health (ASH) 80
Acute infarction ramipril efficacy (AIRE) 348, 349
Adolescent cardiac unit 283—4
Aitken, Robert 105
Albany, Duke of 87
Alder Hey Hospital 282
Alexander, Earl 75
Allbutt, Sir Clifford 4, 11
Alteplase 244
American Heart Association 10
Amiodarone 139
Amyl nitrite 12
Angina 10–12
  and intermittent claudication 12
  pacing in 220
  stable 351–3
  treatment 12, 350, 352–3
  unstable 349–51
  variant 351
Angiocardiography 270
  see also Coronary angiography
Angioplasty, percutaneous transluminal coronary 140–3, 238–9, 338
  in myocardial infarction 152, 348
Angiotensin 311–12
Angiotonin 311
Anglo-Scandinavian study of early thrombosis (ASSET) 244
Anistreplase 347
Anistreplase intervention mortality study (AIMS) 244
Antiarrhythmics 139
Anticoagulants 242–3, 344, 350
Antiplatelet Trialists' Collaboration 244
Antithrombotic therapy 244–5, 347–8
Aortic balloon valvuloplasty 153
Aortic root replacement 206–7
Aortic valve
  replacement 206
  stenosis 112, 301–2
Arnott, Sir Melville 79
Arrhythmias 7–8
  prevention and treatment 345–6
  warning 345
  see also Electrocardiography
Arterial wall in atherosclerosis 328–9, 336
Aschoff bodies 255
ASPIRE study 235
Aspirin 243–4, 330, 338, 350
Association of British Cardiac Nurses 61
Association for European Paediatric Cardiologists 274
Astley, Roy 270
Asymmetric hypertrophy of Teare 112
Atherosclerosis 256–63
  arterial wall 328–9
  Atherosclerosis Discussion Group 257–8
  cardiovascular survey 333
  Central Middlesex Hospital 261
  clinical trials 336–8
  foam cells 257
  increasing incidence 260, 324–5
  lipid/lipoprotein research 331–2
  monocytes 257
  organisational developments 332–3
  plaque disruption 262–3
  plaque rupture 263
  post-war history 323–42
  research developments 333–6
  risk factors 325–8
  St George's Hospital 261–2
  thrombosis research 258–9, 329–31
Atherosclerosis Discussion Group 257–8, 332

Athlone committee 103
Atrial fibrillation 7–8
Atrial flutter 8
Atrial septal defect 204
Atromid 331

B

Bain, Curtis 12
Baker, Charles 62
Balcon, Raphael 150
Balloon atrial septostomy 148
Balloon valvuloplasty 153
Batten, John 99
'Battle of the knights' 312–14
Bayliss, Sir William 7
Bed rest
  in cardiac failure 5
  in myocardial infarction 343–4
  in rheumatic fever 297
Bedford, Evan 12, 13, 58, 66, 67, 74, 88, 94, 281
  Library of Cardiology 72
Bedside diagnosis 111–22
  early systolic sounds 120–1
  first heart sound 118–20
  phonocardiogram 112–15
  principles of examination 111–12
  second heart sound 115–18
Benign hypertension 315–16
Bentall, Hugh 108, 207
Beta-blockers 139, 220, 245–6
  angina 350
  hypertension 319–20
Birmingham Children's Hospital 272
Black, Sir James 319–20
Blalock, Alfred 55, 144, 198, 281
Blood pressure
  measurement 314–15
  sphygmomanometry 18
  see also Hypertension
Bousfield, Guy 12
Bradford Hill, Austin 179
Braimbridge, MV 205
Bramwell, Byron 52, 64
Bramwell, Crighton 66
Breckenridge, Alistair 319
Brigden, Wallace 88, 96, 98
British Association for Cardiac Rehabilitation 237
British Association of Paediatric Cardiologists 274
British Cardiac Society 47, 54–61, 167, 185
  affiliated groups 61
  growth of 55
  international role of 58–9
  meetings 60–1
  named lectures 58
  organisation and offices 59–60
British Cardiovascular Intervention Society 151
British Heart Foundation 61, 74–82, 347
  cardiac care 80–2
  education 78–80
  founding committee 74–5
  fundraising 75–7
  governance 77
  medical department 77
  nurses 82
  professorial chairs 78, 79
  research 77–8
  statement of purpose 75
British Heart Journal 66
British Journal of Cardiology 68
British Nuclear Cardiology Society 159
British Pacing and Electrophysiology Group 60
British Postgraduate Medical Federation 96
British Postgraduate Medical School *see* Royal Postgraduate Medical School
British regional heart study 182–3
Brock, Lord Russell Claude 31, 55, 192, 200, 281, 357–9
Brompton Hospital 31, 33
  adolescent unit 285
  paediatric cardiac unit 271–2, 278
Brompton Magnetic Resonance Unit 164–6
  dedicated mobile scanner 165–6
  functional aspects of cardiac imaging 165
Brown, James 20
Browns Club 199
Brunton, Sir T Lauder 3, 15

C

Calcium antagonists 246
Calomel 6
Cambridge, Duke of 87
Camm, John 58, 148
Campbell, Maurice 14, 67, 71, 73, 74, 88, 94, 98, 125
Campbell, Ronald 58
Canadian Adult Congenital Heart (CACH) 287

Canadian Red Cross Memorial Hospital 294–6
cardiac enlargement and pericarditis 294–5
cardiac output studies 296
closure of 296
murmurs 295, 296
phenylephrine 295
phonocardiography 295–6
Captopril 246
Cardiac care 80–2
cardiac rehabilitation 81–2
defibrillators in ambulances 81
Heartstart UK 81
Cardiac catheterisation 89–90, 105–6, 143–54
angioplasty 150–3
basic technique 149
and cardiac radiology 128–9
catheter based techniques 147–8
congenital heart disease 148
coronary angiography 146–7, 148
current role of 150
early work 143–4
equipment manufacturers 146
in general hospitals 149
left heart studies 146
manometry 147
Cardiac Club 18, 20, 52–4
meetings of 53–4
Cardiac dilatation 1, 127–8, 291, 294–5
Cardiac imaging 156–8
Cardiac nurses 61
Cardiac output 296
postural changes 6–7
Cardiac pacing *see* Pacing
Cardiac radiology 123–132
Cardiac rehabilitation 81–2, 232–41
and cardiology 234–5
consumer involvement 239
as developing speciality 233–4
expansion of services 236–8
mobilisation 232–3
national audit 237–8
programmes and self help packages 237
psychosocial factors 235
review of service provision 238, 238–9
safety and effectiveness 235–6
Cardiac Society 10
Cardiac surgery 98, 192–213
conflict and quality 209–11
coronary artery 208–9
development of 30–2
hypothermia and stopping circulation 202–5
mitral stenosis 194–5, 200–1
paediatric 282
pulmonary valve stenosis 199–200
register 208–9
Royal Postgraduate Medical School 107–8
specialisation 197–9
transplantation 207–8
valvular 205–7
Cardiff, Ereld 77
Cardiology
development of 30–2
ethics and quality 36
geographical equity 34–5
history 71
increasing demand for 35
learning curve 36
private sector 35
rationing by waiting list 35
regional service 30
and rehabilitation 234–5
Cardiomyopathy 264, 304–8
dilated 305
hypertrophic 306
restrictive 307–8
Cardioplegia 205
Cardiopulmonary bypass 205
Cardiothoracic Institute, deans of 98
Cardiovascular pathology 255–68
academic pathology 256
atherosclerosis 256–63
cardiomyopathy and myocarditis 264
morphology 255–6
Cardiovascular research 67
Cardiovascular surgery 89–90
Cardiovascular survey 333
Carrel, Alexis 64
Cassidy, Sir Maurice 54
Central Middlesex Hospital 261
Chapman, Carleton 4
Charlies Club 199
Chest and Heart Association 75
Chest X-ray 123–32
cardiac catheterisation 128–9
cardiac enlargement 127–8
early use of 123–4
fluoroscopy 125–6
heart failure 128

improvements in radiological methods 124
kymography 126–7
orthodiagraphy 127
pulmonary blood flow and oedema 129–30
pulmonary hypertension 130–1
teleradiography 127
Cholesterol, and heart disease 179
Cholestyramine 338
Chorea 292
Christopher Robin Club 199
Churchill Hospital 31
Circulatory arrest 202–5
atrial septal defect repair 204
cardiopulmonary bypass 205
myocardial protection 205
profound hypothermia 204
Circus movement 8
Claquement protosystolique 120
Cleland WP 31, 107–8
Clinical trials 242–54
atherosclerosis 336–8
beta-blockers 245–6
calcium antagonists 246
coronary artery bypass surgery and angioplasty 248–9
coronary care unit 248
heart failure 247–8
hypertension 246–7
intravenous magnesium 246
lifestyle, diet and lipid modifying drugs 249–50
methodology 250–2
nitrates 246
prevention/treatment of thrombosis 242–5
Clinical Trials Service Unit (CTSU) 233, 241
Clofibrate 331, 337
Coats, Andrew 100
Cochrane, Archibald 232, 242
Compensation 1
Conduction defects 8–9
Congenital heart disease 20, 148, 281–3
see also Paediatric cardiology
Conybeare, Sir John Josias 195, 200
Cookson, Harold 18, 19
Coombs, Carey 15, 17, 53, 66
CORDA 164
Coronary angiography 146–7, 148
paediatric 270
Coronary artery bypass revascularization investigation (CABRI) 249
Coronary artery bypass surgery 208–9, 248–9
Coronary artery surgery studies (CASS) 249
Coronary care unit 248, 345
Coronary heart disease 177–8, 343–56
decreasing mortality 186–7
family/genetic studies 334
increasing incidence of 324–5
myocardial infarction *see* Myocardial infarction
prevalence 183–4
prevention *see* Prevention of heart disease
stable angina 351–3
unstable angina 349–51
variant angina 351
see also Atherosclerosis
Coronary perfusion imaging 166–7
Coronary Prevention Group 80
Coronary thrombosis *see* Myocardial infarction
Cotton, Thomas 16, 53, 58, 88, 94
Cowan, John 53, 71
Crawford, Theo 260, 261–2
Cushing, Harvey 64
Cushny, Arthur 2, 5, 7
Cutler, Elliott 194

D

Da Costa's syndrome 20–2
Dave's Club 199
Davies, Michael 67
Decompensation 2
Defibrillators 81, 346
Demand pacemakers 221
Dewar, Hewan 62
Dexter, Lewis 94
Diagnosis
bedside *see* Bedside diagnosis
myocardial infarction 13–14
Diet 249–50
and atherosclerosis 327–8
Diet and reinfarction trial (DART) 250
Digitalis 5–6
Dilated cardiomyopathy 305
Diltiazem 139
Diphtheritic myocarditis 17–18
District hospitals, planning for 28–9
Ditzen, Gerda 143
Dodson, Captain Portlock 85

Doll, Sir Richard 179
Dollery, Sir Colin 107, 319, 320
Doppler echocardiography 172
Drew, Charles 204
Dual chamber pacing 222

E

East, Terence 12, 124
Ebstein's anomaly 119, 145
Echo-planar imaging 164
Echocardiography 170–5
in cardiology 174
Doppler 172
linear array and sector scanners 172–3
M mode 171
paediatric 275
in paediatric cardiology 173
transoesophageal echo 173–4
Education
cardiac rehabilitation 238–9
patient leaflets 80
postgraduate 78–80
of public 79–80
see also Training
Effort syndrome 21, 300, 376
Einthoven's string galvanometer 133–5
Ejection murmurs 117
Ejection sounds 120–1
Electrocardiography 9–10, 133–8
analysis 137
chest leads 10, 147
Einthoven's string galvanometer 133–5
exercise testing 137
intracardiac 138
limb leads 136
recording methods 136–7
surface 138
Emanuel, Richard 53, 98
Emission tomography 159
Encrustation hypothesis of atherosclerosis 328–9
English, Sir Terence 207
Enterococcus faecalis 304
Environmental factors, and heart disease 180
Erythrocyte sedimentation rate, in rheumatic fever 297–8
European Society of Cardiology 59, 67, 167
Evan Bedford Library of Cardiology 72
Evans, Lord Horace 75
Evans, William 60, 74, 88, 94
books of 70
Evelina Hospital 33
Examination, principles of 111–12
Exchanges 77–8
Exercise
lack of, and atherosclerosis 328
testing 137
External pacemakers 214–15

F

Factor P 12
Familial hypercholesterolaemia 333, 334
Fatigue 4–5
Fellowships 77–8
Fetal origins hypothesis of hypertension 315
Fibrates 331
Fibrinogen 330–1
Fibrinolytic therapy 347–8
Fibrinolytic Therapy Trialists' Collaborative Group 244
First heart sound 118–20
splitting 118–20
First responder defibrillation 81
Flack, Martin 9, 18
Fleming, Hugh 62
Fleming, PR 71
Fluoroscopy 125–6
Foam cells 257
Forbes, Sir John 59
Forssmann, Werner 143
Forward failure 2
Frank, Otto 4
Fraser, Francis 92, 104
Fundraising 75–7
legacies, shops and investments 76–7
national and international events 76
public appeal 75–6

G

Gamma cameras
mobile 157
with X-ray source 159
Ganglion blockers 317
Gaskell, Walter 1, 2, 8, 52, 64
Gavey, Clarence 6
Gender differences in lipid levels 331
Genetic factors, and heart disease 180, 334
George, Sir Charles 77

Gibson, Alexander 53
Gibson, Derek 171
Gilchrist, Rae 14, 344, 348
GISSI-1 trial 244
GISSI-2 trial 347
GISSI-3 trial 246, 248
Glasgow, Earl of 86, 87
Global utilization of streptokinase and tissue plasminogen activator for occluded coronary arteries (GUSTO) 244, 347
Glyceryl trinitrate 12, 352
Goldblatt hypertension 316
Goodall, J Strickland 88
Goodall, Strickland 58
Goodenough report 29
Goodwin, John 58–9, 107
Grampian Region early anistreplase (GREAT) study 347
Grant, Ronald 22
Great Ormond Street Hospital 33, 271, 275–6, 278, 282
Grown up congenital heart services (GUCH)
  Brompton Hospital 285
  database 284
  establishment of service 282–5
  failure of national service 286
  first adolescent unit 283–4
  National Heart Hospital 283
  service needs 287–8
  worldwide services 288–9
Grüntzig, Andreas 353
Gruppo Italiano studies *see* GISSI trials
GUCH *see* grown up congenital heart services
Gunn, Marcus 19
Guy's Hospital, 192, 197–8, 281
  paediatric cardiology unit 276–7

H

Haile Selassie lectureship 97
Hall, Roger 67, 68
Hammersmith Hospital *see* Royal Postgraduate Medical School
Hammill, P 93
Hard water, and heart disease 182
Harefield Hospital, paediatric cardiology unit 277
Harken, D 196, 201
Harris, Peter 79, 99, 101
Harrison, Sir James 87
Hay, John 2, 9, 53
Hayward, Graham 88, 96, 98
Headstart UK 81
Heart 64–8, 366
Heart failure 1–7
  clinical trials 247–8
  controversy 3–4
  fatigue 4–5
  nature of 3
  radiology 128
  treatment 5–6
Heart sounds
  early systolic 120–1
  first 118–20
  second 115–18
Heart strain 124
Heart transplantation 207–8
Heartstart UK 81
Heredity in hypertension 312–13
Hertz, Arthur *see* Hurst, Sir Arthur
High density lipids, beneficial role of 332
Hill, Anselm Bradford 179, 251
Hill, Ian 14
Hollman, Arthur 71
Horder, Sir Thomas 16, 53, 303
Howarth, Sheila 66, 106, 302
Howell, Joel 9
Hoyle, Clifford 19
Hudson, Reginald 98, 264–6
Hugh's Club 62
Hume, Sir William 18, 53, 62
Hurst, J Willis 71
Hurst, Sir Arthur 2, 8
Hyperpiesia 18
Hypertensin 311
Hypertension 187–9, 310–22
  angiotensin 311–12
  and atherosclerosis 325–6
  benign 315–16
  beta-blockers 319–20
  clinical trials 246–7
  epidemiology 314–15
  fetal origins hypothesis 315
  Goldblatt hypertension 316
  heredity in 312–13
  hypertension clinic 317
  malignant 315–16
    surgical reversal of 316
  meta-analysis 321
  mild 319, 320–1
  prevention 318

prognosis 319
pulmonary 130
renin 310–11
salt restriction 188–9
treatment 189, 316–17
mild hypertension 319, 320–1
trial ethics 317–18
Hypertensive heart disease 18–19
see also Hypertension
Hypertrophic cardiomyopathy 306
Hypothermia 202–5

I

Inactivity, and heart disease 179
Indomethacin 330
Infective endocarditis 16–17, 303–4
and dental hygiene 304
Institute of Cardiology 89, 94–8, 377
academic unit 96–7
deans of 98
initiation of cardiac surgery 98
international reputation 97
Interhospital meetings 63
Intermittent claudication 12
International study of infarct survival *see* ISIS trials
Intracardiac electrocardiography 138
Intracoronary stenting 151
Ionescu, Marion 206
Irritable heart *see* Soldier's heart
Ischaemic heart disease 10–15
ISIS-1 trial 245, 347
ISIS-2 trial 243, 347
ISIS-3 trial 244, 347
ISIS-4 trial 246, 248

J

Jefferson, Keith 98
Journal of Atherosclerosis Research 332
Journals 63–8
see also individual journals
Julian, Desmond 77, 345
Junior Cardiac Club 63

K

Kay-Cross oxygenator 276
Keith, Arthur 2, 9, 20
Keith Jefferson Lecture 58
Kerley, Sir Peter 98, 127, 131
Khellin 352
Korotkov sounds 18
Krikler, Dennis 67, 108
Kymography 126–7

L

Late assessment of thrombolytic efficacy study (LATE) 244
Latham, Peter 10
Lawrie, Veitch 79, 178
Leatham, Aubrey 88, 96, 98
Leech, Graham 171
Levine, Samuel 13, 58, 94
Lewis, Sir Thomas 3, 5, 7, 8, 21, 53, 54, 64–6, 88, 94, 123–4, 343, 360–3
biography 71
electrocardiogram 135–6
monographs of 68–9
Lifestyle 249–50
LIMIT-2 trial 246
Linear arrays 172–3
Lipids
and atherosclerosis 326–7
beneficial role of HDL 332
fibrate development 331
gender differences 331
and heart disease 180–1
lowering of 185–6, 250
metabolism 333
research 331–2
Lipoproteins 326–7
Lisinopril 246
Lithium-iodine batteries 226–7
London Cardiological Club 62
London Chest Hospital 32
London Health Planning Consortium 34
London Hospital 30
Longmore, Donald 165
Lown, Bernard 345

M

M mode echocardiography 171
Macartney, Fergus 278
McCormick's Club 199
McDonald, Lawson 88, 98
Macfarlane, Peter 137
Mackenzie, Sir James 1–5, 7, 8, 9, 11, 13, 15, 52, 88, 364–7
biography 71
books 68
Heart journal 366
The study of the pulse 2, 68–9
work on heart 365

McMichael, Sir John 6–7, 58, 76, 99, 105–7, 143, 302, 368–70
McNee, Sir John 13, 14, 178
Magnesium 246
Magnetic resonance 163–9
  Brompton Magnetic Resonance Unit 164–6
  CORDA 164
  coronary and myocardial perfusion imaging 166–7
  early days 163–4
  echo-planar imaging 164
  specialist societies 167–8
Magnetic resonance spectroscopy 166
Mair, Alex 71
Malignant hypertension 315–16
Manometry 147
Mansfield, P 163–4
Maseri, Attilio 79, 107–9, 351
Medical Research Council, 242, 294, 320
Melrose, Denis 107, 205
Mersalyl 6
Meta-analysis 321
Middlesex Hospital 31, 202, 204
Mitral valve
  balloon valvuloplasty 153
  floppy 265–6
  prolapse syndrome 302
  regurgitation 205–6
  stenosis 15, 117, 193
    Brock's operation 358
    Souttar's operation 194
    surgery 200–1, 205–6
Mitral valvotomy 144–6
Mobile gamma cameras 157
Monckeberg's sclerosis 255
MONICA project 184
Monocytes 257
Monographs 68–70
Moore, Foster 19
Moore, Stuart 9
Moorfields Eye Hospital 33
Morris, Jeremy 14–15, 179
MRC Atheroma Research Unit 332–3
MRC medical cyclotron unit 156
MRC trial of drug treatment for mild hypertension 320–1
Murmurs
  ejection 117
  rheumatic fever 291, 295, 296
  systolic 117
Myocardial infarction 12–15, 343–9
  angioplasty in 152
  anticoagulant therapy 242–3
  anticoagulants and pressor drugs 344
  bed rest 343–4
  coronary care unit 345
  diagnosis 13–14
  fibrinolytic therapy 347–8
  limiting infarct size 347
  percutaneous transluminal coronary angioplasty 348
  platelet active agents 243–4
  pre-hospital coronary care 346
  prevalence 14–15
  prevention/treatment of arrhythmias 345–6
  pump failure 346
  recognition of 14
  secondary prevention 348–9
  thrombolytic drugs 244–5, 347–8
Myocardial perfusion imaging 166–7
Myocardial protection 205
Myocarditis 264

N

National Health Service
  specialist services 32–3
  training within 38–42
National Heart Forum 80
National Heart Hospital 31, 33, 58, 83–91, 117–18
  adolescent unit 283
  cardiac catheterization and cardiovascular surgery 89–90
  closure and rebirth 90
  Dr Eldridge Spratt 85–6
  establishment of 87–8
  and Institute of Cardiology 89
  London hospitals prior to special hospitals 83–4
  origins 85
  pacing at 219–25
    demand pacemakers 221
    dual chamber pacing 222
    non-atrial responsive generators 222–5
    quality assurance and coding systems 225
    research 220–1
  paediatric cardiac unit 271–2
  postgraduate education 93–4
  recognition of special hospitals 84–5

rise of special hospitals 84
St Cyres Lecture 58
Second World War 88
National Heart and Lung Institute
amalgamation 99–100
deans of 98
formation 98–9
National Hospital for Diseases of the Heart 29–30
Nationalisation 28–9
Newcastle Cardiac Club 62
Nifedipine 353
Nitrates 246, 350
Non-atrial responsive generators 222–5
Non-coronary interventions 153
Norman, John 90
Nuclear medicine 155–62
British Nuclear Cardiology Society 159
cardiac imaging 156–8
cost-benefit analysis 159–60
early scanners 155
emission tomography 159
mobile gamma cameras 157
MRC medical cyclotron unit 156
new tracers 158
radionuclide ventriculography 157
risk stratification 158
scintigraphy 157
Nursing profession 61
Nutrition, and atherosclerosis 327–8

O

Oakley, Celia 107
Oligaemia 125
Oliver, Michael 79, 178
Oram, Samuel 70
Orthodiagraphy 127
O'Shaugnessy, Laurence 196
Osler, Sir William 2, 3, 10, 11, 16, 52, 64, 103

P

Pacing 139–40, 214–31
National Heart Hospital 219–25
dual chamber pacing 222
improvement of demand pacemakers 221
non-atrial responsive generators 222–5
quality assurance and coding systems 225
research themes 220–1
regional centres 225–9
batteries 226–7
development of service 227
early pacemakers 225–6
management of 228–9
pacing techniques 228
St George's Hospital
external pacemaker 214–15
pacing rate 217–19
permanently implantable devices 216
Paediatric cardiac units 271–4
Paediatric cardiology 269–80
academic units 278
angiography 270
echocardiography in 173
establishment of consultant posts 274
investigations 275
paediatric cardiac service 275–7
paediatric cardiac units 271–4
pioneering procedures 269–70
professional associations 274
see also Congenital heart disease and Grown up congenital heart services
Paediatric Cardiology Group 274
Pantridge, Frank 346
Papworth Hospital 30
Pardee, Harold 14
Parkinson, Sir John 2, 6, 14, 19, 53, 60, 66, 88, 94, 128, 371–4
Parsons-Smith, BT 88, 94
Patent ductus arteriosus 55
Pathology *see* Cardiovascular pathology
Peacock Club 198–9
Peart, Sir Stanley 311–2
Peel, Fitzgerald 343-4
Pentaerythritol tetranitrate 12
Pentecost, Brian 77
Percutaneous transluminal coronary angioplasty 348, 353
Perhexilene 352
Pericarditis 294–5
Permanently implantable pacemakers 216
Perry, Bruce 293
Pete's Club 199
Peto, Sir Richard 251, 315
Phenylephrine 295
Phonocardiography 112–15, 295–6, 302
Pickering, Sir George 4, 12, 33, 243, 310–12
Plaque disruption 262–3
Plaque rupture 263
Platelet active agents 243–4

Platelets 330
Platt, Sir Robert 312–14
Pomerance, Ariela 261
Poole-Wilson, Philip 100
Postgraduate education 78–80
  National Heart Hospital 93–4
  special institutes for 92–3
Postgraduate Medical School of London *see* Royal Postgraduate Medical School
Potassium arrest 205
Pravastatin 185
Pre-hospital coronary care 346
Prenylamine 352
Pressor drugs 344
Prevention of heart disease 176–91
  coronary thrombosis 177–8
  decreasing mortality 186–7
  epidemiological studies 179–84
  hypertension 187–9
  lipid lowering 185–6
  rheumatic heart disease 176–7
Price, Frederick 88
Pridie, Ron 171
Prinzmetal, Myron 310, 351
Private sector 35
Professorial chairs 78, 79
Pronethalol 320
Propranolol 320
Psychosocial aspects of rehabilitation 235
Pulmonary blood flow 129–30
Pulmonary blood vessels 127–8
Pulmonary heart disease 19–20
Pulmonary hypertension 130
Pulmonary oedema 129–30
Pulmonary valve stenosis 199–200
Pulsus irregularis perpetuus 7, 135
Purkinje fibres 255

Q

Quinidine 139

R

Radcliffe Infirmary 31, 33
Radiology 123–32
Radionuclide ventriculography 157
Randomised intervention treatment of angina (RITA) 249
Read, Gay 59
Rehabilitation *see* Cardiac rehabilitation
Renin 310
Restrictive cardiomyopathy 307–8
Rheumatic fever 290–9
  aetiology 292
  bed rest 297
  Canadian Red Cross Memorial Hospital 294–6
  cardiac dilatation 291
  changing prevalence 292–4
  chorea 292
  history 290
  murmurs 291
  prophylaxis 177
  treatment 297
Rheumatic heart disease 15, 176–7
  see also Rheumatic fever
Rickards, AF 150
Risk factors for atherosclerosis 325–8
  cigarette smoking 325
  hypertension 325–6
  lipids 326–7
  nutrition 327–8
  physical inactivity 328
Ritchie, William 8, 53
Roberson-Aikman, Colonel 87
Romanes, George 8
Rose, Geoffrey 181
Ross, Donald 90, 97, 99, 206, 283
  work on oxygen consumption 203
Ross, Keith 90
Ross operation 90, 206
Rowlett, Sue 261
Royal Brompton Hospital *see* Brompton Hospital
Royal Colleges of Physicians 39
Royal Liverpool Children's Hospital 271
Royal Marsden Hospital 33
Royal Postgraduate Medical School 103–10, 368–70, 375
  cardiac catheterisation 105–6
  cardiac surgery 107–8
  foundation 103–4
  hypertension clinic 317, 318–19
  research 104–5, 108–9
  Second World War 106
  voluntary hospitals 104–5
Royal Society of Medicine 52
Russell-Wells, Sir Sydney 85, 87

S

St Cyres Lecture 58, 93–4
St George's Hospital
  cardiovascular pathology 261–2

pacing 214–19
external pacemaker 214–15
good outcomes 219
pacing rate 217–19
permanently implantable devices 216
St Thomas's solution 205
Salicylates, in rheumatic fever 297
Scadding, Guy 105
Scarlet fever 292
Scintigraphy 157
cost-benefit analysis 159–60
Scotland, paediatric cardiac units 273
Scott, Sir Ronald Bodley 80
Second heart sound 115–18
Second World War 27–37, 88
development of cardiology 30–2
hospitals and specialists before 27–8
NHS organisation 32–3
planning for district hospitals 28–9
speciality development 29–30
Sector scanners 172–3
Sellors, Sir Thomas Holmes 55, 97, 199–200, 204
Sharpey-Schafer, Peter 105, 143, 302
Shillingford, John P 58, 77, 105, 108
Simon, M 130
Simon Marks chair 78
Sleight, Peter 79
Smith, Fred 3
Smith, Shirley 67
Smoking, and atherosclerosis 325
Social class, and heart disease 180, 183
Societies *see individual societies*
Society of Cardiological Technicians 60
Society for Cardiovascular Magnetic Resonance 167
Society of Cardiovascular Science and Technology 60
Sodium nitrite 12
Soldier's heart 21–2, 300, 361
Somerville, Jane 58, 71, 98
Somerville, Walter 63, 67, 90
Souttar, Sir Henry 194–5, 210–11
Sowton, Edgar 98, 150, 220
Special hospitals 27–8
recognition of 84–5
rise of 84
Specialised units 27–8
Specialist services
development of 29–30
geographical distribution 49–50
location of 32–3
regulation of numbers 45–8
training for 40
Sphygmomanometry 18, 314–15
Spratt, Sir Eldridge 85–6
Stable angina 351–3
Starling, Ernest 4, 7, 64
Steell, Graham 2, 3
Steiner, Robert 107
Stents 151
Steroids, in rheumatic fever 297
Streptokinase 152, 243, 244, 347
Stress, and heart disease 179
Stuart-Harris, Sir Charles 20, 105
Surface electrocardiography 138
Survival and ventricular enlargement (SAVE) 348, 349
Sutherland, George 3
Swan-Ganz catheter 147
Syndrome X 22
Syphilitic heart disease 17
Systolic murmurs 117

T

Taussig, Helen 55, 144, 198
Teaching hospitals 33
Technetium-99m 158
Teleradiography 127
Textbooks 70–1
Thallium-201 158
Theophylline 6, 352
Thomas Lewis Lecture 58
Thrombolytic drugs 244–5, 347–8
Thrombus 258–9
Thursby-Pelham, Christopher 77
Tissue plasminogen activator 244, 347
Total body cooling 204
Training 38–42
cardiac rehabilitation 238–9
first steps 39
formal 42–5
geographical distribution 49–50
membership 39–40
new UK guidelines 44–5
pattern of 41–2
pressure for change 46–7
progression into specialities 40
proposals for 43–4
regulation of numbers 45–8

Trandolapril cardiac evaluation (TRACE) 348, 349
Transoesophageal echo 173–4
Transplantation 207–8
TRENT trial 246
Tricuspid closure 118–20
Tubbs, Oswald 16, 31, 55, 197

U

Ultrasound *see* Echocardiography
United Kingdom cardiac registers 208–10
University College Hospital 31, 63, 360
Unstable angina 349–51

V

Valve register 210
Valvular heart disease 300–3
  mitral valve prolapse syndrome 302
  non-cardiac origin 301
  phonocardiogram 302
  soldier's heart 21–2, 300
  see also individual heart valves
Vectorcardiography 137
Verapamil 139, 353
Vineberg operation 353
Voluntary hospitals 104–5

W

Wales, paediatric cardiac units 273–4
Walkabout UK 76
Waller, Augustus Desiré 52, 87, 133
Warburg, Erik 7
Warning arrhythmias 345
Wassermann reaction 17
Water-hammer pulse 112
Waterston, David 275, 282
Wayne, Sir Edward 12
Wells, Peter 171
Wells, Russell 87
Wenckebach, Karel 2, 94
West, John B 107
West of Scotland coronary prevention study (WOSCOPS) 185–6, 250, 338
White, Paul Dudley 94, 176
Whitney, Captain Robert 85, 86, 87
Wilkinson KD 53
Wilson, Frank 10
Wilson, R Macnair 71
Wolff-Parkinson-White syndrome 8, 139, 372
Wood, Paul 4, 20, 22, 74, 88, 94, 96, 105, 375–9
  cardiac catheterisation 144–6
  Diseases of the heart and circulation 70, 376
  lectures 377–8
  Paul Wood lecture 97
  research 377
  valvular heart disease 303
Wooller, Geoffrey 205–6
Wynn Institute of Metabolic Research 100

X

X disease 22
X-ciser 152

Y

Yacoub, Sir Magdi 79, 99, 204, 206, 207–8, 277

Z

Zipper Club 239

MIX
Papier aus verantwortungsvollen Quellen
Paper from responsible sources
FSC® C105338

If you have any concerns about our products,
you can contact us on
ProductSafety@springernature.com

In case Publisher is established outside the EU,
the EU authorized representative is:
Springer Nature Customer Service Center GmbH
Europaplatz 3, 69115 Heidelberg, Germany

Printed by Libri Plureos GmbH
in Hamburg, Germany